Atlas of Chest Wall Reconstruction

Alan E. Seyfer, M.D., F.A.C.S.
Colonel, Medical Corps U.S. Army
Chief, Plastic Surgery Service
and Hand Surgery Section
Orthopaedic Surgery Service
Walter Reed Army Medical Center
Washington, D.C.;
Associate Professor of Surgery,
Chief, Division of Plastic Surgery
Uniformed Services University of
the Health Sciences
Bethesda, Maryland

Geoffrey M. Graeber, M.D., F.A.C.S.
Lt. Colonel, Medical Corps U.S. Army
Thoracic Surgery Service
Walter Reed Army Medical Center
and Chief, Department of Surgery
Walter Reed Army Institute of Research
Washington, D.C.;
Associate Professor of Surgery
Uniformed Services University of the Health Sciences
Bethesda, Maryland

Gary G. Wind, M.D., F.A.C.S.
Associate Professor of Surgery
and Assistant Professor of Anatomy
Uniformed Services University of
the Health Sciences
Bethesda, Maryland

AN ASPEN PUBLICATION® • Rockville, Maryland • Royal Tunbridge Wells • 1986

Library of Congress Cataloging in Publication Data

Seyfer, Alan E.
Atlas of chest wall construction.

"An Aspen publication."
Includes bibliographies and index.
1. Chest—Surgery. 2. Flaps (Surgery) I. Graeber, Geoffrey M. II. Wind, Gary G. III. Title. [DNLM: 1. Surgical Flaps—atlases. 2. Thoracic Surgery—atlases. WF 17 S519a]
RD536.S48 1986 617′.54 86-3439
ISBN 0-87189-352-5

Editorial Services: M. Eileen Higgins
Production and Manufacturing: Debbie Collins

The authors have made every effort to ensure the accuracy of the information herein. However, appropriate information sources should be consulted, especially for new or unfamiliar procedures. It is the responsibility of every practitioner to evaluate the appropriateness of a particular opinion in the context of actual clinical situations and with due consideration to new developments. Authors, editors, and the publisher cannot be held responsible for any typographical or other errors found in this book.

The opinion or assertions contained herein are the private views of the authors and are not to be construed as official or as reflecting the views of the Uniformed Services University, The Department of the Army, or the Department of Defense.

Library of Congress Catalog Card Number: 86-3439
ISBN: 0-87189-352-5

Printed in the United States of America

1 2 3 4 5

To our families and teachers:

Especially Major General Lewis A. Mologne, M.D., F.A.C.S., Commanding General, Walter Reed Army Medical Center and Norman M. Rich, M.D., F.A.C.S., Professor and Chairman, Department of Surgery, Uniformed Services University of the Health Sciences.

All of the illustrations and color plates in this book were created by Gary G. Wind, M.D., F.A.C.S.

Contents

List of Color Plates

Foreword

It has been a privilege to have the opportunity to review this outstanding Atlas on a subject of increasing significance. Reconstruction of the chest wall has assumed additional importance in recent years for many reasons, particularly the expanding role of surgical management of a number of disorders by techniques not previously available. The authors have provided a remarkably clear and skillfully written exposition of the basic anatomical features including embryology, surgical anatomy, and pulmonary physiology. The significance of the blood supply to the involved muscles and skin of the chest wall is uniquely written about with appropriate emphasis. A particularly outstanding feature of this work is the quality of the illustrations, a number of which are in color and make a penetrating impression both for their accuracy and attention to detail. Careful consideration is given the preoperative preparation of the patient, especially those in whom the chest wall defect is the result of a complication, particularly since the latter may be serious.

The authors deserve high commendation for the section describing the planning of the reconstruction, specifically the choosing of flaps, providing structural support, and the use of multiple flaps in achieving an optimal result. Similarly, the section on resection and debridement of the chest wall includes the approaches designed to manage neoplasms, infection, trauma, radiation necrosis, and the status following removal of large segments of the chest wall. The description of postoperative management of these often complex surgical procedures is very well done and forms an important part of this much needed text.

Finally, this text is edited by three contributors, each of whom represents a different discipline within the field of surgery. This is both important and fortunate. Dr. Seyfer is Chief of Plastic Surgery and the Hand Surgery Section at Walter Reed and is on the faculty of the Uniformed Services University of the Health Sciences. He has a very gifted background of training and experience. His colleagues, Dr. Graeber, of the Thoracic Surgery Service, and Dr. Wind, of the General Surgery Service, who is also Assistant Professor of Anatomy, have impressive backgrounds fully qualifying them as being very knowledgable in this field. It can be predicted that this important work will rapidly gain wide acceptance and find a receptive audience among those who are participating in this increasingly important segment of surgery.

David C. Sabiston, Jr., M.D.

James B. Duke Professor of Surgery and
Chairman of the Department
Duke University Medical Center

Foreword

To write a foreword for this Atlas on Chest Wall Reconstruction by Alan Seyfer, Geoffrey Graeber, and Gary Wind is both a privilege and pleasure. Highly practical and richly illustrated, it will be very useful to those surgeons who treat patients with a need for reconstruction of the integrity of the chest wall.

This Atlas is timely because the approach to chest wall reconstruction has changed substantially in the past decade, but no definitive text has yet been written. That change occurred with the rediscovery that a regional transposition flap of muscle, with or without its overlying skin, is not only safe and reliable to use but also provides the surgeon with highly desirable and versatile reconstructive options for any given defect of the chest wall.

The techniques are not new. Muscle transposition has been known for at least a century, but like many other advances in medicine and surgery, its acceptance required a perceived and compelling need. Muscle, when transposed, remains richly vascularized (in contrast to transposition flaps of skin and subcutaneous tissue). Accordingly, any ischemic phase attendant upon that transposition ordinarily is transient, and, thus, the surgeon has a powerful biologic tool for use in the therapy of his patient. Muscle flaps not only provide bulk to seal off defects of one sort or another, but also provide the elements for repair and host defense.

This Atlas is unique. It is written and illustrated by three surgeons. All are active faculty members within the Uniformed Services University of the Health Sciences and at the Walter Reed Army Medical Center. One of this trio of surgeons directs the division of plastic surgery, another is director of the division of surgery of the Walter Reed Army Institute of Research and a staff surgeon on the cardiothoracic surgical service, and the third is not only an active surgeon but a clinical anatomist and medical illustrator. Thus, the translation of what is in the mind's eye of a surgeon to that of the medical illustrator and the rendering of a drawing did not need to take place. All of the important steps in the procedures are well known to all three individuals who coauthored this book.

It is detail, the richness and accuracy of the particular, that is the mark of this Atlas. The surgeon using it for his education should have no doubt as to its authenticity and reliability. The broad principles that are so well documented in this Atlas and the wide applicability of the reconstructive techniques illustrated reflect the broad experience and dedication by the authors to the total care of surgical patients. As a longtime consultant to the Walter Reed Hospital it is no small pleasure for me to have played a very small role in the genesis of this book.

M.J. Jurkiewicz, M.D., F.A.C.S.

Professor of Surgery
Chief of Plastic Surgery
Emory University School of Medicine

Introduction

This atlas is intended for the busy clinical surgeon and his team who must deal with surgical problems of the chest wall. Its concise atlas format, with abundant illustrations, is designed for quick assimilation. Four major musculocutaneous flaps, which are currently the most useful for chest wall reconstruction, are described in detail: These are the pectoralis major, rectus abdominis, latissimus dorsi, and lower trapezius flaps. The omentum is also described as another source of richly vascularized tissue for filling chest wall defects. Two of us (one a plastic surgeon, the other a cardiothoracic surgeon) have jointly treated a large number of patients requiring chest wall reconstruction. Using these flaps, along with certain ground rules, we describe our approach to some of the more common lesions we have encountered and offer guidelines that have been useful to us in minimizing morbidity and disability. The techniques are by no means original with us, and the real credit goes to those surgeons and teachers who developed these safe means of dealing with large, full-thickness chest wall defects. There seems to be a need, however, for a handy reference of this type. Our experience and the perceived need, combined with the expertise of the third author who is a surgeon, anatomist, and medical artist, prompted this endeavor.

The Team Concept

There are few fields where close cooperation among many medical and surgical disciplines can be as rewarding and as critical to good patient care as that of chest wall surgery. The patient with an affliction that requires removal of a large full-thickness segment of the thorax faces a formidable operation, a challenging period of rehabilitation, time lost from work, and depending on the occupation, a real threat to his very livelihood. In addition to the expected perioperative recovery, there may be a long period of anticancer therapy as well. The mission of the team is to return the individual to the mainstream of life as soon as possible with a minimum of risk and disability. This means a thorough preoperative evaluation, teamwork during the operative procedure, and close follow-up care.

The patient is admitted to the thoracic or plastic surgery service, depending on the referring physician, and the evaluation is initiated (see Chapter 4). The thoracic surgeon and plastic surgeon examine the patient and the preliminary clinical data together and begin to formulate the plan of treatment. The anticipated extent of the final defect is matched against the available options for the reconstruction of that defect. The need for special testing and consultation with other disciplines is discussed. Gradually, the nature of the lesion is characterized and specific plans are developed to deal with it.

There is no doubt that for certain lesions either the thoracic surgeon or the plastic surgeon would feel perfectly competent to treat the problem without this team effort and to do everything alone. However, it is in the patient's best interest if experience is pooled and efforts are combined to formulate a plan for each specific clinical problem. Indeed, when such consultation and teamwork is available, the question should be, Why not take advantage of it in the interest of the patient? This philosophy does not in any way question the competence of the other team member but welcomes it. In dealing with malignancies, some authors have made the point that the surgeon who resects the tumor should not be the surgeon who reconstructs the defect. The reason for this is that during the ablative procedure, the surgeon may not take as wide a margin as desired if he is constantly concerned about how to reconstruct such a massive defect. There may or may not be merit to this philosophy. On the other hand, there is something to be said for allowing the thoracic surgeon to perform such resection and perform it with the resectional margins that he considers appropriate for the pathology. He is, in general, more familiar on a day-to-day basis with operations in this region than most plastic surgeons and, therefore, should be able to perform this portion of the procedure with less operative risk to the patient. As a corollary, the thoracic surgeon is often happy to defer the reconstruction to the plastic surgeon after a lengthy extirpative effort. In this way, a fresh team member is available for the reconstructive portion of the operation, which may also take a long time to complete.

Our method usually involves both team members during the entire operation. The plastic surgeon assists the thoracic surgeon with the debridement or excisional effort. Later, the thoracic surgeon, after a short break, assists the plastic surgeon with the reconstruction. Admittedly, there have been times when one of us was unavailable and the other member was responsible for both phases of the operation. However, it is preferable to utilize the team effort whenever possible in the interests of saving time, pooling available experience, and increasing the margin of safety for the patient. After the operation, one surgeon is responsible for directing postoperative care while consulting with the other members of the team. Each member is responsible for the specific aspects of care referable to his specialty.

Preoperatively, the anesthesiologist is also consulted and made aware of pertinent details of the upcoming operation. When dealing with a neoplasm, it is also advisable to discuss the problem with the pathologist so that he can be available for frozen sections or have the opportunity to assess the need for special studies such as electron microscopy. He should also have the opportunity to review any available histological sections before the operative procedure. This is usually done simultaneously with a member of the surgical team. In this way, the pathologist and surgeon get a chance to confirm the diagnosis and collaborate on the plan of treatment. This confirmation of the histology of the tumor is invaluable before embarking on any operative procedure. The diagnostic radiologist, medical oncologist, and radiation therapist may in a similar fashion contribute information that could refine the diagnosis or allow for later chemotherapy or radiotherapy. Such an informal tumor board can be effective in the absence of a formal committee.

The key is to gain as much information as possible before completing the treatment plan. When the options are developed, they can then be presented to the patient along with the recommended course of treatment. This is done by the primary surgeon, usually with the other members of the surgical team present, in an honest and compassionate manner. Next of kin and family are usually present and any questions are answered at that time.

The Scope of the Book

The book is divided into three parts. The first section establishes the basics that must be understood to reconstruct the chest wall successfully. These include the details of the regional anatomy and physiology along with various aspects of perioperative care. As the resection must precede the reconstruction, this aspect of the surgery is dealt with in Section I.

Section II provides careful anatomical descriptions of the major flaps mentioned in the introduction and shows the technique of mobilizing the flaps in a step-by-step manner. A case study that illustrates an additional aspect is provided for each flap. While the first two sections of the book are oriented toward the more common, straightforward cases, Section III addresses special problems such as intrathoracic flap transfer.

We have attempted to cover some of the more common problems related to the chest wall and to offer some general methods of treatment that can be used for a wide variety of problems and that are within the scope of the community hospital setting and most thoracic and plastic surgeons. Those patients requiring special treatment facilities or procedures (such as microsurgical operations) should be referred to centers where such therapy is routinely available. It is hoped that this atlas will be of value to all surgeons who are faced with lesions of the chest wall.

SECTION I

General Principles

1

Some Historical Aspects of Chest Wall Reconstruction

The roots of chest wall reconstruction can be traced to early experiences in the management of penetrating wounds and full-thickness neoplasms. Patients with these conditions presented many challenges, but their early survival was directly linked to the success (or failure) of the surgeon in his efforts to maintain adequate ventilation. For the patient with a sucking chest wound, this meant prompt closure of the defect. For the individual with a tumor, the surgeon had to avoid entering the pleural space and be ready to repair such an opening quickly.

For most of these lesions, a simple closure was performed. This maneuver usually restored the pleural seal and prevented an early demise. However, the use of this method severely limited the safe resection of large portions of the chest wall and could result in a catastrophic dehiscence if the tension on the suture line was excessive. With the advent of later techniques, more satisfactory reconstructions gradually became available; these extended the limits of safe excision, debridement, and reconstruction. This review is intended to highlight some of the more interesting developments in the treatment of both neoplasms and injuries.

Primary Chest Wall Neoplasms

Meade, in his extensive history of thoracic surgery, credits Parham with authoring the first important paper on chest wall neoplasms in the North American literature.[1] In his report, published in 1899, Parham described two patients:[2] In the first individual, during the removal of a tumor, a large rent developed in the pleura. Shortly thereafter, the patient became hypoxic, and his condition began to deteriorate rapidly. Parham was able to mobilize the soft tissues of the chest wall and to close them over the entire defect. The patient survived.

In another patient, the operation began under chloroform anesthesia, which was administered by direct inhalation. Parham was removing a large tumor and assiduously avoiding entry into the chest cavity when a small hole developed in the pleura. The rent was initially controlled with gauze packing, but the patient nearly expired when the defect was suddenly enlarged and the lung collapsed. Control was finally established by using a larger pack and converting to a crude form of endotracheal anesthesia. The patient's ventilation was stabilized, and the wound was closed in layers by soft tissue mobilization.

Both cases demonstrate the lethality of the open pleural space and its difficult management in the early history of chest wall reconstruction. During these years, the primary axiom of chest wall surgery was maintenance of a closed pleural space to assure pulmonary expansion.

In addition to avoidance of the pleural space, other modalities were attempted. In 1906, Rhen reported three cases in which he sutured the lung to the parietal pleura and was able to maintain lung expansion while pursuing wider resections.[1] Dollinger successfully used staged preoperative pneumothorax to prevent the acute respiratory embarrassment of an uncompensated open pneumothorax during the operation.[3] Another novel, though cumbersome, approach involved placing the patient and the operative team in a negative pressure chamber (Sauerbruch's technique) to keep the lung from collapsing.[4]

The emphasis during these early years was on the problem of maintaining normal pulmonary mechanics. Secure closure of the chest wall was a necessary step toward this goal. The use of endotracheal anesthesia, early in this century, solved many intra-operative problems.

"Avenues of Exit"

Early attempts at managing patients with penetrating chest wounds usually met with disaster since the open thorax and subjacent lung injuries rarely allowed adequate ventilation. Meade credits Hewson (1767) with the observation that patients were unable to breathe well with an open chest wound but could do so if the wound was promptly closed.[4] This knowledge went unnoticed until the principle was again quite accidentally noted by Napoleon's great military surgeon, Baron Larrey.[4] A soldier was brought to his field hospital with a large, sucking chest wound. Larrey sized up the situation and fully expected the injury to be rapidly fatal. He quickly closed the wound to prevent the other soldiers from seeing the injury and to spare them the sight of what was to be a horrible death. Much to his surprise, the wounded soldier improved markedly and survived. After this success, Larrey adopted primary closure as the method of choice in handling open chest wounds. He emphasized the need for drainage to allow retained blood and other material to egress from the wound and onto the dressing.

A half century later, during the American Civil War, Billings also employed early closure of open chest wounds since this approach usually caused a marked improvement in the patient's ventilation and permitted survival in some.[4] He despaired of the long-term results of this approach since many of his patients later developed empyema and a dehiscence of their wounds. What Billings had failed to note (which Larrey had observed and recommended) was that blood clot and retained material within the wound must be allowed an "avenue of exit." For Larrey, the avenue was through a small portion of the wound and onto the dressing. For Billings, there was no avenue since he closed the margins tightly. Hence, suppuration often followed.

Despite these battlefield successes, the controversy over whether to close the chest continued until the First World War. During this conflict, further experience led to a general agreement that open chest wounds should be closed to enhance early survival. Any subsequent infection would have to be drained if it emerged. Meade relates that the British issued orders early in the war directing that all chest wounds would be closed.[4] By the end of the conflict, this approach was adopted by virtually all allied medical services. Success in avoiding lethal postoperative infection was related to whether retained material was allowed an avenue of exit; whether thoracentesis was performed aggressively for any early empyema; and seemingly a large element of pure luck. A legacy of open empyema cavities ensued for those fortunate enough to survive successful drainage in this preantibiotic era. Once open, the large defects were allowed to granulate in and eventually to be closed by secondary intention (Figure 1.1).

The Second World War

The magnitude of such wounds has been reviewed by Lyman Brewer, who compared the results obtained in the First World War to his experience in the Second World War.[5] Much of the success in the Second World War can be attributed to surgical principles recognized and developed in the period between the two conflicts.

An important trend during this time was the emergence of surgeons who had a primary interest in the practice of thoracic surgery. This was also occurring in plastic surgery, largely as a result of the experience in reconstructing maimed individuals from the First World War. At the outset of the Second World War, the U.S. government gathered surgical specialists to develop standard procedures for treating battle injuries. A manual for thoracic surgery was published in 1943,[6] and centers for reconstructive plastic surgery were established in the same year. Four thoracic surgeons were selected to prepare the thoracic surgical manual: Evarts A. Graham, Issac M. Bigger, Edward D. Churchill, and Leo Eloesser. It was fitting that Graham was selected as the chairman because of his substantial contributions to pulmonary resection in the previous decade.

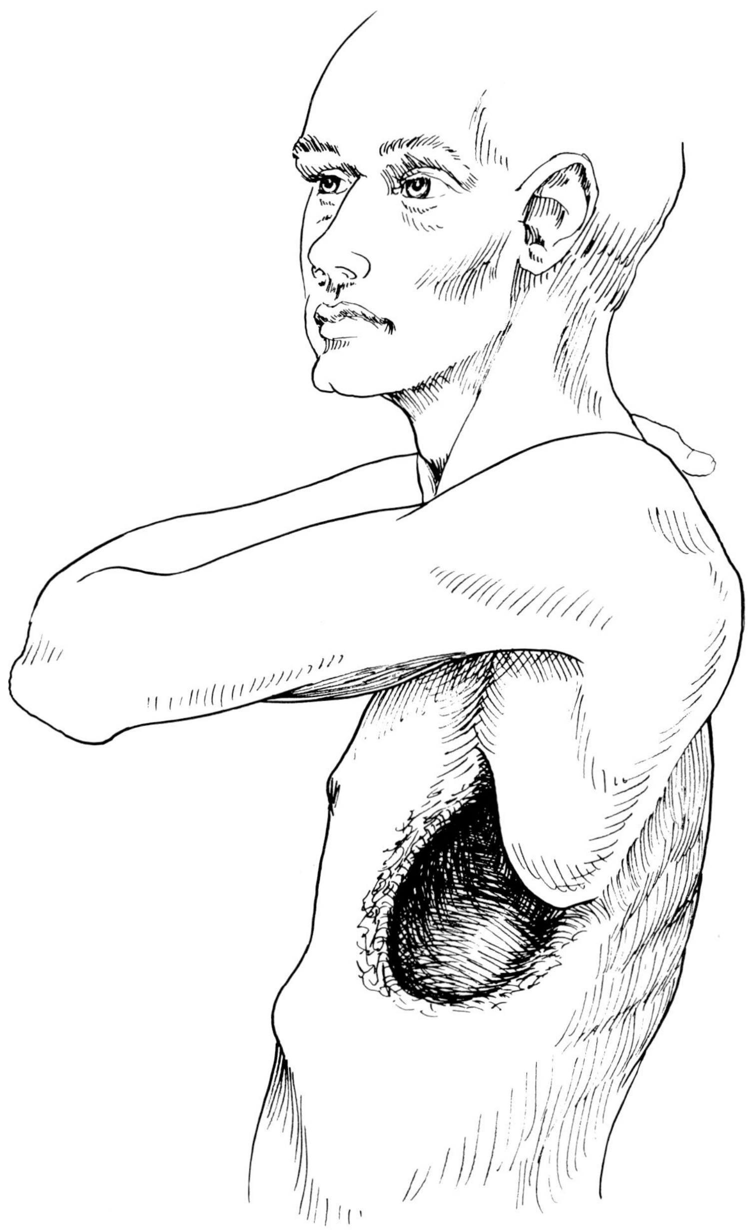

FIGURE 1.1 This patient sustained an open chest wound by artillery shell fragments in the First World War. After initial closure, empyema developed and the cavity was drained. The resulting cavernous defect, like so many during this era, was then allowed to heal by secondary intention. (Drawn from a photograph in *Surgery in WWII. Thoracic Surgery.* Dept. of the Army, 1963.)

The manual listed therapy for all types of wounds. Some of the methods prescribed were notable.

The gravity of the sucking chest wound was again recognized, and immediate closure to maintain ventilation was strongly recommended. However, several different methods of closure were presented. The first was simple debridement followed by direct suture. If approximation without tension were impossible, then mobilization of the tissues at the margins of the wound was advocated. The authors stressed that the local soft tissues (including nearby muscles or even segments of muscles) may be pressed into service to achieve a tension-free closure (Figures 1.2 and 1.3). Thus, the use of muscle flaps and segments was evident long before our present era.

If mobilization of surrounding tissues was insufficient, then transposition of the diaphragm after crushing the phrenic nerve could be considered. As a last resort, suturing the pulmonary parenchyma to the chest wall (as Rhen had described) was recommended. Those were great steps toward the modern concept of a tension-free muscular closure.

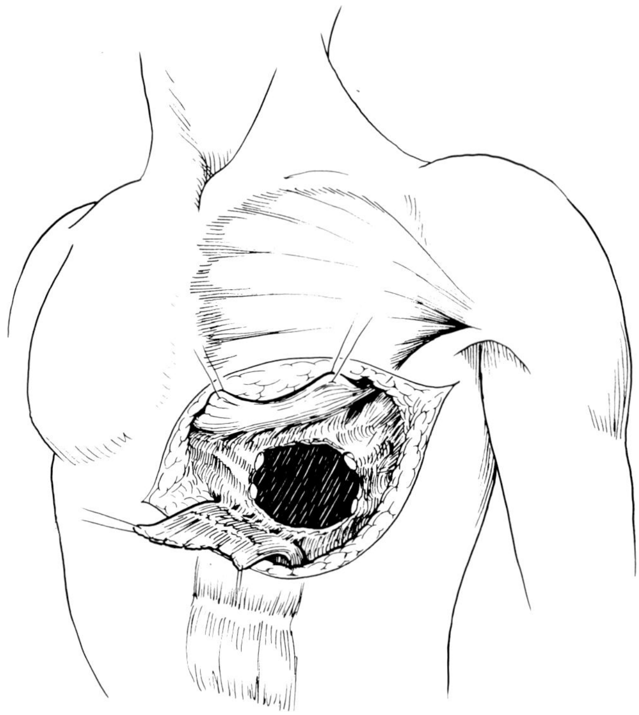

FIGURE 1.2 This figure illustrates the closure of a full-thickness chest wall injury due to a bullet wound during the Second World War. After debridement, adjacent muscles are mobilized to close the defect. (Drawn from a photograph in *Surgery in WWII. Thoracic Surgery.* Dept. of the Army, 1963.)

The authors also recognized the lethality of the untreated pneumothorax and recommended initial aspiration followed by tube thoracostomy for control. Thus, a solid foundation was established for treating open (and closed) chest injuries for the duration of the conflict. These early precepts took into account the restoration of normal ventilatory physiology as well as provision for thorough debridement, tension-free closure, and a reliable means of drainage (tube thoracostomy). Such principles had

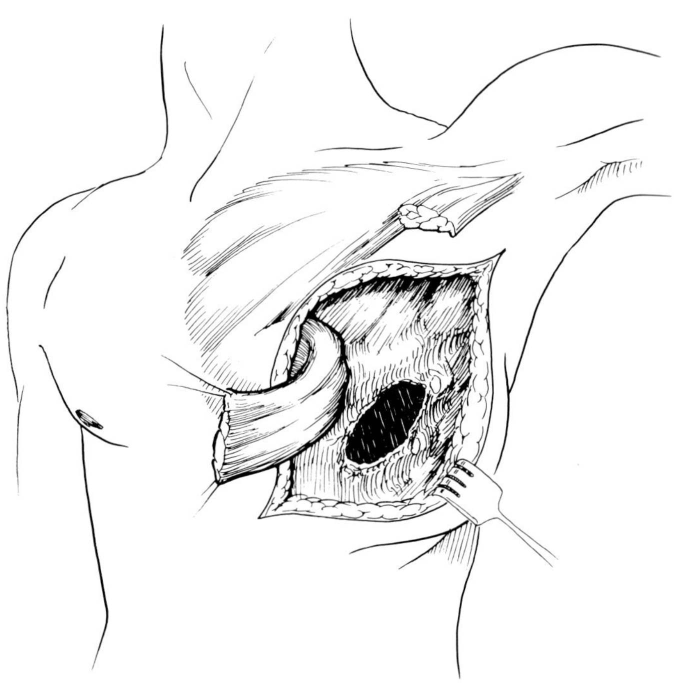

FIGURE 1.3 This figure illustrates the closure of a gunshot wound during the Second World War. Surgeons used muscles and segments of muscle, which were mobilized to allow a tension-free closure. Thus, muscle flaps (and segmental muscle flaps) were used long before today's era of rediscovery. (Drawn from a photograph in *Surgery in WWII. Thoracic Surgery.* Dept. of the Army, 1963.)

useful application in caring for the many casualties encountered. Brewer and others have documented their successes with the Second Auxiliary Surgical Group.[5,7–9] Two volumes subsequently published by the U.S. Army describe in detail the application of these principles and their maturation through the course of the War. They provide valuable insight into the principles governing the management of chest wounds today.[10,11]

The Era of Flap Reconstruction

The techniques learned during the Second World War and subsequent conflicts (Korea, Vietnam) continued into the 1970s, when the use of pedicled flaps became the preferred approach to chest wall reconstruction. The use of these flaps emerged from previous studies which showed that large parcels of muscle and skin could be safely moved from one area of the body to another while still attached to their vascular pedicle. Their employment in the reconstruction of the chest wall was a logical extension of their earlier use in head and neck surgery and extremity operations because many of these flaps are located on the thorax or torso.

Since the reports of Orticochea and McCraw,[12,13] much has been rediscovered about the blood supply to the skin and the application of this knowledge to difficult plastic surgical problems. In their continued quest for reliable, well-vascularized flaps, innovative surgeons have also extended their armamentarium by reaching into the abdomen for pedicled tissue.

Use of the omentum was initially reported by Kiricuta in the 1950s. He successfully employed it to treat vesicovaginal fistulae and used it both inside and outside the chest to repair bronchopleural fistulae, as well as to reconstruct the postmastectomy deformity. He also used this versatile tissue to treat other chest wall lesions and to palliate lymphedema of the upper extremity.[14] The arterial anatomy and practical techniques for omental lengthening were later described by Goldsmith.[15] Larger series were subsequently reported by Jurkiewicz and others; these included the more common problem of invasive chest wall malignancy, its extirpation, and reconstruction with omental flaps.[16,17]

The latissimus dorsi muscle, initially described by Tansini in 1906,[18] was used by Campbell in 1950 for chest wall reconstruction.[19] Since then it has become the workhorse for restoration of the parietes in all sectors of the thorax.[20]

Although described in the Second World War[1,4,6,7] (Figure 1.3), the pectoralis major muscle was again recognized as a potential myocutaneous unit in 1968.[21] Arnold and Pairolero described its use as an island flap for reconstruction of the anterior thoracic wall[22] and subsequently defined its use for other defects.[23]

In 1946, Shaw and Payne, still serving in the Army after the War, described flaps based on the inferior epigastric and circumflex iliac arteries.[24] Almost three decades later, two Japanese surgeons described the use of an upper abdominal flap based on the superior epigastric vessels to reconstruct chest wall defects caused by recurrent breast cancer.[25] Further application of these concepts (of using portions of the abdominal wall based on the epigastric arcade) was advanced by the group at Emory University and has greatly extended the margins of safety in chest wall reconstruction.[26] Hartrampf, also at Emory, has defined the use of the rectus abdominis musculocutaneous flap.[27]

The flaps described by these surgeons have revolutionized the treatment of chest wall lesions, both congenital and acquired. They afford the clinician with reliable, durable, and tension-free closures that are within the scope of most clinical surgeons and preserve the ventilatory mechanics that often eluded earlier practitioners. It is these flaps that are described in this book.

Notes

1. Meade RH: *A History of Thoracic Surgery*. Springfield, Ill, Charles C Thomas, 1961, Chap 2, Surgery for Tumors of the Chest Wall.
2. Parham DW: Thoracic resections for tumors growing from the bony chest wall. *Trans S Surg Ass* 1899;II:223–363.
3. Dollinger J: Der artificielle pneumothorax als vorberein vorberieten der operation zur exstirgsation durchgreifender brustwand tumoren. *Z Chir* 1902;29:82–83.
4. Meade RH: *A History of Thoracic Surgery*. Springfield, Ill, Charles C Thomas, 1961, Chap 1, The Management of Wounds of the Chest.
5. Brewer LA III: The contributions of the Second Auxiliary Surgical Group to Military Surgery during World War II with special reference to thoracic surgery. *Ann Surg* 1983;197:318.
6. Graham EV, Bigger IA, Churchill ED, Eloesser L: *Thoracic Surgery*. Philadelphia and London, WB Saunders, 1943.
7. Brewer LA III: Late results in war wounds of the chest, in Daughtry DC (ed): *Thoracic Trauma*. Boston, Little, Brown & Co, 1960.
8. Brewer LA III: Long-term (1943–1961) follow-up studies in combat-incurred thoracic wounds, in Ahnfeldt AL (ed): *Surgery in World War II. Thoracic Surgery*. Washington, DC, Office of the Surgeon General, Department of the Army, 1965, vol. 2.
9. Cox WA, Feltis JM, Jr: The management of war wounds of the chest, in Daughtry DC (ed): *Thoracic Trauma*. Boston, Little, Brown & Co, 1960.
10. Ahnfeldt AL, Berry FB (eds): *Surgery in World War II. Thoracic Surgery*. Washington, DC, Office of the Surgeon General, Department of the Army, 1963, vol. 1.
11. Ahnfeldt AL, Berry FB (ed): *Surgery in World War II. Thoracic Surgery*. Washington, DC, Office of the Surgeon General, Department of the Army, 1965, vol. 2.
12. Orticochea M: Musculo-cutaneous flap method: immediate and heroic substitute for the method of delay. *Brit J Plast Surg* 1972;25:106.
13. McCraw J, Vasconez L, Madden J: Experimental free transfer of "island" myocutaneous flaps. Presented before the Plastic Surgery Research Council, New Haven, Conn, April 1975.
14. Kiricuta I: L'emploi du grand epiploon dans la chirugie du sein cancereux. *Presse Med* 1963;71:15–17.
15. Alday ES, Goldsmith HS: Surgical technique for omental lengthening based on arterial anatomy. *Surg Gynecol Obstet* 1972;135:103–107.
16. Jurkiewicz MJ, Arnold PG: The omentum: an account of its use in the reconstruction of the chest wall. *Ann Surg* 1977;185:548–554.
17. Dupont C, Menard Y: Transposition of the greater omentum for reconstruction of the chest wall. *Plastic Reconstr Surg* 1972;49:263–267.
18. Tansini I: Sopro il mio nuovo processo di amputazione della mamella. *Gaz Med Ital* 1906;57:141.
19. Campbell DA: Reconstruction of the anterior thoracic wall. *J Thorac Surg* 1950;19:456–461.
20. Seyfer A, Graeber G: The use of latissimus dorsi and pectoralis major musculocutaneous flaps for chest wall reconstruction. *Contemp Surg* 1983;22:29.
21. Hueston JT, McConchie IH: A compound pectoral flap. *Aust N Zeal J Surg* 1968;38:61–63.
22. Arnold PG, Pairolero PV: Chondrosarcoma of the manubrium: resection and reconstruction with pectoralis major muscle. *Mayo Clin Proc* 1978;53:54–57.
23. Arnold PG, Pairolero PC: Use of pectoralis major muscle flaps to repair defects of anterior chest wall. *Plastic Reconstr Surg* 1979;63:205–213.
24. Shaw DT, Payne RL: One stage tubed abdominal flaps. *Surg Gynec Obstet* 1946;83:205–209.
25. Tai Y, Hasegawa H: A transverse abdominal flap for reconstruction after radical operations for recurrent breast cancer. *Plastic Reconstr Surg* 1974;53:52–54.
26. Brown RG, Vasconez LO, Jurkiewicz MJ: Transverse abdominal flaps and the deep epigastric arcade. *Plastic Reconstr Surg* 1975;55:416–421.
27. Elliott L, Hartrampf C: Tailoring of the new breast using the transverse abdominal island flap. *Plastic Reconstr Surg* 1983;72:887.

2

Embryology, Anatomy, and Physiology of the Chest Wall

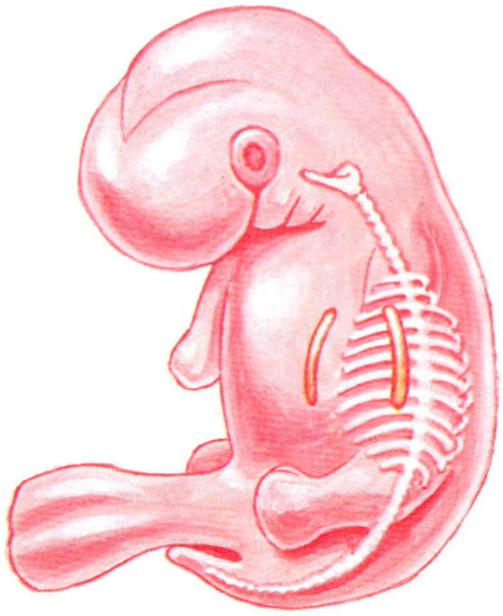

A

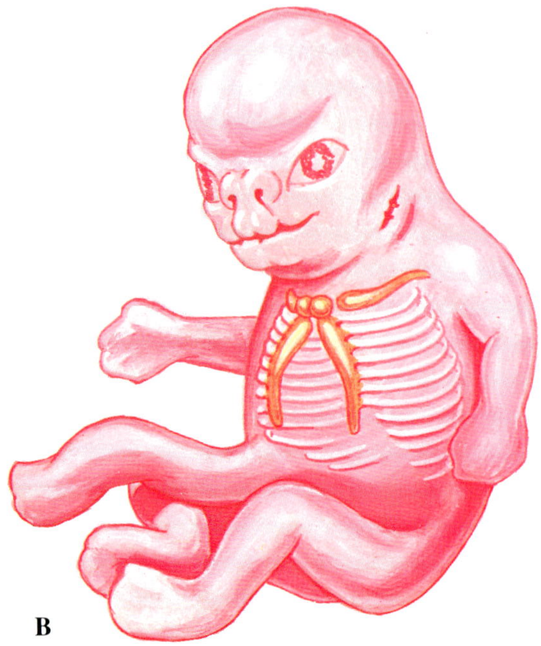

B

PLATE 2.1, FIGURE A This drawing presents the developing sternum and ribs as they appear in a 5½-week (9-mm) embryo. The two sternal primordia exist as lateral bars emerging from the appendicular skeleton while the ribs, arising from the axial skeleton posteriorly, are beginning to grow anteriorly in conformity with the body wall. There is no fusion between the ribs and the sternal primordia at this point.

PLATE 2.1, FIGURE B This drawing shows the development of the sternum and ribs by 7 weeks (17-mm embryo). The fusion of the two sternal primordia is beginning at the cephalad end of the emerging sternum. The cephalad medial mesenchymal mass and the two variable lateral suprasternal elements have fused to form the primitive manubrium. The primitive structures that will become ribs and costal cartilages are just reaching the sternal primordia.

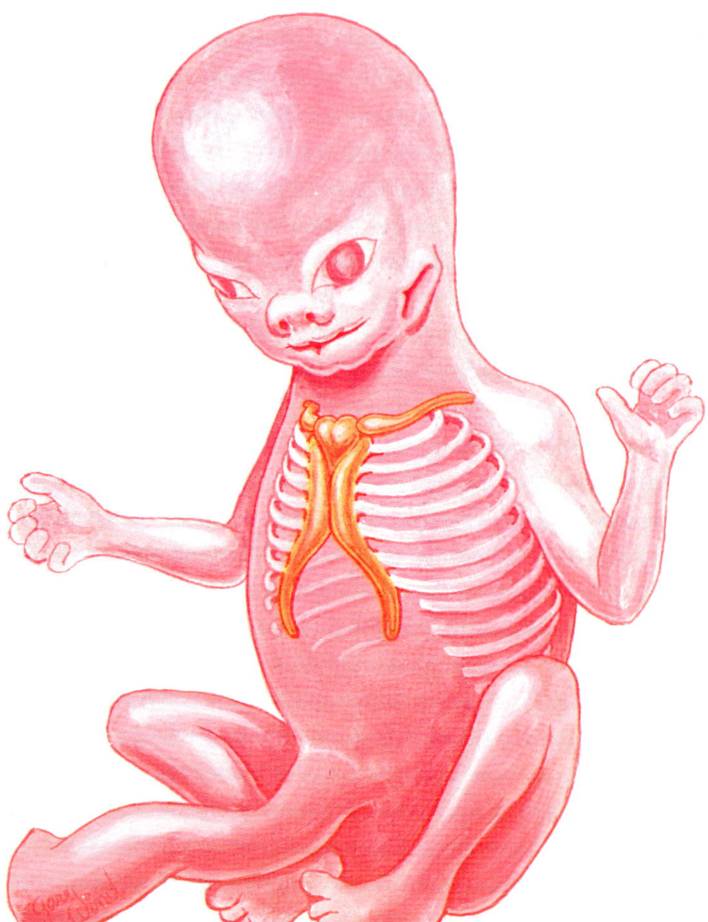

C

PLATE 2.1, FIGURE C This drawing depicts the nearly completed fusion of the sternal elements that has occurred by the beginning of the ninth week (23-mm embryo). Note the further development of the manubrium, the fusion of the two sternal bars, and the attachment of the upper costal cartilages bilaterally to the sternum. The development of the costal arches is continuing. By this time, the sternum and ribs are cartilaginous.

Embryology

The ribs, their costal cartilages, and the sternum arise relatively early in embryonic development during the sixth week of gestation. The ribs and costal cartilages are derived from the axial skeleton while the sternum arises from the appendicular skeleton. Errors in the maturation of the developing primordia account for observed chest wall anomalies.

The primitive sternum originates from two lateral mesenchymal bands that arise in the appendicular skeleton in close association with the emerging pectoralis major muscles. These bands, which lie ventrolaterally in the body wall, share no common connection initially. The thoracic ribs, which have arisen from the posterior common vertebral mass of the axial skeleton, grow anteriorly, laterally, and then ventrally in conformity with the emerging musculature of the body wall (Plate 2.1, Figure A). The ribs, costal cartilages, and intercostal muscles continue their growth and maturation independent of sternal development. The two lateral sternal primordia migrate ventrally and begin to fuse in a progressively craniocaudad fashion (Plate 2.1, Figure B). During fusion, the emerging sternum incorporates a smaller, cephalad mesenchymal medial mass (which corresponds to the presternum of lower animals) and two variable suprasternal elements. These three mesenchymal precursors are fused into the emerging manubrium. By nine weeks, sternal fusion is complete, the sternum has become cartilaginous, and the ribs and costal cartilages have matured so that costal cartilages 1–7 have joined the sternum. The corresponding costal arches are still emerging and soon incorporate cartilages 8–10 (Plate 2.1, Figure C). At five months, sternal ossification centers appear but all are not present until childhood.

Anomalies of sternal development lead to the recognized clinical entities known as *sternal clefts*. A complete sternal cleft is the result of a total lack of fusion, wherein the two primitive sternal bars remain in their lateral positions. A superior sternal cleft follows a deficiency in cephalad fusion, while a distal sternal cleft results from an early cessation of fusion. This distal cleft is also associated with other midline and cardiac developmental anomalies (Cantrell's pentalogy).

The emerging ribs are also subject to errors in the developmental sequence, which present clinically as anomalies. Agenesis and hypoplasia occur; the former accounts for absence of ribs, while the latter leads to rudimentary ribs. Hypoplasia of costal cartilages is also associated with Poland's Syndrome, in which cartilages 2, 3, 4, and occasionally 5 may be absent. Supernumerary ribs, which occur most commonly in the first cervical and first lumbar positions, are a result of overdevelopment of the rib primordia. Ventral bifurcation of developing ribs leads to forked or bifid ribs and costal cartilages.

Chest Wall Anatomy

Skeletal Framework

The ribs and cartilages of the chest wall have an inherent flexibility; they also possess latitude for movement by virtue of their articulations. These factors allow the excursion necessary for respiration and also provide a semirigid capsule to protect the thoracic and upper abdominal viscera. The head of each rib is bound to one or two

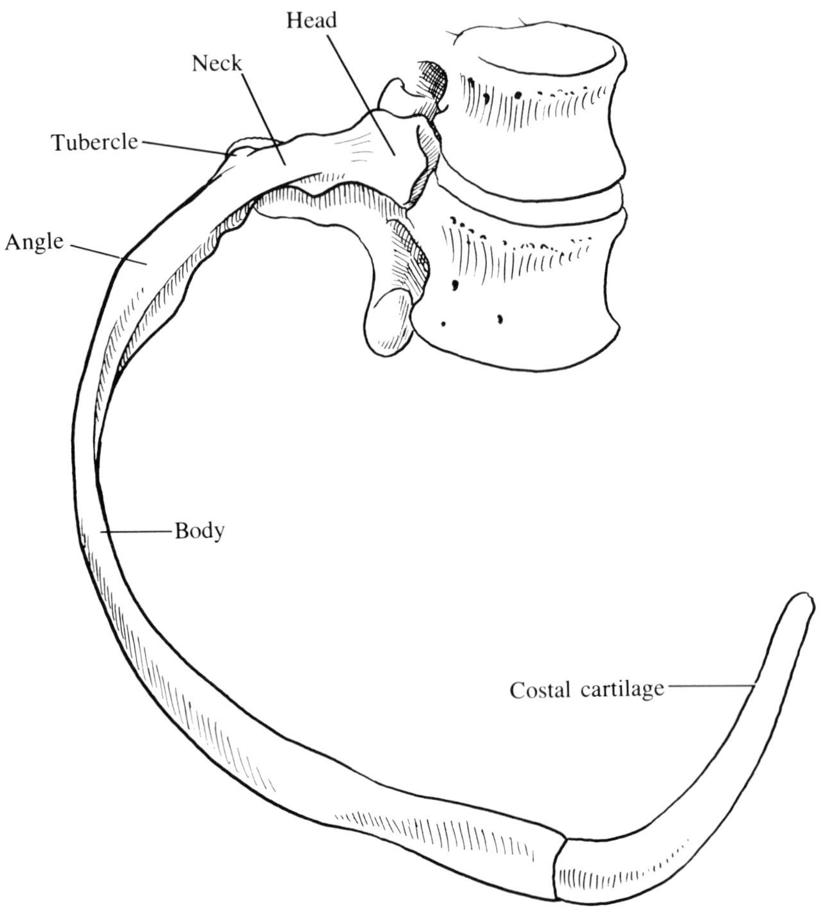

FIGURE 2.1 The ribs articulate with both the adjacent vertebral bodies and the transverse process of the vertebral body below. These attachments allow for the hinge-like motion during ventilation.

vertebral bodies by flexible ligaments. The tubercle distal to the short neck of the rib articulates with the transverse process of the vertebra below. Beyond the tubercle, an angulation turns the body of the rib anteriorly (Figure 2.1). The ribs increase in length as the rib cage expands caudally and then taper again toward the inferior aperture of the thorax (Figure 2.2). The first seven ribs end in cartilages that connect directly to the sternum. The cartilages of the next three ribs join to the one above, forming the anterior costal margin. The last two have no sternal connection.

The sternum consists of a manubrium, body, and xiphoid process. The junction of manubrium and body is angulated, forming a palpable landmark for locating the attachment of the second costal cartilages. The movement of the manubrium and ribs is discussed in the section dealing with respiratory physiology.

Superimposed on the intrinsic framework of the chest wall is the pectoral girdle formed by the clavicles and scapulae. The sternoclavicular joint is the sole point of skeletal attachment between these systems, giving the pectoral girdle great mobility.

Visceral Relationships The skeletal framework of the chest wall encloses the thoracic viscera and much of the region occupied by the upper abdominal organs (Figure 2.3). The thoracic and abdominal cavities are separated by the diaphragm,

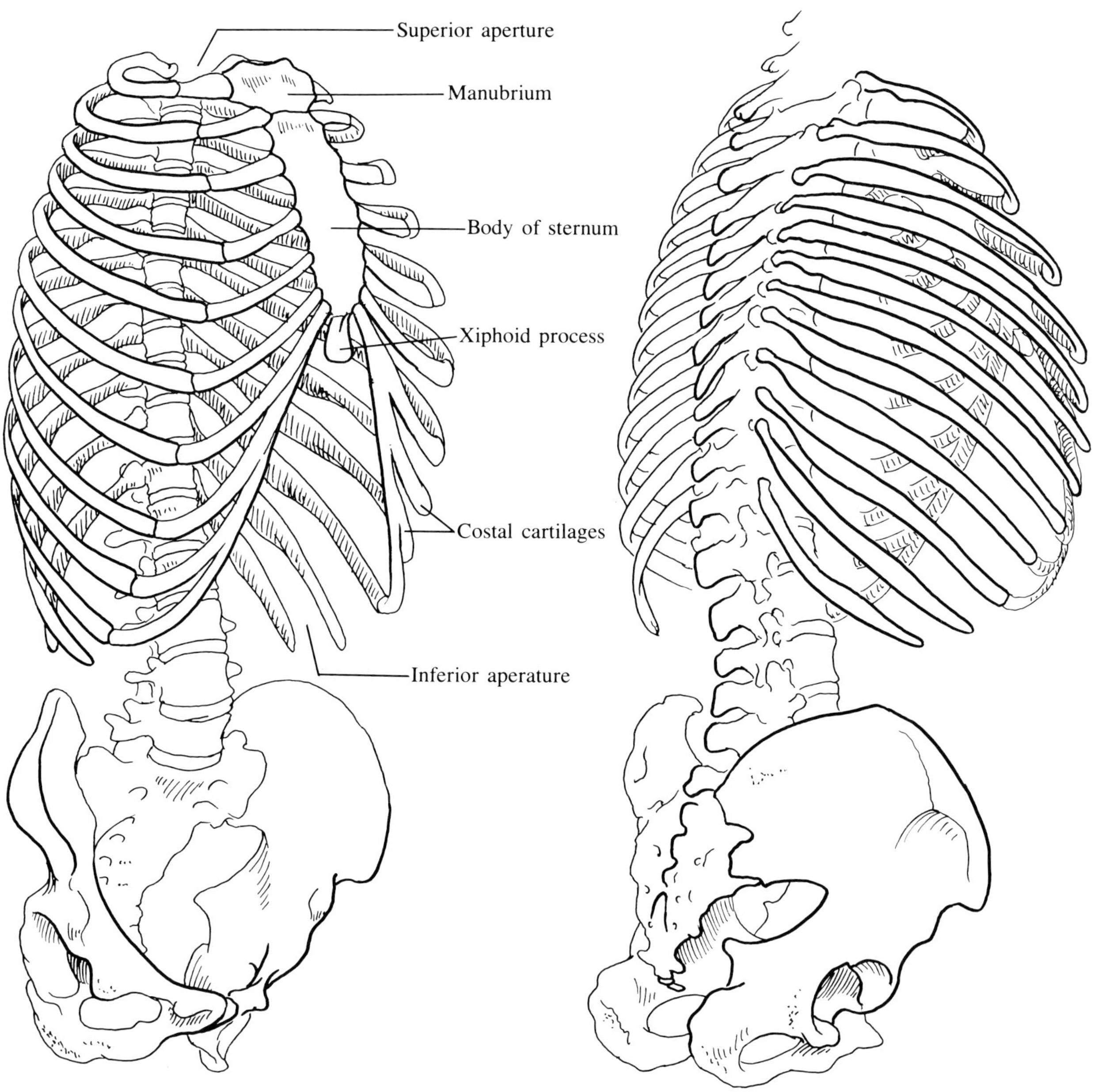

FIGURE 2.2 The rib cage forms a semirigid shell that affords effective protection for thoracic and abdominal viscera, yet allows for expansion and contraction of the intrathoracic volume.

which originates around the rim of the inferior thoracic aperture. Above the diaphragm, the heart, great vessels, trachea, and esophagus occupy the central part of the chest cavity between sternum and vertebral column. The pleural cavities conform to the remaining space, extending into the recesses at the rim of the diaphragm and around the heart. The lungs extend only part of the way down into the costophrenic recesses, leaving room for excursion with respiration. Below the diaphragm, the spleen and most of the stomach are covered by the left lower rib cage, while the right lower rib cage covers the majority of the liver. Posteriorly, the upper poles of the kidneys lie deep to the lower two ribs.

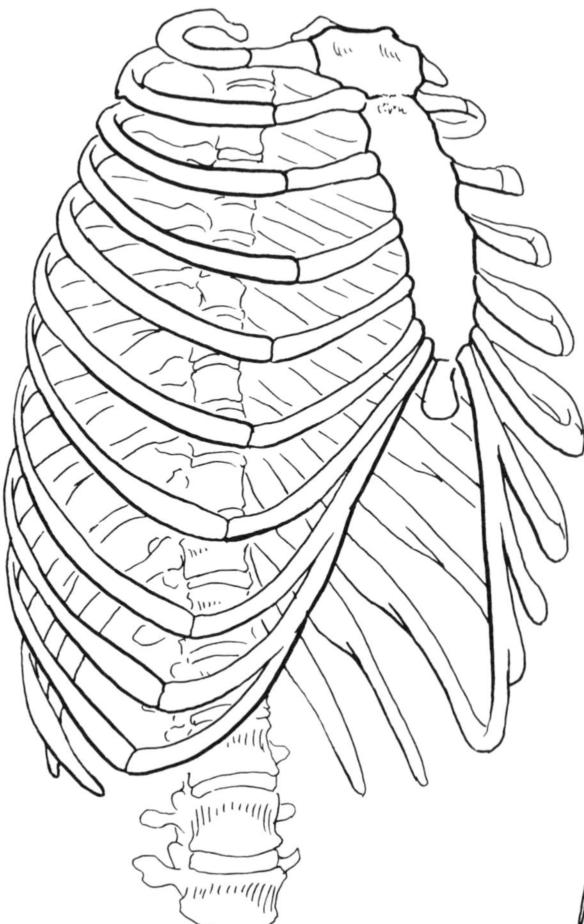

FIGURE 2.3 Both thoracic and upper abdominal viscera (shown below) are covered by the chest wall skeleton (left). These relationships become important when large sections of the chest wall must be removed and reconstructed.

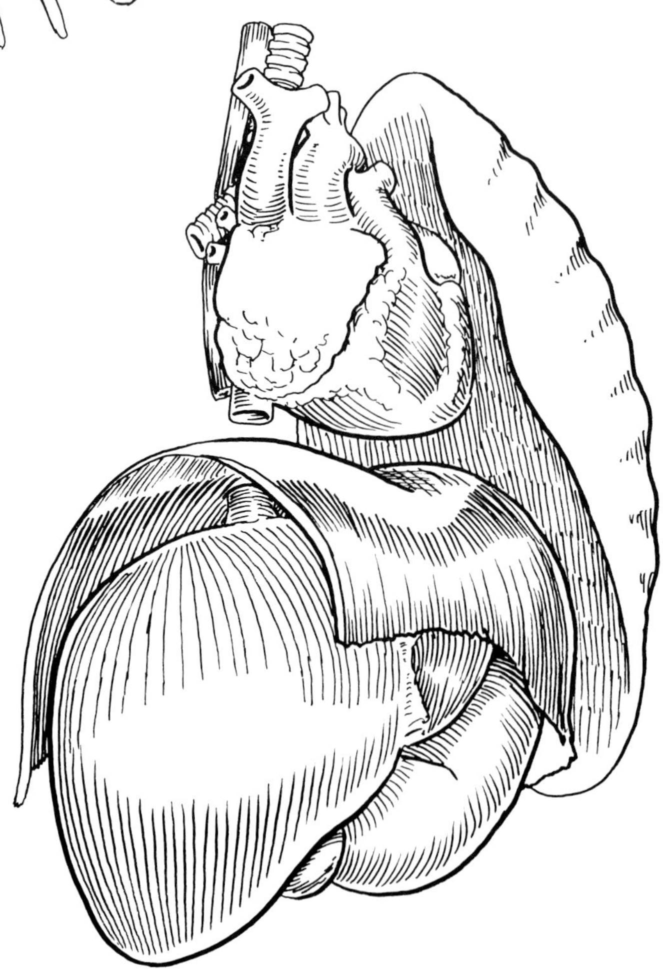

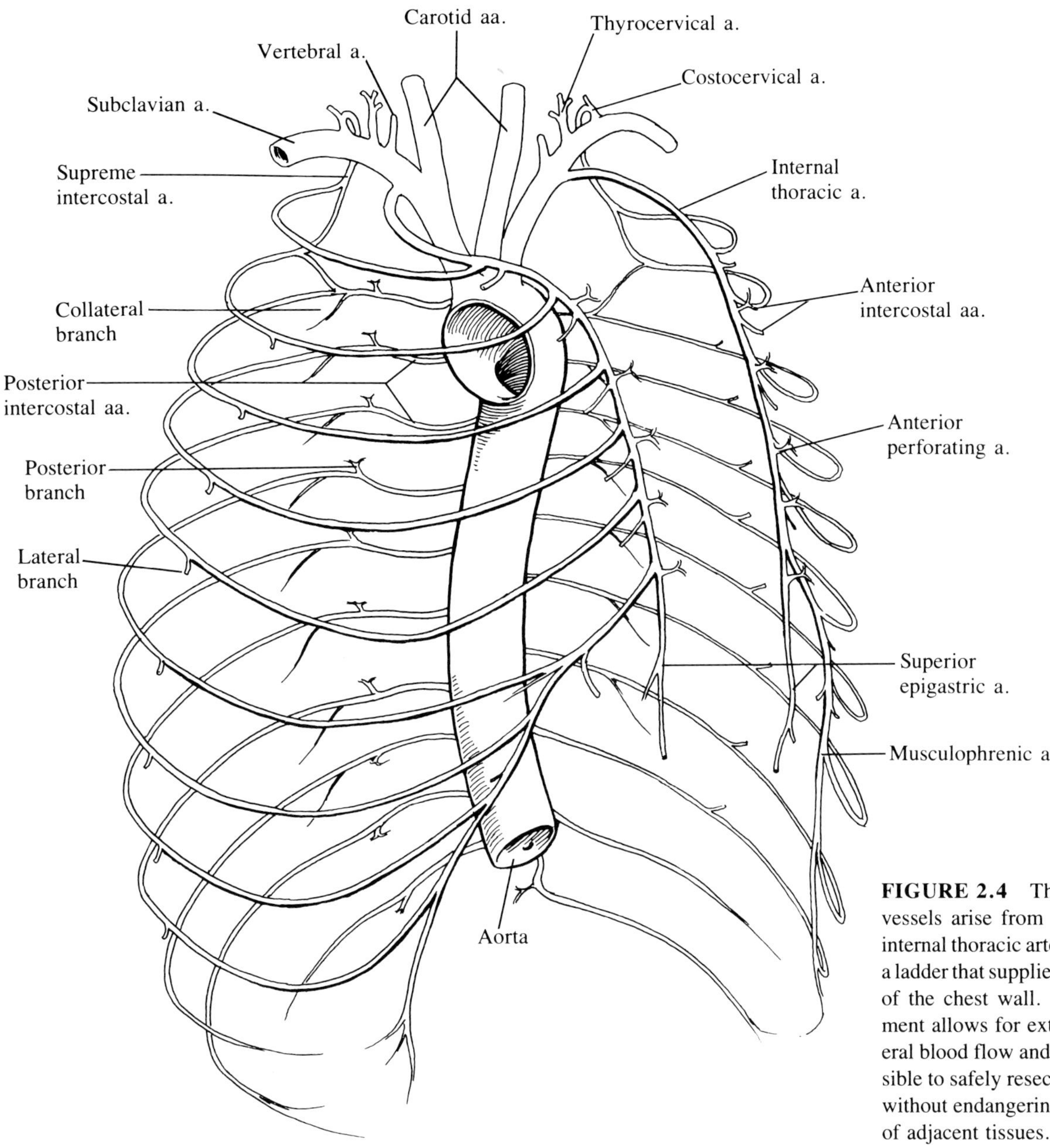

FIGURE 2.4 The intercostal vessels arise from the aorta and internal thoracic arteries and form a ladder that supplies large sectors of the chest wall. This arrangement allows for extensive collateral blood flow and makes it possible to safely resect certain areas without endangering the viability of adjacent tissues.

Neurovascular Pattern

The intrinsic arterial supply to the chest wall consists of paired vessels originating from the aorta posteriorly (except for the first one or two that come from the costocervical artery) and from the internal thoracic complex anteriorly (Figure 2.4). From the dorsal wall of the aorta, the posterior intercostal vessels pass around the vertebral bodies to reach the intercostal space. There they continue in the groove beneath the cephalad rib and lie in a plane between the intercostal muscles. At the neck of the rib, each posterior intercostal gives rise to a branch that provides segmental blood supply to the contents of the spinal canal, the vertebrae, and the muscles and skin of the medial back. Lateral branches provide regional blood supply to chest wall muscles, skin, and the breast in the

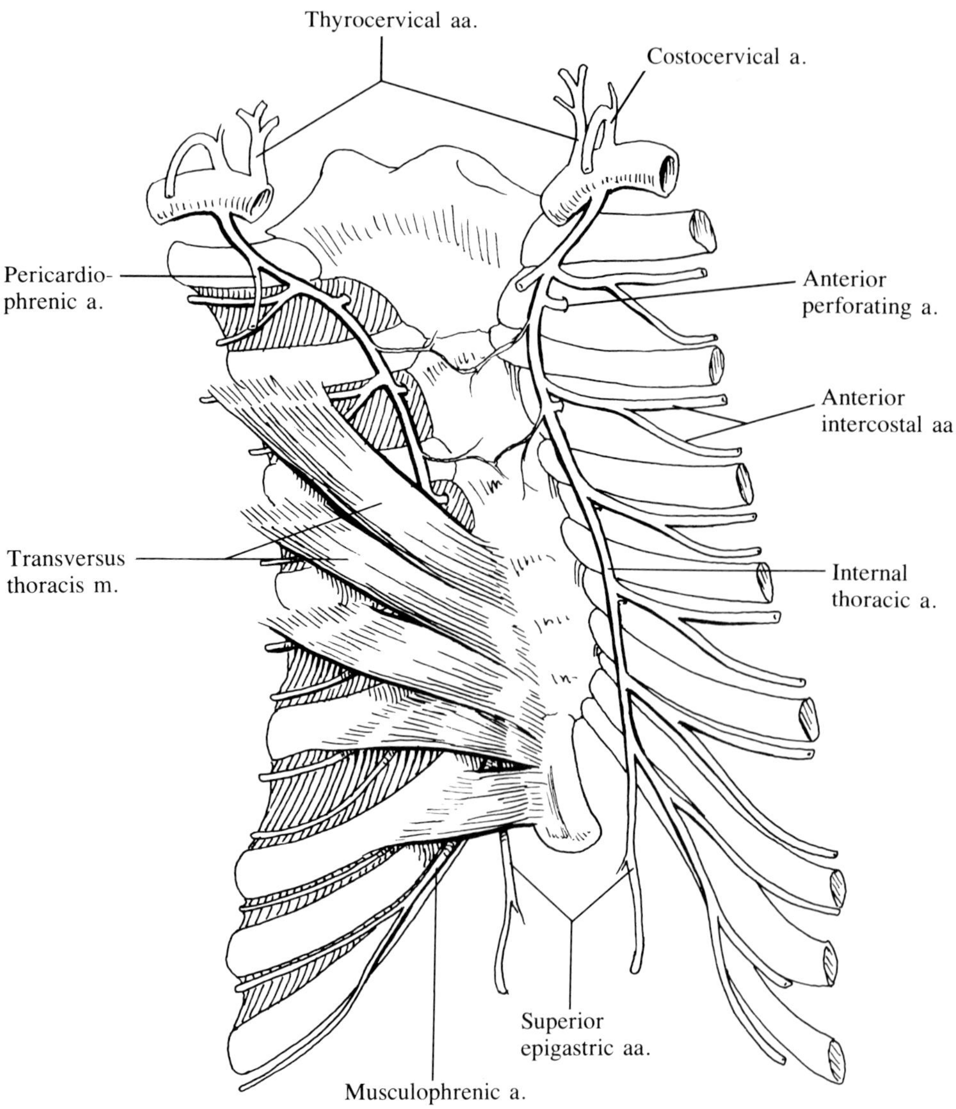

FIGURE 2.5 In an inside view of the sternum, the internal thoracic vessels are seen to lie deep to the costal cartilages and parallel to the borders of the sternum.

female. Posteriorly, the intercostal gives rise to a smaller collateral branch. The collateral and the dominant posterior intercostal artery anastomose with the two anterior intercostals that arise in each space from the internal thoracic and its musculophrenic branch.

The internal thoracic arteries arise from the first portion of the subclavian and run along the inside of the anterior chest wall parallel to the sternum (Figure 2.5). The caudal portions of the vessels lie between the transversus thoracis muscle slips and the costal cartilages. Pericardiophrenic branches arise from the proximal part of the internal thoracics. Along with the anterior intercostals in each interspace, the internal thoracic gives rise to anterior perforating branches that supply the sternal part of the pectoralis major muscle and the overlying skin. At the inferior margin of the costal cartilages, the internal thoracic splits: the musculophrenic branch gives rise to the lower anterior intercostal vessels and supplies the rim of the diaphragm; the superior epigastric continues in the direction of the internal thoracic to enter the posterior rectus sheath (Chapter 11).

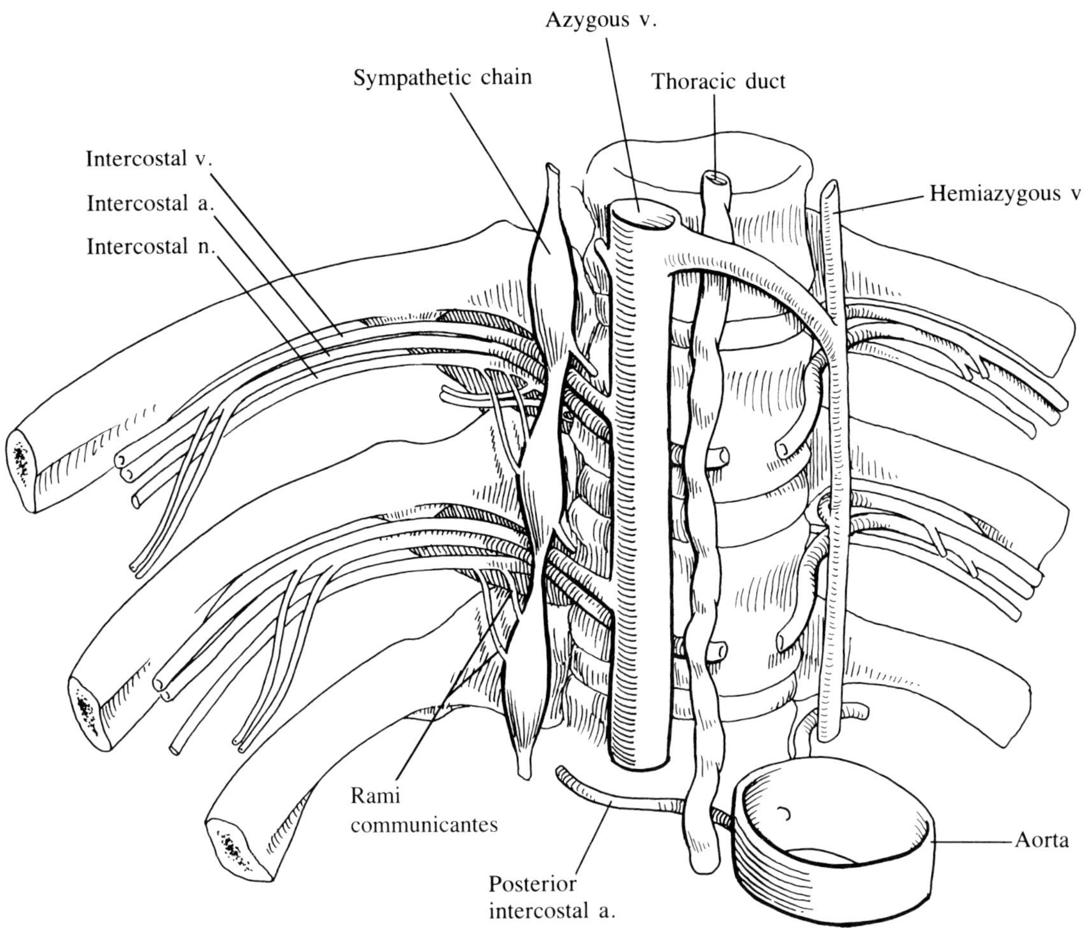

FIGURE 2.6 A complex of vascular channels and neural structures surrounds the vertebrae.

The venous drainage of the chest wall is variable but follows the same general pattern as the arterial supply. From cephalad to caudad, the triad of structures in each interspace consists of vein, artery, and nerve. The branching pattern of the intercostal nerves closely follows that of the arterial structures. Figure 2.6 shows the relationships of arterial, venous, nervous, and lymphatic structures at midthorax level. The rich, intimately connected lymphatics of the chest wall should be noted but are not dealt with in detail here.

Chest Wall Muscles

The muscles of the chest wall can be conceptualized as belonging to three groups (Figure 2.7): (1) the intrinsic intercostals and transversus thoracis; (2) the muscles attaching at the superior and inferior apertures of the thorax that provide the power for forced respiratory movement; and (3) the muscles related to the upper extremities. The diaphragm is considered separately.

The external and internal intercostals connect adjacent ribs and sandwich the intercostal neurovascular bundle between them. Laterally, where the neurovascular bundles seem to lie within the internal intercostal muscle, some authors designate the deep portion of the muscle as a separate innermost intercostal layer. The two major layers are analogous to the external and internal oblique muscles of the abdomen, and the obliquity of their fibers corresponds to these muscles. The external intercostals become

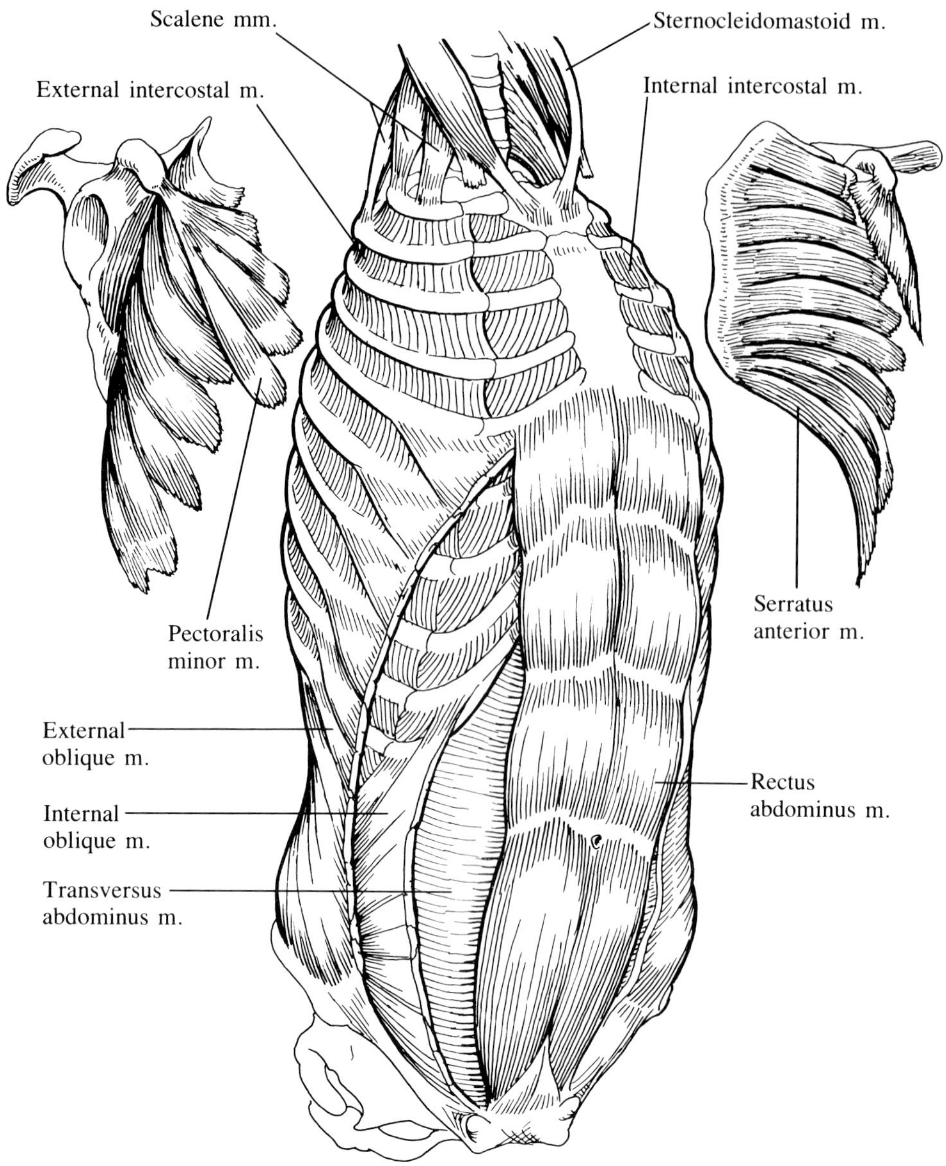

FIGURE 2.7 The muscles of the chest wall include an intrinsic group; the muscles of forced respiration that attach at the superior and inferior apertures; and the group of muscles related to the upper extremities. Some of the anterior muscles are shown here. The clavicles and subclavius muscles that attach the clavicles to the chest wall are not shown.

membranous at their anterior end about the costochondral junction, while the internal intercostals are membranous posteriorly. The innermost layer, the transversus thoracis, is found anteriorly and corresponds with the transversus abdominis with which it is continuous below. Often, these layers are credited with acting more prominently in one phase of chest wall motion than another. As a whole, they probably act most significantly to stabilize the bony framework in inspiration and to narrow the intercostal spaces and depress the rib cage during expiration.

The two muscles that attach the scapulae to the anterior chest wall are the serratus anterior and the pectoralis minor. These muscles play a minor role in elevating the rib cage.

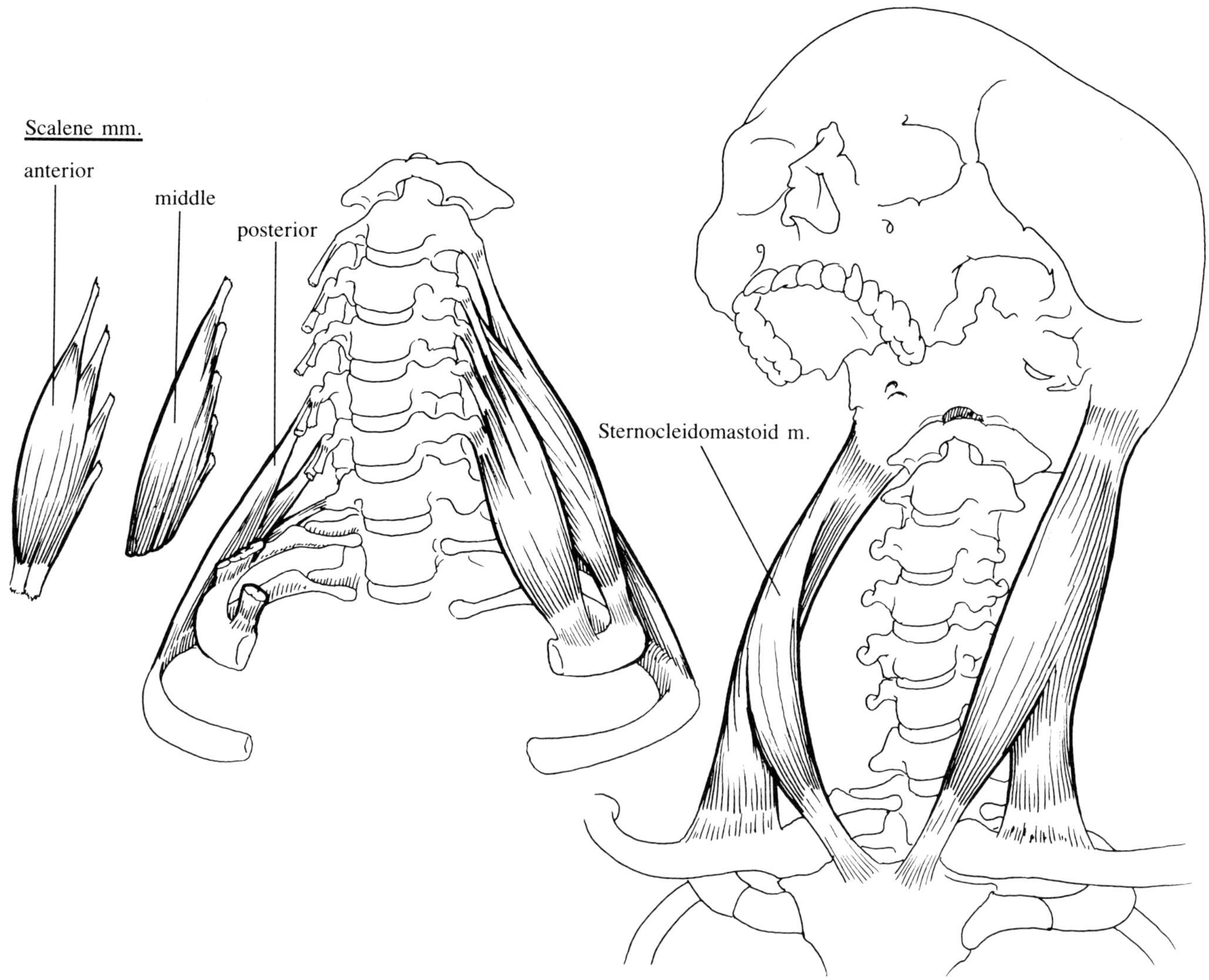

FIGURE 2.8 The scalene and sternocleidomastoid muscles elevate the rib cage during forced inspiration and are part of the group of muscles located about the superior thoracic aperture.

Around the inferior aperture of the thorax are attached the broad flat muscles of the abdominal wall: the external oblique, internal oblique, transversus abdominis, and rectus abdominis (Chapter 11). Posteriorly, the quadratus lumborum also anchors the lower rib cage. The contraction of these muscles depresses and compresses the thorax and squeezes the abdominal viscera up toward the diaphragm. Both actions push air out of the lungs in forced expiration.

At the superior thoracic aperture, the scalene muscles and sternocleidomastoids help provide power to elevate the rib cage and expand the chest during forced inspiration (Figure 2.8). The most superficial and largest muscle of the anterior chest wall is the pectoralis major (Figure 2.9), which attaches to the proximal part of the humerus (Chapter 9).

Posteriorly, the erector spinae complex fills the groove between the angles of the ribs and the vertebral spinous processes (Figure 2.10). The serratus posterior superior and serratus posterior inferior are thin, flat muscle groups that provide minor aid in elevating and depressing the ribs respectively.

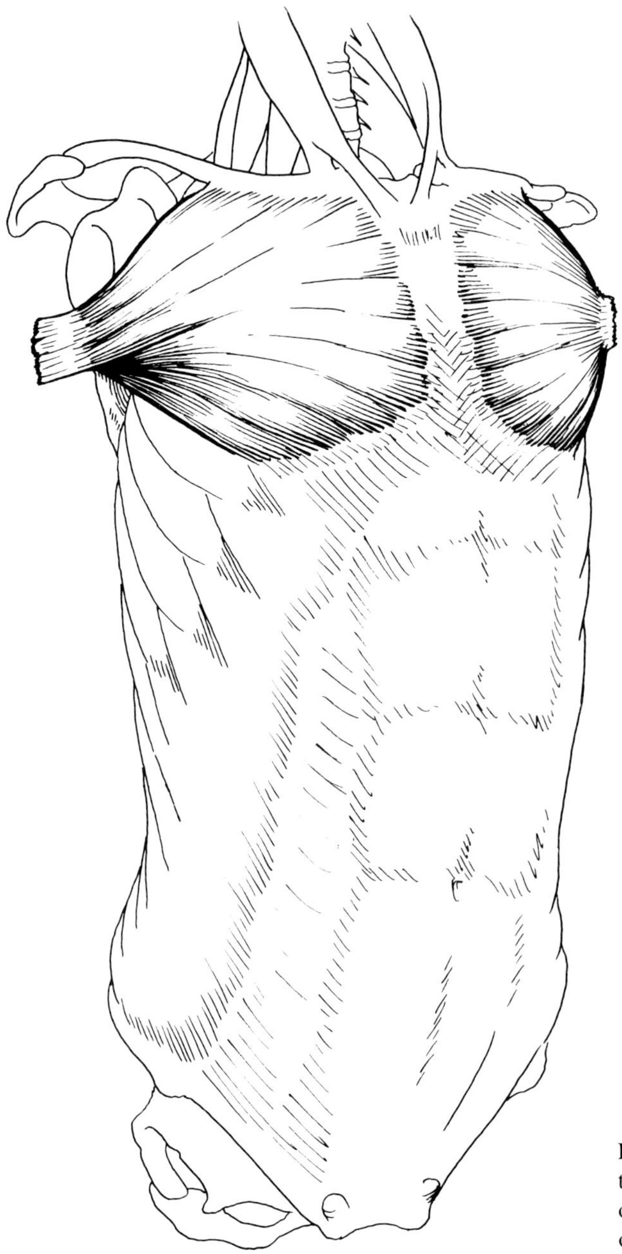

FIGURE 2.9 The large pectoralis major, although the largest of the anterior group, is a muscle of the upper extremity.

The deep muscles connecting the scapulae to the axial skeleton posteriorly are the rhomboids and the levator scapulae. The large superficial back muscles (Figure 2.11) are the trapezius (see Chapter 12) and the latissimus dorsi (Chapter 8), both muscles of the upper extremity.

Superior Thoracic Aperture

It is important to note the tight embrace of the first ribs around major visceral structures (Figure 2.12). The arch of the aorta and brachiocephalic veins lies directly beneath the manubrium. The subclavian vessels straddle the insertion of the anterior scalene muscle on the first rib, and the brachial plexus trunks accompany the subclavian artery between the anterior and middle scalene muscles. The phrenic nerves cross the anterior scalene muscles to reach the chest.

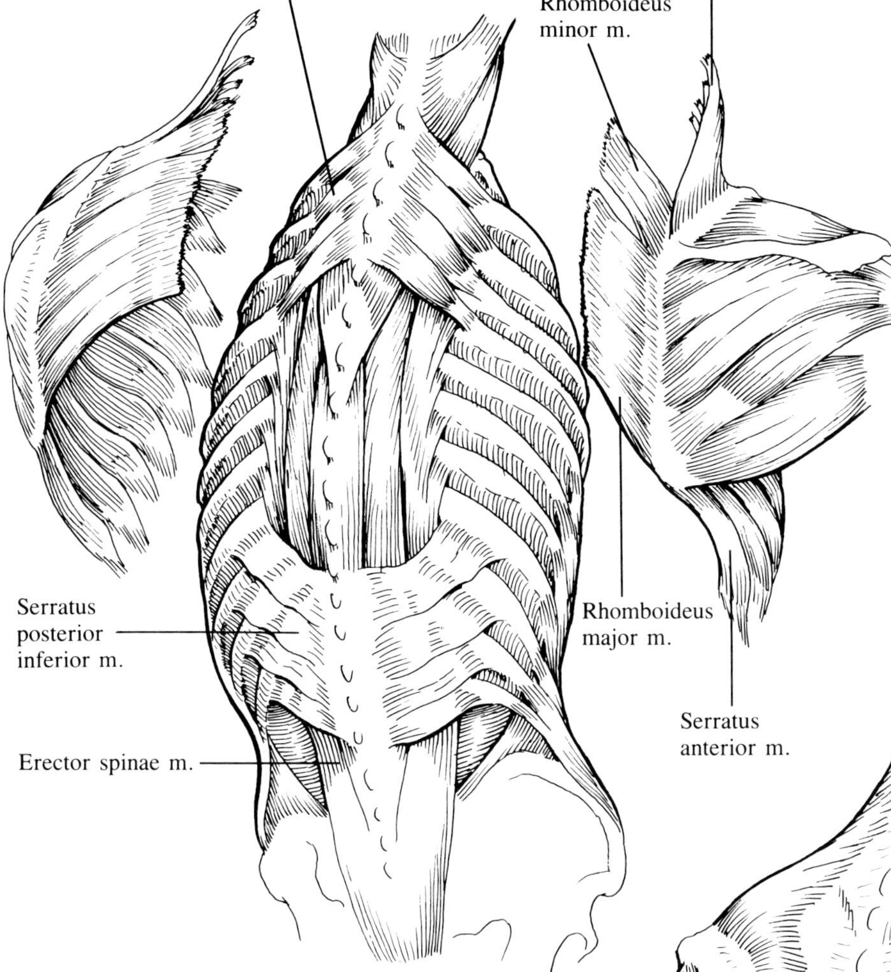

FIGURE 2.10 The deep muscles of the posterior chest include members of the intrinsic group that acts on the axial skeleton as well as members of the group that moves the upper limb.

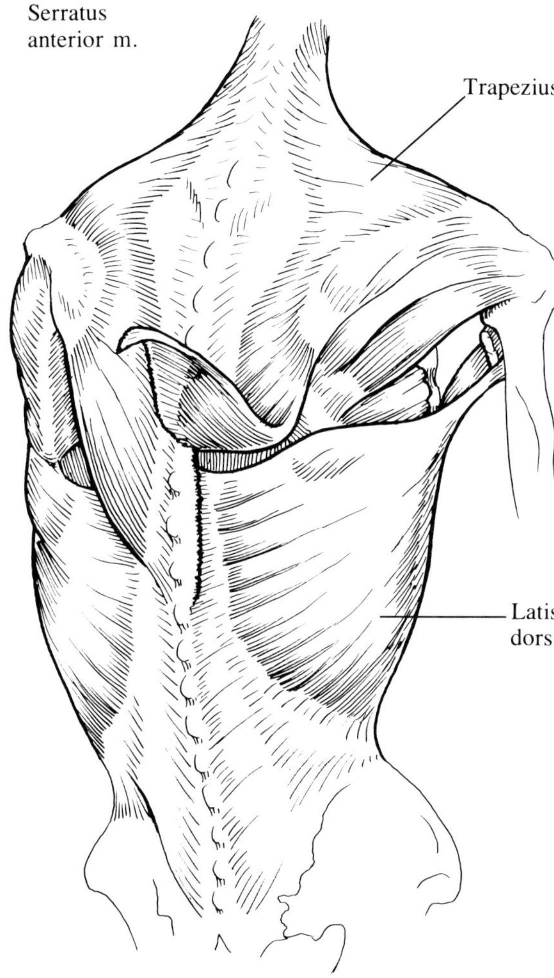

FIGURE 2.11 The trapezius and latissimus dorsi constitute the superficial muscle layer that covers most of the back and function in upper extremity movements. These muscles are useful in chest wall reconstruction.

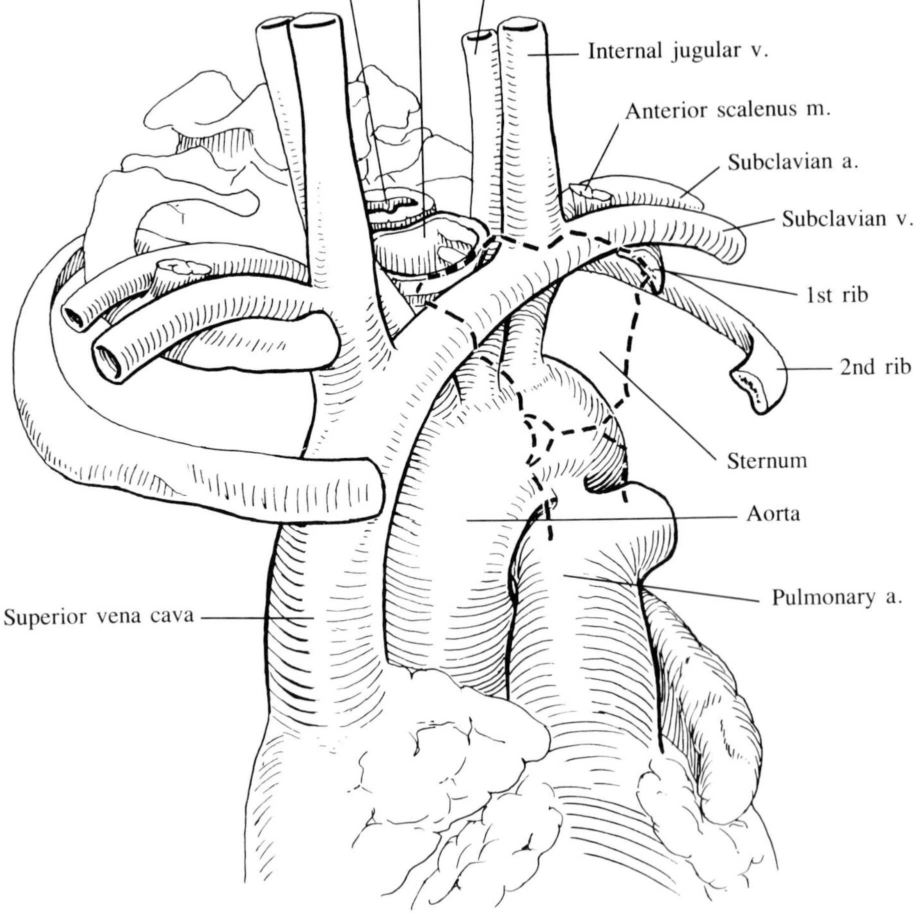

FIGURE 2.12 The superior thoracic aperture hugs a complex of vital structures and forms a protective ring around these important neurovascular, tracheal, and esophageal tissues.

Diaphragm

The diaphragm separates the thoracic from the abdominal cavity and forms a double dome over the upper abdominal organs (Figure 2.13). Its muscular fibers arise around the inner rim of the inferior thoracic aperture and converge in a flat, three-lobed tendinous aponeurosis of interlacing fibers. The base of the pericardium and the middle leaflet of this tendon are partially fused. The sternal and costal muscular fibers of the diaphragm arise from the inner surfaces of the xiphoid process and the costal margin. Posteriorly, two fibrous arches on each side span from the tip of the twelfth rib to the transverse process of L1 and from there to the body of L1 or L2. These lateral and medial lumbocostal ligaments, which cross the quadratus lumborum and psoas muscles respectively, give rise to the posterior muscular fibers of the diaphragm. The sympathetic trunks pass posterior to the medial lumbocostal arches. On either side of the upper two to three lumbar vertebrae, thick bands of muscle fibers arise to form the diaphragmatic crura, which arch upward toward the central tendon.

The medial crural fibers from each side cross and blend anterior to the aorta forming an arch. This aortic hiatus lies just cephalad to the celiac trunk at about the level of T12. Through this arch, the azygous vein and thoracic duct also enter the chest. The right crus divides and contributes the majority of muscle fibers that surround the esophageal hiatus at the level of T10. The last major hiatus, through which the vena cava

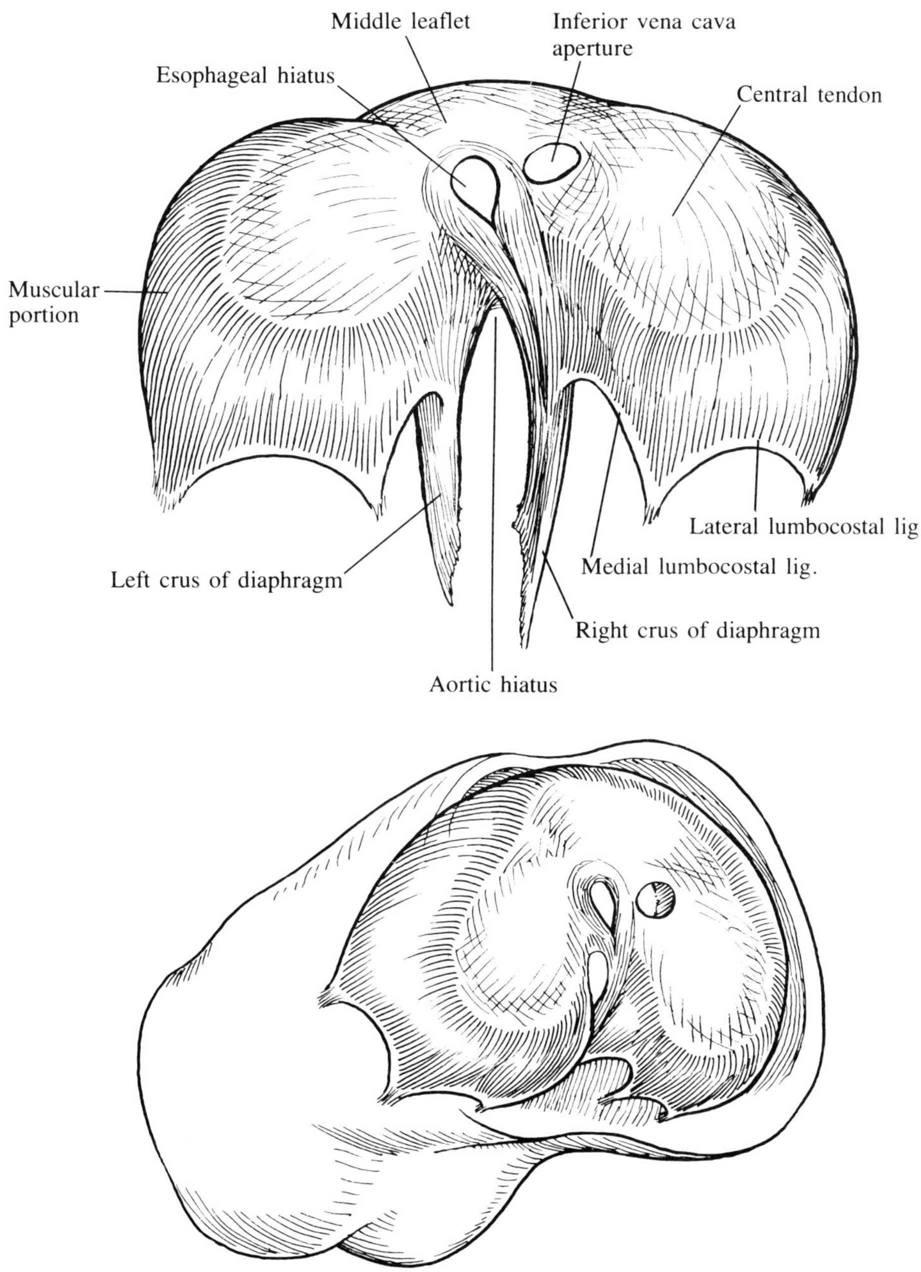

FIGURE 2.13 The domes of the diaphragm (viewed from above and posteriorly) are formed by a corona of muscle fibers arising at the inferior thoracic aperture and inserting into a central tendon.

passes, lies about the level of T8–9 at the junction of the right and middle leaf of the central tendon. The splanchnic nerves and hemiazygous vein penetrate the crura.

The blood supply to the diaphragm comes from two pairs of small arteries exiting the aorta just above and below the aortic hiatus. Additional circulation is supplied by the pericardiophrenic and musculophrenic arteries.

The diaphragm is innervated by the phrenic nerves, which are derived primarily from the fourth cervical nerve roots with contributions from roots 3 and 5. The phrenics traverse the chest cavity between the superior thoracic aperture and diaphragm, accompanied by the pericardiophrenic vessels. They lie between pericardium and pleura bilaterally. Contraction of the muscular elements of the diaphragm flattens the domed contour and constitutes one of the key elements of the respiratory mechanics discussed next.

Respiratory Physiology

Successful chest wall resection and reconstruction requires a thorough knowledge of respiratory physiology especially as it relates to the process of ventilation, that is, how the inspired air is conveyed to and from the alveoli. This complicated function is dependent on the neuromuscular integrity of the chest wall as well as the bony and cartilaginous articulations through which it works. Although secondary effects may occur in diffusion and blood flow, the primary derangements following removal of a full-thickness chest wall segment are due to altered ventilation. The following is a brief review of basic concepts and common abnormalities that can affect the patient undergoing chest wall surgery.

Ventilation is most easily understood by considering the mechanical model of breathing. A spirometer can be used to evaluate these respiratory mechanics. With this device, the patient exhales into a chamber that is inside a slightly larger container filled with water. By inhaling and exhaling into this closed system, the patient causes upward and downward motions of the container, which activates a pen on a recording cylinder. By following these recordings during the inspiratory and expiratory phases of breathing, one can gain an understanding of the volumes of air that make up the total lung capacity.

Total lung capacity is that volume of gas that completely fills the lungs to their maximum expansion from a state of maximal collapse (Figure 2.14). A small component of this is the *tidal volume*. This is the volume of air in each breath drawn in by the patient while at rest. When the patient takes in a maximal inspiration and then exhales that breath to the endpoint of forced maximal expiration, the patient has demonstrated vital capacity. The vital capacity and the residual volume in the lung after maximal forced expiration make up the total lung capacity. The functional residual capacity includes the residual volume and the expiratory reserve volume. The inspiratory capacity includes the tidal volume and the inspiratory reserve volume (see Figure 2.14 for these latter parameters).

Each of these portions of the spirometric curve is generated by the muscles of the chest wall and diaphragm. During quiet respiration, the normal tidal volume is governed

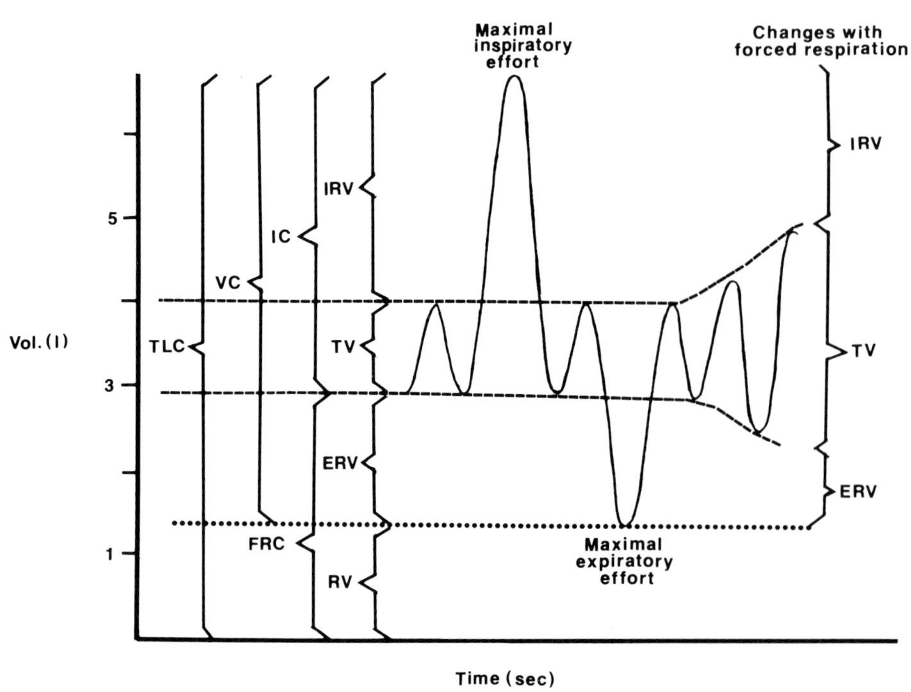

FIGURE 2.14 This diagram depicts some important volumetric measurements in ventilatory physiology. Key: TLC—total lung capacity; VC—vital capacity; IC—inspiratory capacity; FRC—functional residual capacity; IRV—inspiratory reserve volume; TV—tidal volume; ERV—expiratory reserve volume; RV—residual volume.

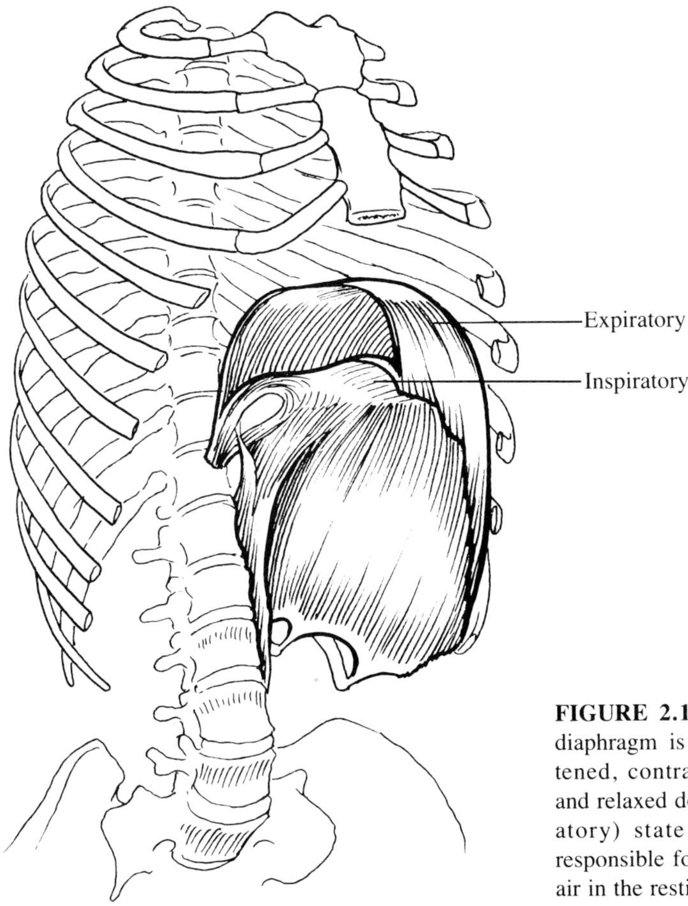

FIGURE 2.15 The left hemidiaphragm is shown in its flattened, contracted (inspiratory) and relaxed dome-shaped (expiratory) state. This motion is responsible for the movement of air in the resting state.

by the diaphragm and by the intrinsic elastic forces of the lung. With simple inspiration, the diaphragm contracts and hence moves downward (Figure 2.15). This creates a negative intrapleural pressure, the lung remains in continuity with the chest wall, and air moves into the alveoli. During quiet expiration, the diaphragm relaxes and the lung returns toward its resting station due to its intrinsic elastic forces. Tidal volumes in resting adult individuals are generally around 600–800 cc per breath. The accessory muscles of respiration are not necessary to generate the tidal volume except in individuals who have exceptional restrictive or obstructive components that limit the inflow and outflow of air.

The inspiratory reserve volume is proportional to the individual's capabilities in using these accessory muscles of inspiration. After a maximal depression (contraction) of the diaphragm, the pleural space can be expanded further by the elevation of the ribs. This lifting of the ribs occurs in anteroposterior and lateral directions and causes an elevation of the sternum as well. The ribs are, in effect, hinged posteriorly to the spine and anteriorly to the sternum. They move upward in a bucket-handle fashion so that both the anteroposterior and lateral diameters of the thoracic cavity are increased in relation to the fixed spine. The sternum is elevated more at the xiphoid than at the sternal notch, somewhat like a pump handle. This bucket-handle mechanism of the ribs and the pump-handle mechanism of the sternum are illustrated in Figure 2.16. The accessory muscles of inspiration are shown separately (Figure 2.17). These include the sternocleidomastoid, which elevates the sternum; the scalene muscles, which elevate and fix the upper ribs; the external intercostals, which elevate the ribs; and the parasternal intercartilaginous muscles, which have a smaller role.

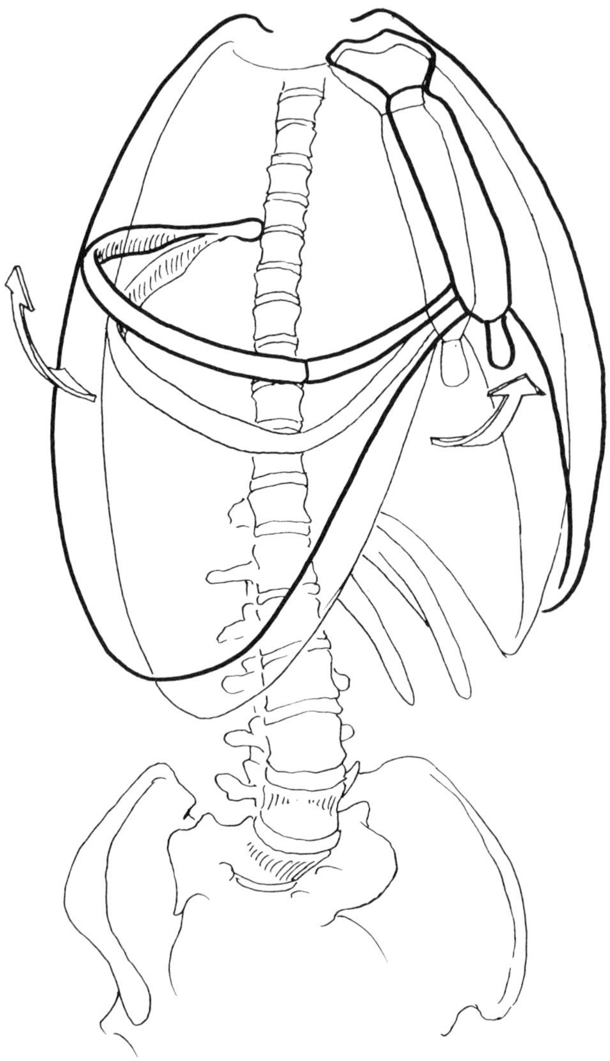

FIGURE 2.16 Forced inspiration depends on the bucket-handle motion of the ribs and the pump-handle motion of the sternum. This energy-consuming effort is mediated through the accessory muscles of respiration and occurs when metabolic demand outstrips ventilatory capabilities at rest. Excessive removal of the chest wall in the wrong patient can activate this response and lead to exhaustion.

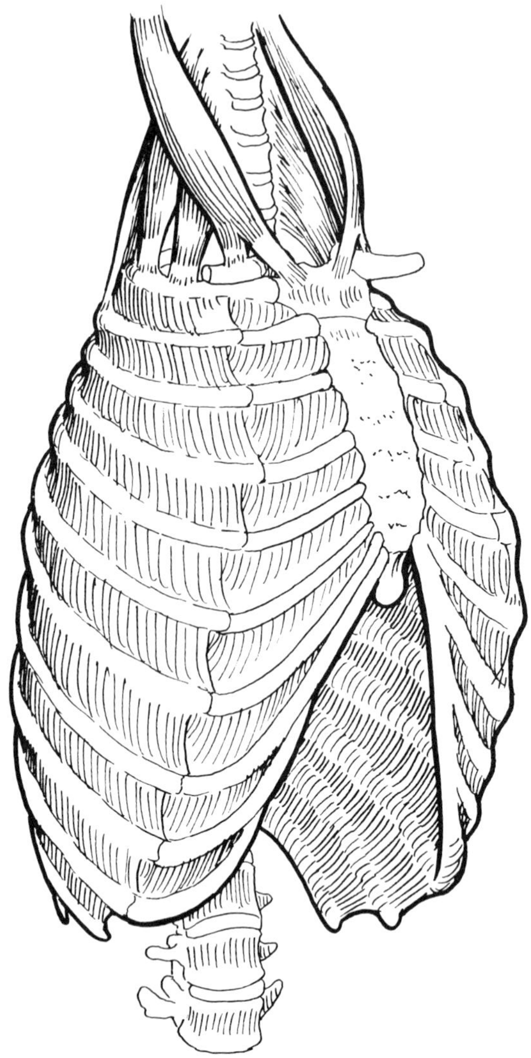

FIGURE 2.17 The accessory muscles of inspiration include the sternocleidomastoids, the scalene muscles, the external intercostals, and the parasternal intercartilaginous muscles. These muscles activate the bucket-handle and pump-handle mechanisms.

Forced expiration, beyond that generated by recoil of the chest wall and lung, is effected by contraction of the accessory muscles of expiration (Figure 2.18). These include the internal intercostals, which depress the ribs and decrease the intercostal distances, and the abdominal muscles, which also depress the ribs and compress the abdominal contents, forcing the relaxing diaphragm upward. The latter include the rectus abdominis, external oblique, internal oblique, and transversus abdominis muscles. Maximal contraction of these muscles causes the patient to exhale the expiratory reserve volume and leaves a minimal amount of air in the lung. This remaining volume is the *residual volume,* which resides in the alveolar spaces and airways.

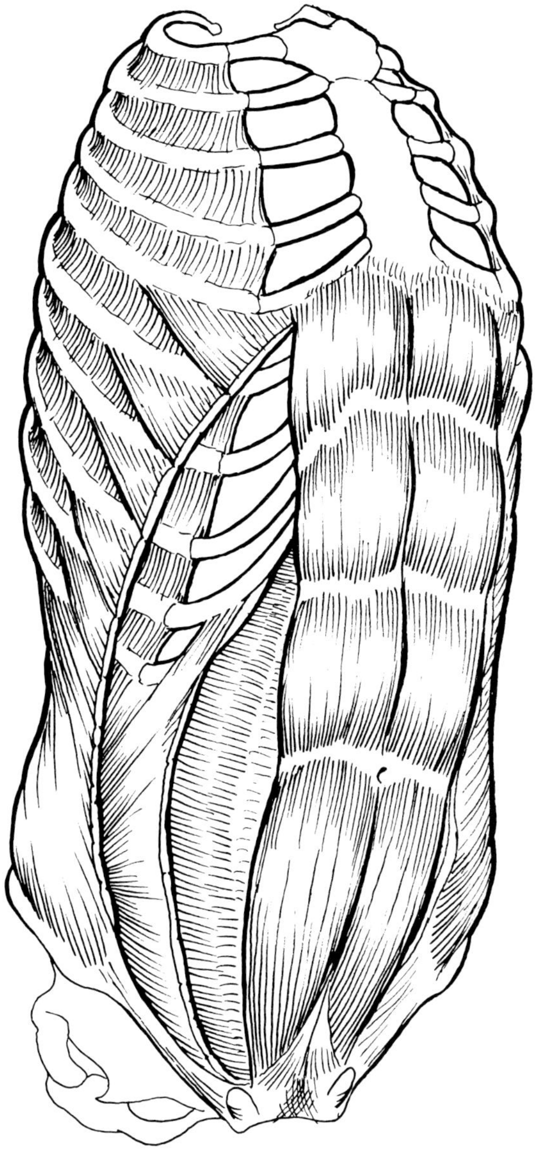

FIGURE 2.18 The accessory muscles of forced expiration consist of the internal intercostals and abdominal wall muscles. Forced expiration, like forced inspiration, can lead to exhaustion and hypoxia in certain patients.

Mechanics of Ventilation in Diseased States

Intrinsic respiratory disease can adversely affect pulmonary mechanics. The two most common types of respiratory illness are obstructive disease, which traps air within the lungs, and restrictive disease, which diminishes the expansile capacity of the lungs.

Patients who have obstructive pulmonary disease have an increased residual volume because of trapped air within the lungs and bronchi. The spirogram shows a decreased expiratory rate (Figure 2.19). Such patients have a decreased inspiratory reserve volume and a decreased vital capacity.

With restrictive diseases, such as pulmonary fibrosis, the lung is rendered incapable of expanding to its full capacity. In such cases, residual volume, total lung capacity, and vital capacity are all decreased. These patients (with pure restrictive disease) can exhale at a normal rate; hence their FEV_1 is normal. Their vital capacity is reduced since the restrictive component prohibits full expansion of the lung (Figure 2.19).

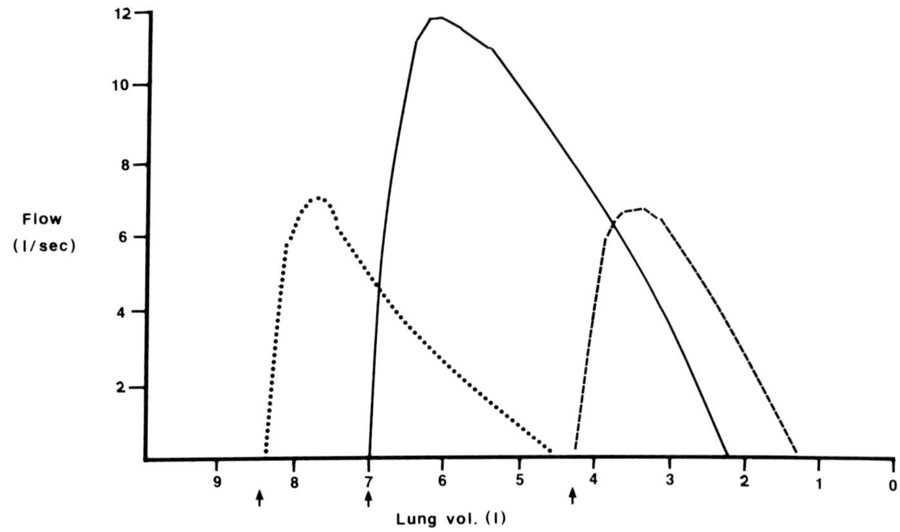

FIGURE 2.19 This figure shows representative maximal expiratory flow-volume curves for a normal individual (solid line), for a patient who has pure restrictive pulmonary disease (dashed line), and for a patient who has pure obstructive pulmonary disease (dotted line). The arrows denote where each of the three patients began to exhale after a maximal inspiration. The residual volume is represented by the second intersection of the tracing with the horizontal axis (at the end of forced expiration). The volume exhaled is the vital capacity; this, plus the residual volume, is the total lung capacity. The patient with obstructive disease does not achieve the flow rate of the normal individual because of airway obstruction. The expiratory phase is prolonged and the residual volume is increased. The patient with restrictive disease cannot achieve the expiratory flow of the normal individual because vital capacity (and total lung capacity) are diminished. The expiratory phase is normal in duration, and the patient's residual volume is markedly diminished.

Restrictive and obstructive pulmonary disease can coexist. Patients presenting with both of these components are generally at greater risk since their ventilatory capabilities are diminished by both processes. Careful preoperative evaluation is mandatory in all individuals to assure that they can tolerate the operation and be successfully weaned from the ventilator after their chest wall resection and reconstruction (Chapters 4 and 7).

References

Embryology

Arey LB: *Developmental Anatomy: A Textbook and Laboratory Manual of Embryology,* ed. 7. Philadelphia, WB Saunders, 1965.

Ravitch MM: *Congenital Deformities of the Chest Wall and Their Operative Correction.* Philadelphia, WB Saunders, 1977.

Respiratory Physiology

Netter FM: *The Ciba Collection of Medical Illustrations, Vol. 7: Respiratory System. Section II: Physiology.* Summit, NJ, Ciba-Geigy Corp., 1979.

West JB: *Respiratory Physiology—The Essentials,* ed. 2. Baltimore, Williams & Wilkins, 1979.

West JB: *Pulmonary Pathophysiology—The Essentials.* Baltimore, Williams & Wilkins, 1977.

3

Blood Supply to the Skin of the Chest Wall

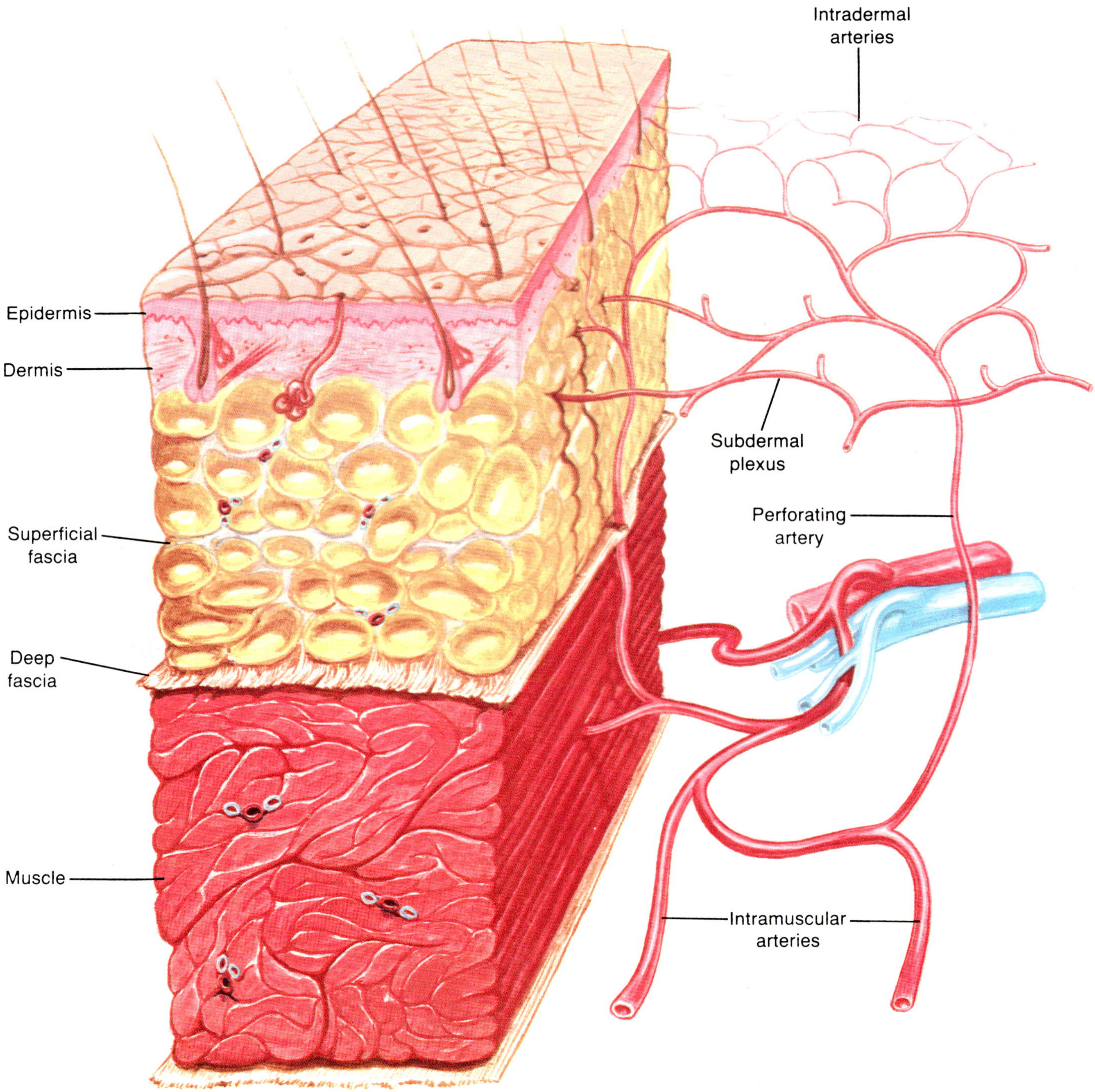

A block of skin, fascia and underlying muscle is shown next to an isolated set of vessels that traverse these layers. Note the deep intramuscular origin of the arteries that feed the subdermal and intradermal plexi.

PLATE 3.1 In this segment of chest wall skin, note the three vascular levels: (1) the large muscular artery and vein at the deepest level, which sends nutrient vessels coursing through the muscle; (2) the medium-sized perforators, which emerge from the muscular fascia into the subcutaneous fat to supply the subdermal net of vessels; and (3) the rich dermal layer of vessels, which supplies the skin.

Over the last ten to fifteen years, a greater understanding of the circulation to the supporting tissues and skin has evolved, and this knowledge has greatly extended the capabilities of those dealing with surgical problems of the chest wall. Based on this understanding, ample segments of skin and muscle can be safely mobilized as flaps, without interruption of blood supply, and shifted to reconstruct large full-thickness thoracic defects. Such techniques have enabled surgical teams to effectively treat extensive tumors in one stage and to reliably repair ablative defects that previously could not be accomplished without grave risk to the patient.

In order to perform such reconstructive operations safely, a thorough knowledge of the range, size limitations, indications, and contraindications for each flap is mandatory. Such knowledge begins with an understanding of the blood supply to the skin and parietes.

General Organization of the Vessels

The network of arterioles and capillaries that support the skin interconnects in a rich plexus within and immediately subjacent to the dermis. The small vessels in and around this layer not only provide nutrition to the adnexal structures (sweat glands, sebaceous glands, nerves, etc.) but, by diffusion through the basement membrane, supply nutrients to the avascular layers of surface cells, the epidermis (Plate 3.1). At the arteriolar level, this plexus performs its important thermoregulatory function. There are two important concepts to keep in mind about this plexus arrangement: it is continuous from one area of skin to the next, throughout the body, and it forms a final common pathway for the blood delivered by the different types of feeding vessels to the skin.

Most of this network is supplied by larger vessels (called *perforators* since they perforate the deep fascia) that travel only a short vertical distance after emerging from the deep fascia of the underlying muscle. From the fascia, the arteries rise through the subcutaneous fat and arborize into the network supplying the overlying skin (Plate 3.1). However, in certain areas (which are less common), the larger vessels do not go directly up into the subdermal plexus but travel parallel to the undersurface of the skin (or horizontally) for some distance, usually above the superficial fascia, while sending small branches up to the subdermal vascular net along the way (Figure 3.1). Whichever of these two major systems is present (the vertical or the horizontal arteries), once the blood enters the dermal and subdermal plexi, it circulates through the rich anastomoses, supplying nutrition and serving the thermoregulatory mechanism before entering the network of veins that drains the skin structures. These veins empty into ever-enlarging tributaries that parallel the incoming arteries before entering the deep venous systems for the return trip to the heart. Certain regional circulatory arrangements determine the type and size of skin flap selected for the reconstruction.

Types of Flaps and Supplying Vessels

If a small rectangle of skin and fat is chosen to reconstruct an adjacent defect, this can be done safely by freeing the skin and fat from the deep fascia but leaving them attached along one side of the rectangle. This ensures that the resulting skin flap will retain an adequate circulation. The flap is then rotated into the recipient defect. However, as the flap is mobilized, it is necessary to divide some of the randomly situated, vertically oriented vessels that perforate the muscular fascia and enter the skin from below (Figure 3.2). The only vessels left to provide circulation to the flap are those near the side that was left intact (the base of the flap). Since these vertical vessels are small, there is a limit to the area of the skin flap that can be moved without necrosis occurring on the side away from the base (Figure 3.3). If the base of the flap contains only one or two

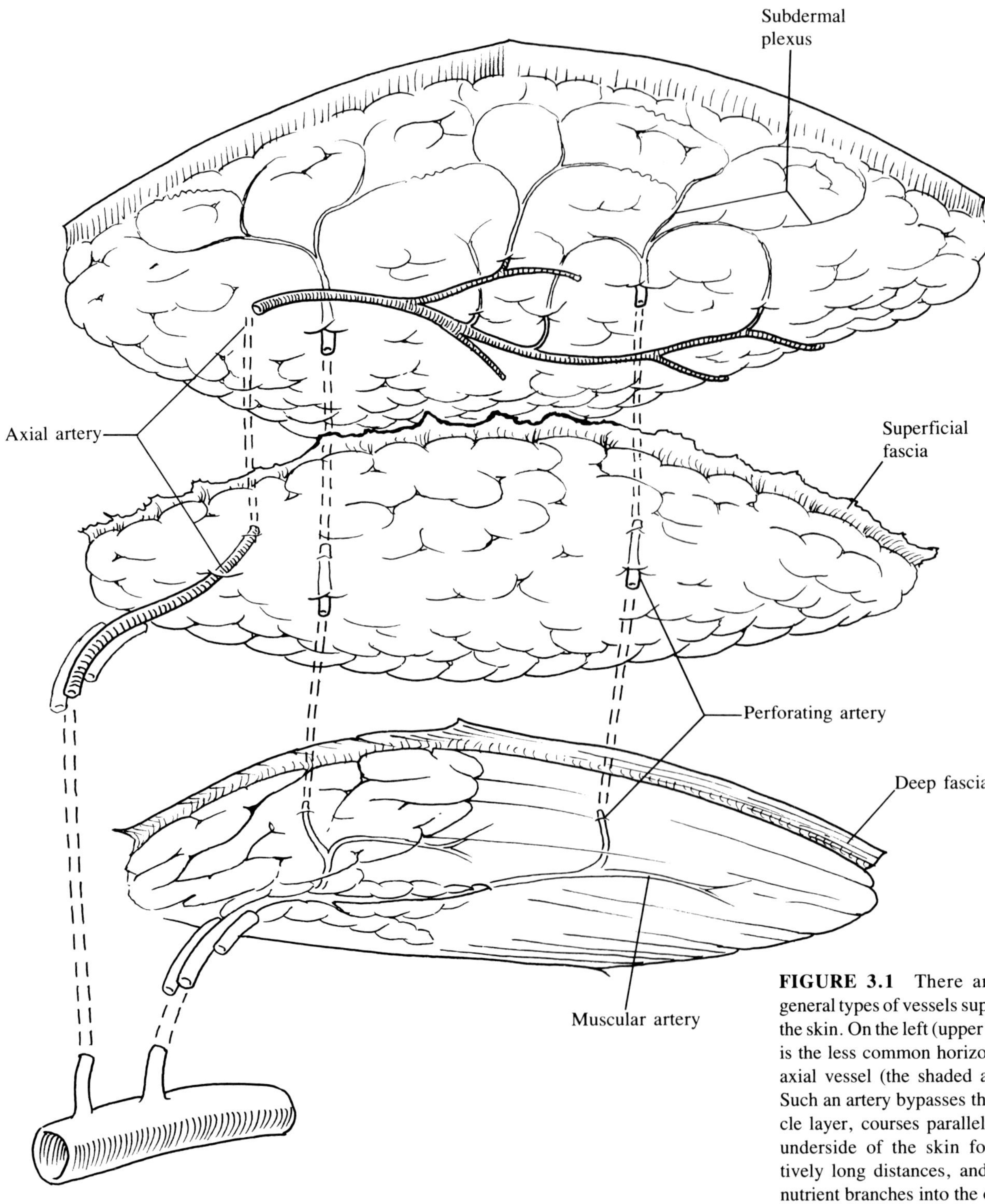

FIGURE 3.1 There are two general types of vessels supplying the skin. On the left (upper figure) is the less common horizontal or axial vessel (the shaded artery). Such an artery bypasses the muscle layer, courses parallel to the underside of the skin for relatively long distances, and sends nutrient branches into the overlying dermal vascular net. On the right (lower figure) is the more common arrangement. These vessels course along the deep aspect of the muscle (and within it) before sending perforating branches up through the fascia and into the dermal plexus.

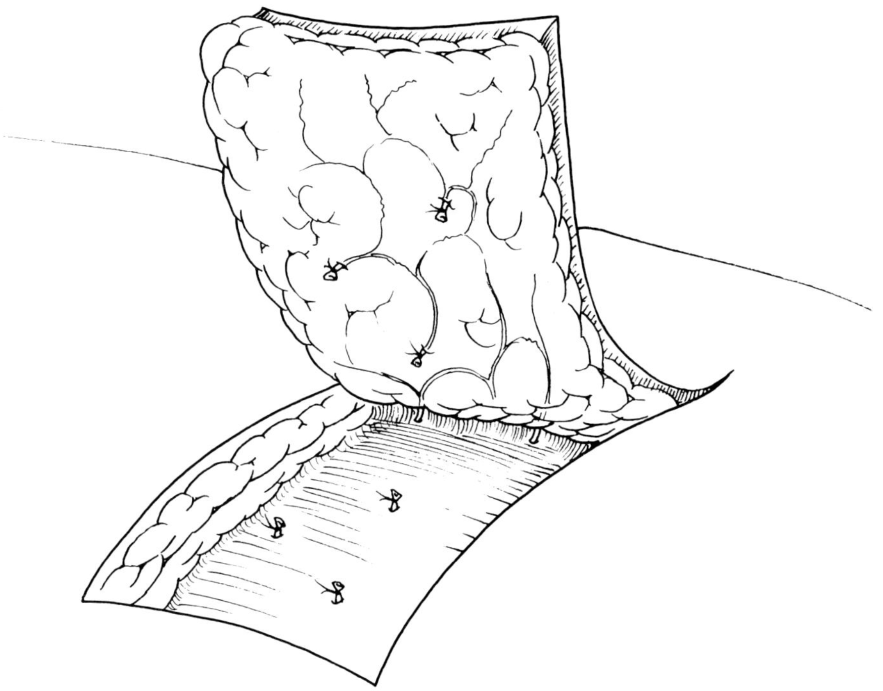

FIGURE 3.2 In a random pattern skin flap, as the flap of skin and subcutaneous fat is mobilized, it is necessary to divide some of the perforators from the underlying muscle that supplies the skin. It then depends on the circulation entering from the remaining perforators along the undisturbed margin. Such a flap must necessarily be relatively short in length due to its limited blood supply.

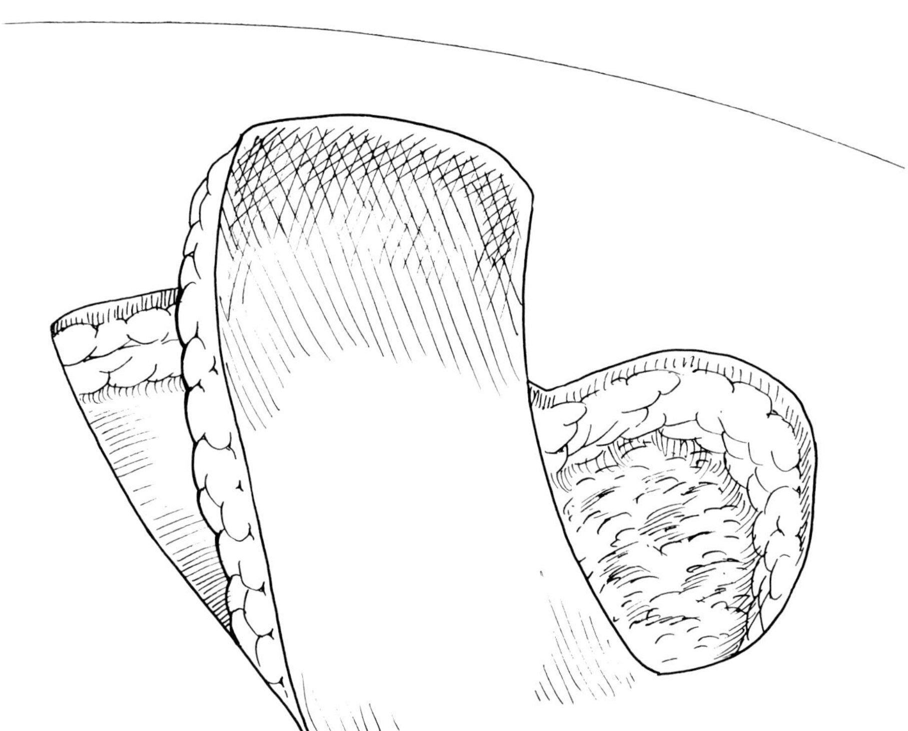

FIGURE 3.3 This random pattern skin flap has been mobilized to fill a nearby defect to the right. Such flaps, due to their limited blood supply, have a short range of coverage and are used primarily for adjacent defects. The cross-hatched area, being at the greatest distance from the base, has the greatest risk of necrosis.

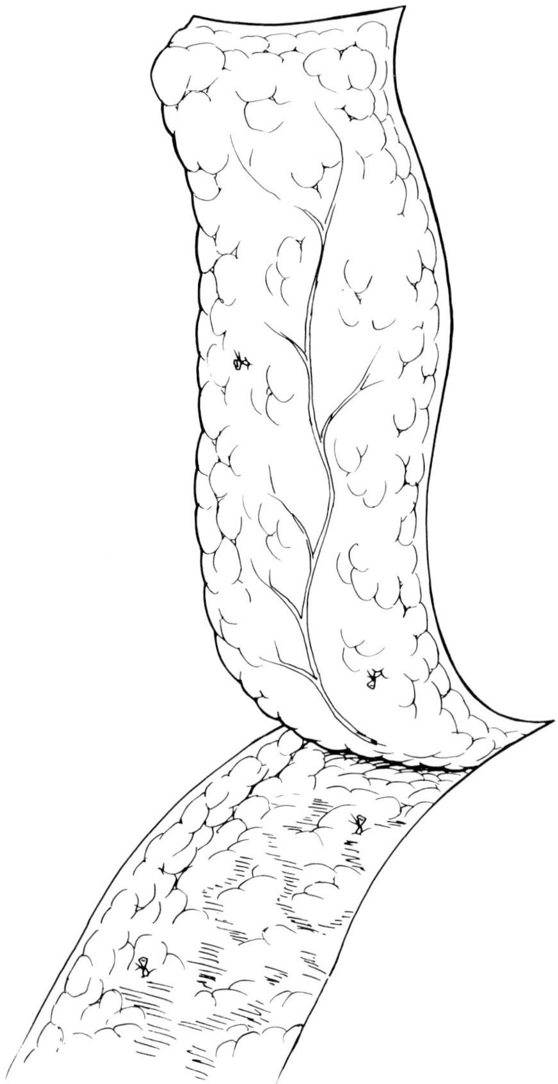

FIGURE 3.4 The axial pattern skin flap has a much greater range of coverage than the random pattern flaps since it carries its blood supply with it. Instead of random perforators from the deep muscle layers, its blood supply is a long artery coursing directly under the skin and running along the axis of the flap.

perforators, the threat of necrosis increases. Since this flap depends on random, perforating blood vessels from below the dermis, it is called a *random pattern skin flap*. The key to remember with this type of flap is that some of the perforating vessels are transected as the flap is elevated. This severely restricts the blood supply, and only a short flap of skin survives for use in any reconstruction.

Another important type of flap depends on a different circulatory arrangement. This type supports the skin not by vertical perforators from the deep muscular fascia but by a vessel that runs parallel to and under the skin in a horizontal direction within the subcutaneous fat as described earlier. Small branches from this vessel supply the overlying skin until the main artery gets so small that it blends into the dermal-subdermal anastomotic network (Figure 3.4). Before fading out, however, the vessel runs superficially for a relatively long distance along a predictable axis or direction. This is of great use since a reliable flap can be designed with this vessel running down the middle, incorporating a long, wide strip of viable skin and a thin layer of subcutaneous fat containing the vascular pedicle. This type of flap is called an *axial pattern flap* since it includes a named artery within its longitudinal axis. Like other major flaps, it has a relatively constant territory of skin that it supplies and that can be used reliably for reconstructive purposes. Such flaps are much longer and thus have a greater range of

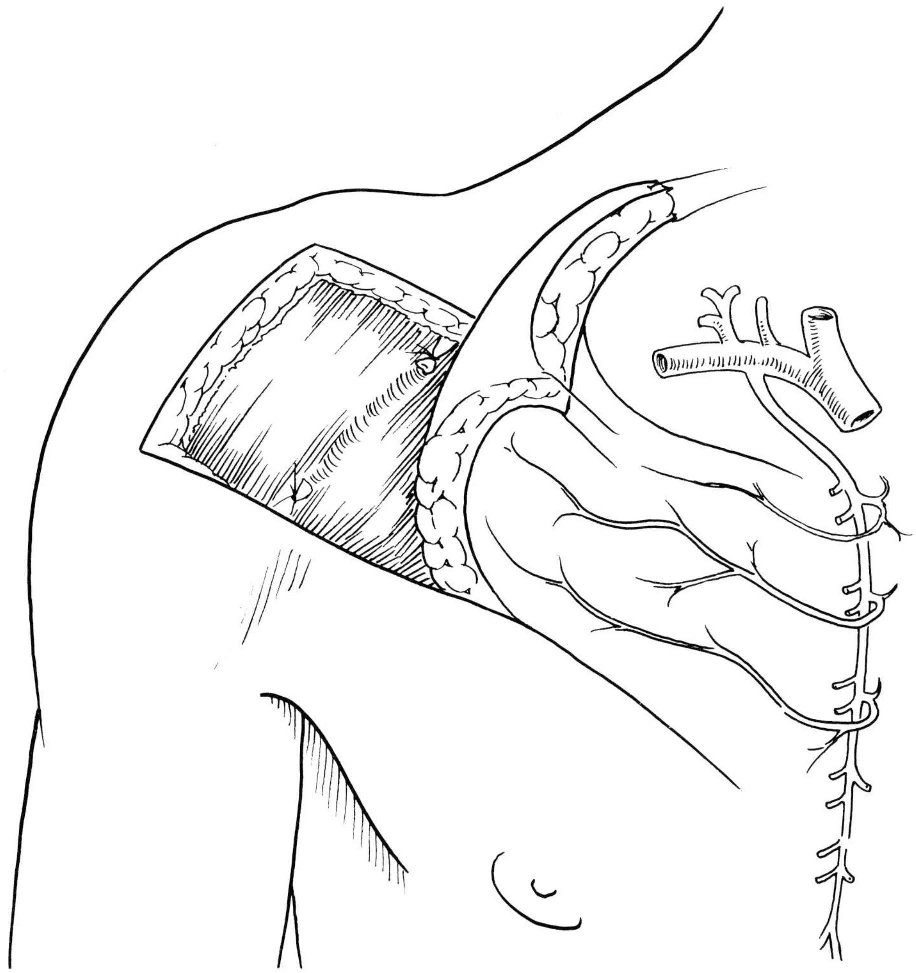

FIGURE 3.5 The deltopectoral axial pattern skin flap is supplied by the long, subcutaneous branches of the internal thoracic artery. A long strip of skin, incorporating this hearty blood supply, can be safely mobilized for reconstructive operations.

coverage than the random pattern flaps. Like the musculocutaneous flaps (discussed next), they can be mobilized so that they are attached only by their vascular pedicle. Only a few axial territories exist in humans. An example of an axial flap on the chest wall is the deltopectoral flap, which is supplied by the cephalad branches of the internal thoracic artery (Figure 3.5).

On the other hand, the majority of the skin of the body (and chest wall) is supplied by the vertical transmuscular type of circulation. If it were possible to preserve a large number of these perforators while mobilizing a specific area of skin, the territory of the skin that could be moved safely and without necrosis would be greatly increased. This can, in fact, be accomplished in many areas of the body by moving not only the skin but the muscle through which the perforators travel. With such a maneuver, the whole system of perforating vessels is moved with the muscle-skin flap as a unit. In effect, the muscle serves as a carrier for the skin. Such a composite flap is called a *musculocutaneous flap* since the muscle and skin move as a unit based on the artery that supplies both of them (Figure 3.6). This artery usually travels on the underside of the muscle and within its substance. The range or reach of these flaps far exceeds the cutaneous random pattern flaps since they are not tethered along one side but can be circumferentially mobilized until attached only by their vascular pedicle. Since the blood supply is carried with the flap, a larger and more reliable flap can be designed. Musculocutaneous flaps may be supplied by single or multiple arteries, depending on the particular muscle. Since the type of vascular pedicle differs from one muscle-skin unit to another, this variation must be taken into consideration in planning the reconstructive effort. For example, the rectus abdominis musculocutaneous flap has two major pedicles

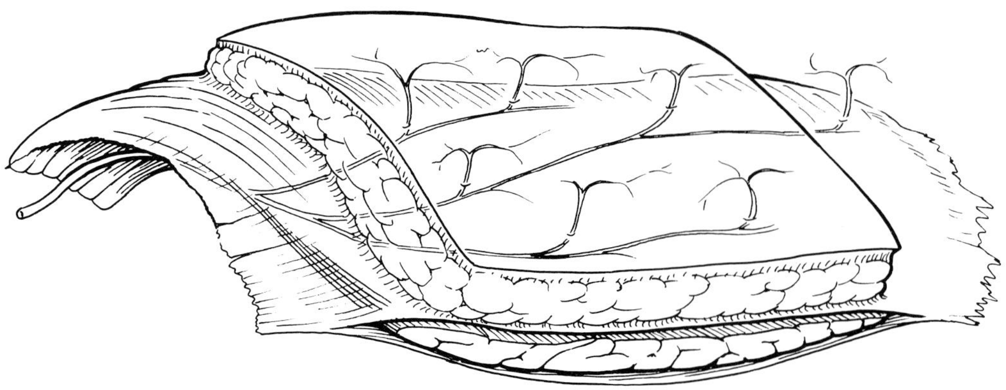

FIGURE 3.6 A musculocutaneous flap is a composite of muscle and skin, both supplied by the same arterial system. The vascular pedicle usually courses on the deep aspect of the muscle and sends branches up through the muscle to perforate the fascia and enter the subcutaneous fat. These perforators then arborize to supply the overlying skin. Such flaps have a great range of coverage since the underlying muscle can be widely mobilized, along with its vascular pedicle, to reach distant defects. The muscle, in effect, acts as a carrier for the skin. The muscle can also be used without the overlying skin and employed as a muscle flap alone.

(Figure 3.7) while the latissimus dorsi musculocutaneous flap has one major pedicle and a smaller, minor system of feeding vessels (Figure 3.8). Also, the muscle selected must be relatively dispensable in terms of function if postoperative disability is to be minimized.

The Concept of Vascular Territories

The pattern of the cutaneous blood vessels has important implications in the design of skin and muscle flaps for reconstructing chest wall defects. For example, if a large flap is required, the factor that limits its size is the blood supply. The surgeon must therefore be able to predict accurately how large an area of skin can be safely moved before ischemic necrosis of the flap occurs. To do this, it is helpful to divide the skin into vascular territories, which can be used to plan the reliable movement of large skin segments based on their blood supply. Such regional maps of the skin circulation have been charted both experimentally and clinically. They provide the surgeon with a reliable estimate of just how much tissue will survive when it is cut loose from its normal surroundings and moved to a new location while still attached to a localized vascular pedicle. This information can be used effectively to plan for the safe reconstruction of defects in specific areas of the chest wall. The territories are defined by the arrangement of arterial feeders to the skin.

When undisturbed, each vascular territory depends on a circulatory equilibrium within the skin, such that the boundaries are at the junction of adjacent areas of arterial runoff. If the pedicle to an in situ area of skin is ligated, adjacent territories expand to provide nutrition to that skin segment (Figure 3.9). This degree of overlap is extensive on the chest wall, such that a specific area of skin may receive collateral circulation from a number of distant sources. As discussed, these are mainly derived from the vertical transmuscular perforators underlying the skin. When an area of skin is circumferentially released from its surroundings and moved to another location, the collateral flow is interrupted and at least one major pedicle (or system of perforators) must remain undisturbed or the skin will not survive. Herein lies the value of the concept of vascular territories: it allows the surgeon to formulate a reliable reconstructive plan before attempting to move a large area of skin. The following discussion describes, in a general way, the territories based on their blood supply.

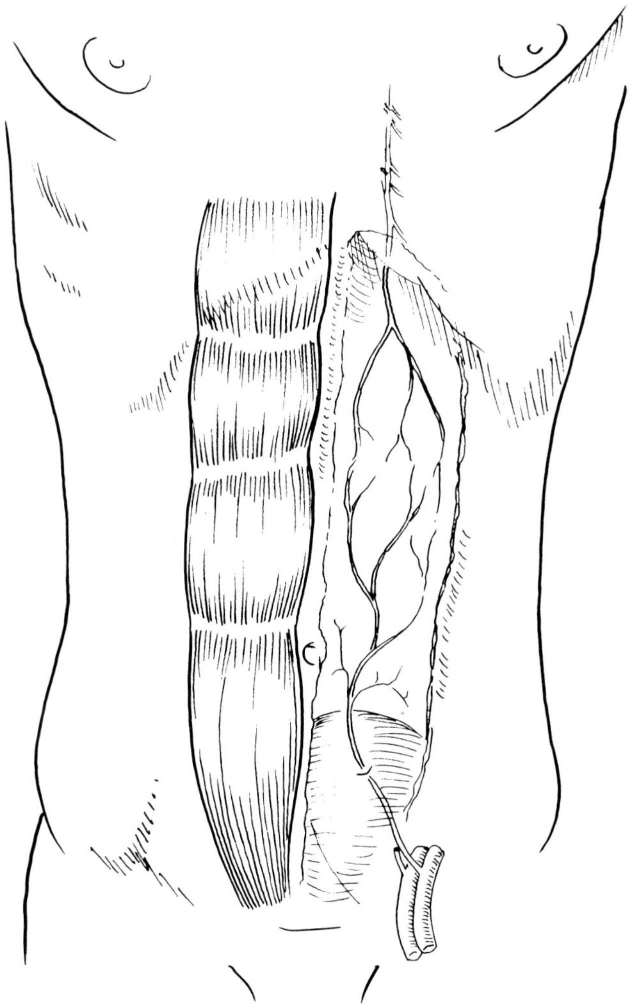

FIGURE 3.7 The rectus abdominis muscle and musculocutaneous flap is an example of a flap with two pedicles, either one of which can be used as the sole vascular supply (Chapter 11).

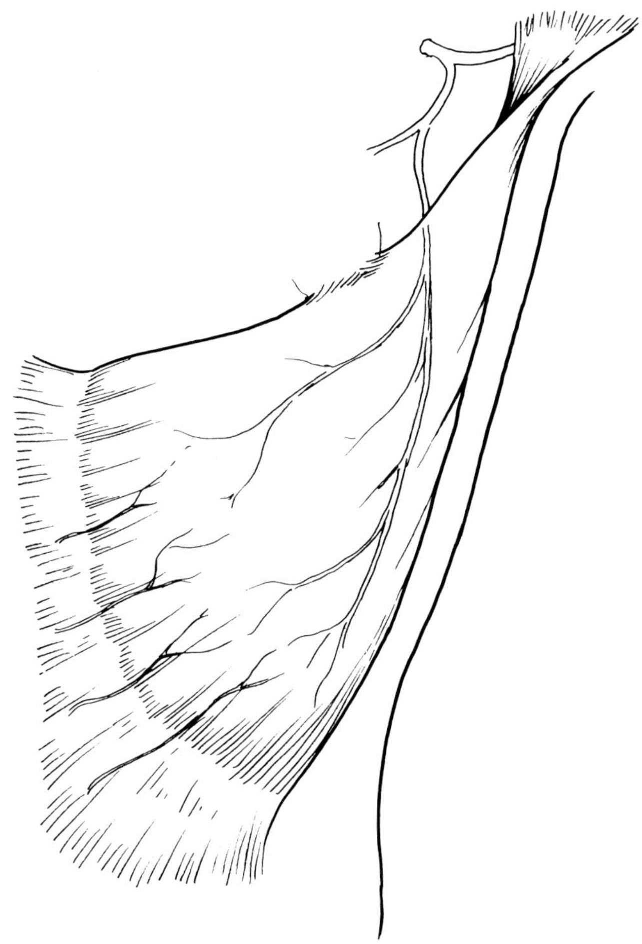

FIGURE 3.8 The latissimus dorsi flap has a major vascular pedicle coming in from the axillary area and a minor system of small feeding vessels entering near the spine (Chapter 8).

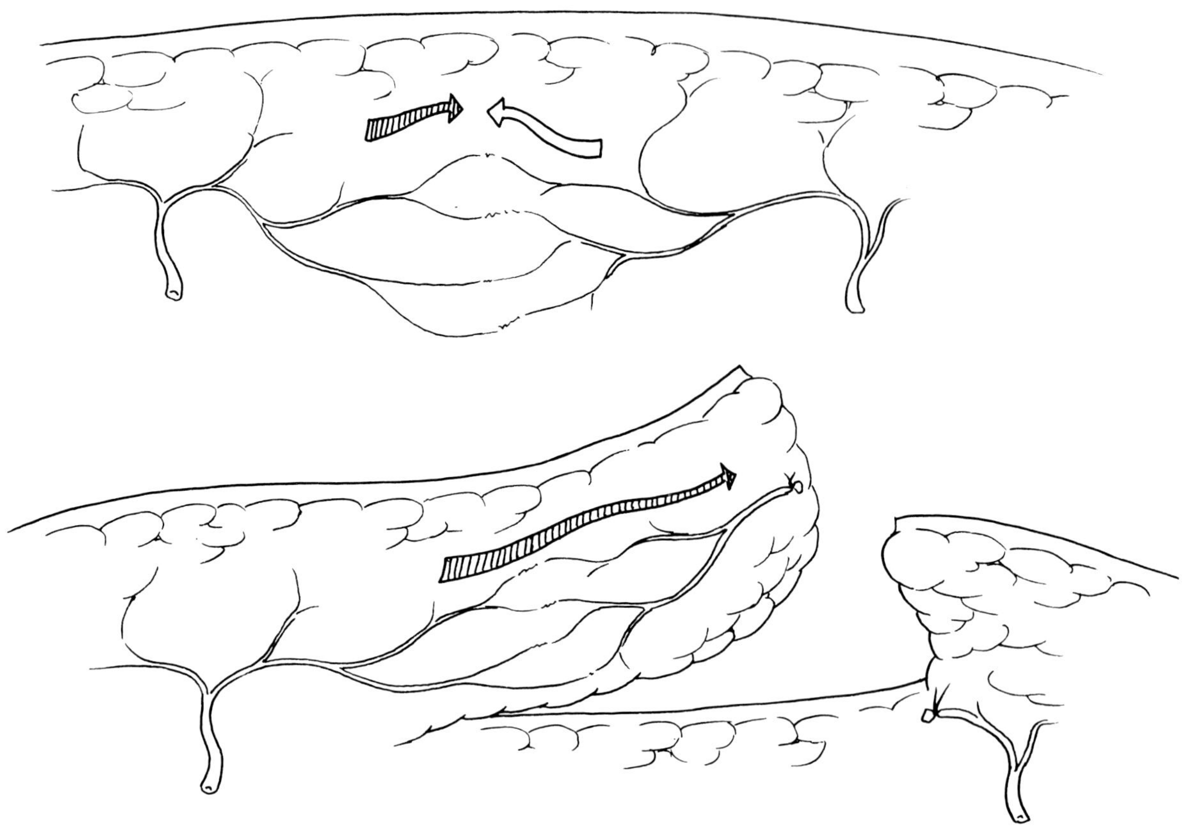

FIGURE 3.9 Each perforating vessel from the underlying muscle has an area or territory it supplies. In the undisturbed state, the circulation is in a dynamic equilibrium between adjacent territories. Here, two perforating vessels anastomose to supply collateral flow to the skin at the boundary of their territories (top illustration). After an incision that interrupts the flow of one system (lower illustration), the equilibrium is upset, and the circulation from an adjacent system must expand its area in order for the skin to survive. There is a limit to this expansion, and if the skin is incised circumferentially, at least one major musculocutaneous system of vessels must be left intact for the skin to survive.

Vascular Territories of the Anterior Trunk

The skin of the anterior abdomen and chest has several arterial sources and overlapping vascular territories of importance in chest wall reconstruction. The largest system is the ventral ladder of the internal thoracic-inferior epigastric system (Figure 3.10). This system links the femoral artery to the ipsilateral subclavian artery in a rich ventral anastomosis, with lateral contributions from the segmentally arranged intercostal vessels. When the skin is intact, anastomoses within this system preserve the viability of the skin territories, even if one of the major feeders to a specific area is interrupted. However, when incisions are made, at least one major vascular contribution must be left intact for the skin to survive.

The internal thoracic-inferior epigastric system runs longitudinally beneath the anterior skeletal and muscular elements and sends arterial branches through these layers to supply the skin from the ventral midline as far laterally as the midaxillary line. A large area of skin, supplied by this ventral system, can be safely mobilized by incorporating the major nutrient vessels with the flap and in so doing vastly increase the range or reach. To do this, the long strip of muscle through which the epigastric vessels send perforators (the rectus abdominis muscle) must be included with the flap. With this technique, a large portion of the ventral abdominal skin becomes available for use in reconstruction.

For example, a wedge of skin from the mid- and lower abdominal regions, based superiorly on the superior epigastric vessels, can be used to resurface the upper anterior

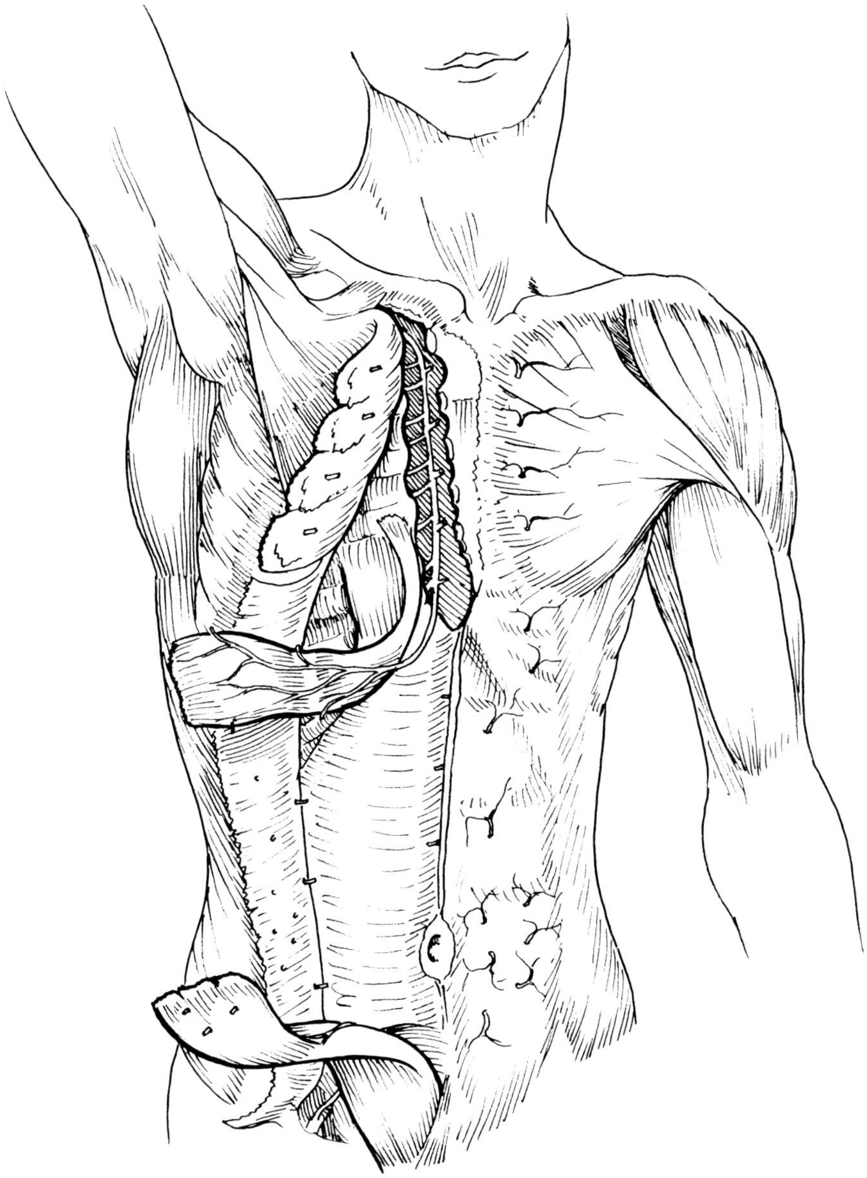

FIGURE 3.10 The internal thoracic-inferior epigastric system connects the subclavian and femoral arteries and provides circulation to large areas of skin on the ventral thorax and abdomen. The rectus abdominis muscle is divided for clarity. Note the numerous perforating branches exiting the deep fascia medially to arborize into the skin. These large branches supply the skin as far as the midaxillary line. By mobilizing the rectus abdominis musculocutaneous flap, this vascular network can be moved as a unit, and a large segment of tissue can be safely used to reconstruct distant defects.

chest wall as far away as the shoulder (Figure 3.11). Conversely, lower chest wall and upper abdominal tissue, based inferiorly on the deep inferior epigastric vessels, can be mobilized to reach the area about the knee (Figure 3.12). The deltopectoral axial skin flap is also supplied by this system and can be based medially on the large second through fourth branches of the internal thoracic artery. It can then reach inferiorly to the costal margin or cephalad to the scalp (Figure 3.13).

In addition to the area supplied by the internal thoracic system, the anterior chest wall skin is supplied by perforators that enter from another direction, through the underlying pectoralis major muscle. These branches originate from the thoracoacromial artery, which in turn arises from the axillary artery. The skin overlying the pectoralis major muscle, with an additional area beyond its inferior border, is nourished by this system (Figure 3.14). In order to take advantage of this arrangement, the thoracoacromial territory can be mobilized by moving the pectoralis major muscle, along with the overlying skin, as a musculocutaneous unit. It is then capable of resurfacing large upper sternal defects as well as areas of the head and neck as high as the supraorbital ridge. Alternatively, the pectoralis major muscle can be mobilized without the skin, again based on the thoracoacromial artery, without jeopardizing the overlying

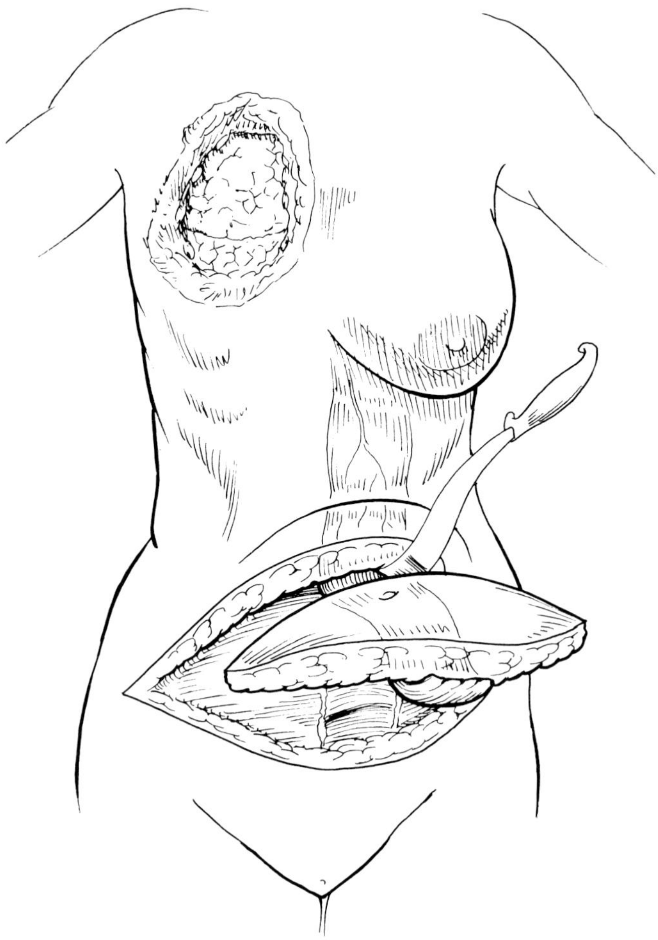

FIGURE 3.11 A left rectus abdominis musculocutaneous flap, based superiorly on the internal thoracic/superior epigastric artery, is shown. It can carry a large flap of lower abdominal wall tissue cephalad to be used for closure of the contralateral full-thickness defect in the chest wall.

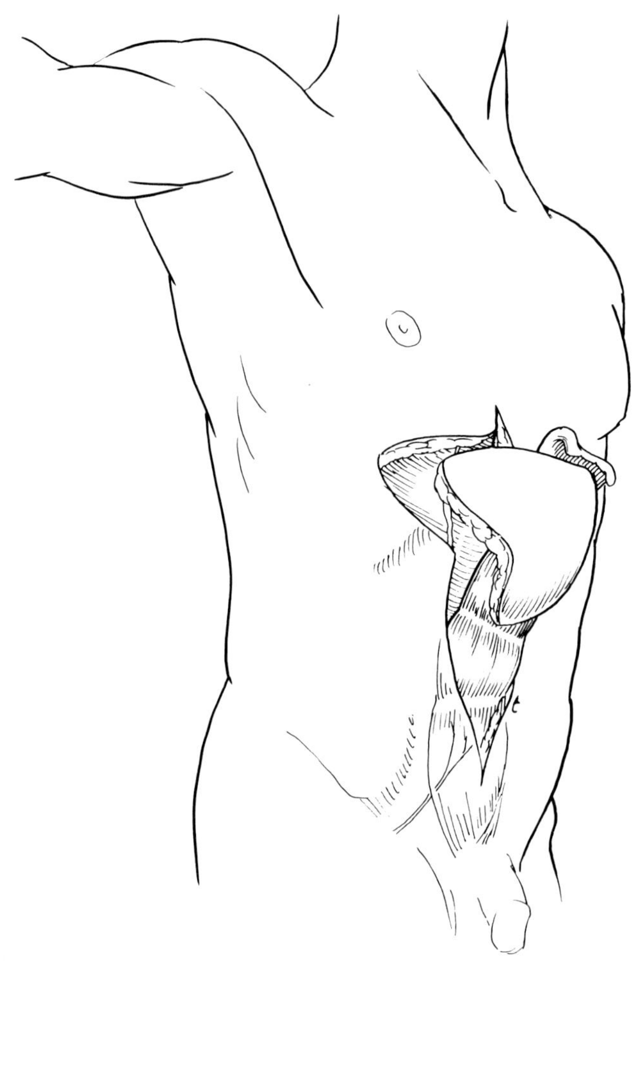

FIGURE 3.12 A right rectus abdominis musculocutaneous flap, based inferiorly on the inferior epigastric artery, is shown. It can be used to reconstruct a variety of lateral thoracoabdominal and caudal defects.

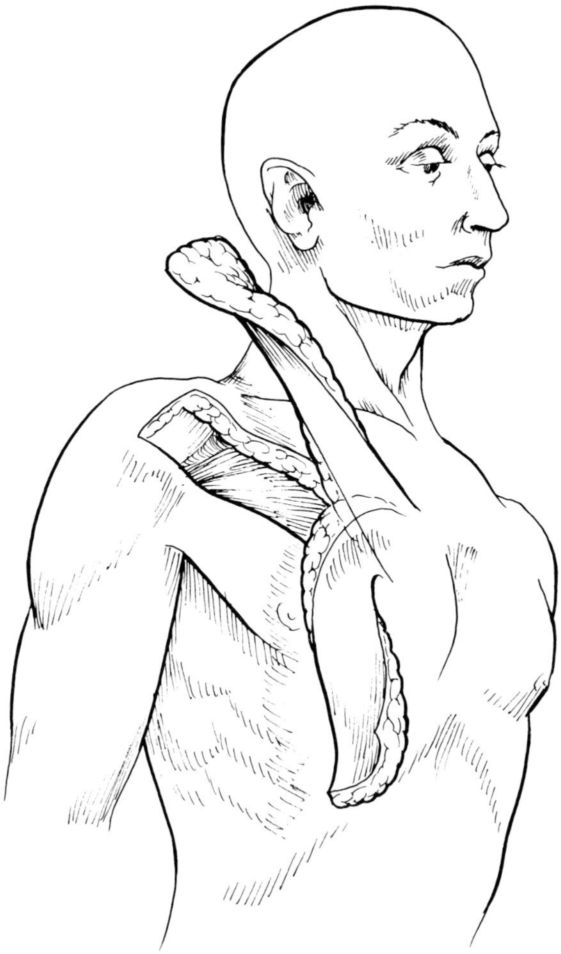

FIGURE 3.13 The deltopectoral axial skin flap, supplied by the internal thoracic artery through large medial branches, has a versatile range of coverage. It, too, is supplied by the internal thoracic/superior epigastric system.

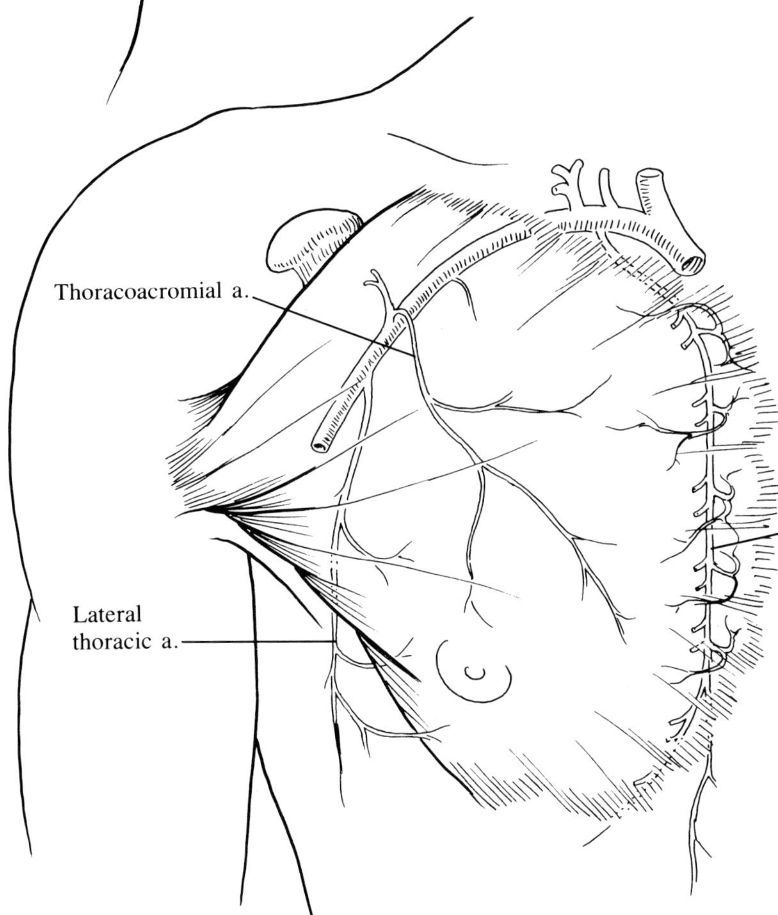

FIGURE 3.14 The skin of the upper lateral chest wall is supplied by several arterial sources: medially, by the internal thoracic system; superiorly, by the thoracoacromial system; and laterally, by the lateral thoracic system. The most valuable of these in chest wall reconstruction is the thoracoacromial vascular pedicle, which supports the pectoralis major musculocutaneous flap.

cutaneous segment. Such a maneuver is possible since the skin of this territory is also supplied by collateral circulation from the lateral thoracic artery, segmental intercostal branches, and branches from the superior epigastric artery (Figure 3.14). As long as a major feeding system to this skin is left undisturbed, the skin remains viable in spite of incisions that interfere with other systems.

Thus, there is a wide degree of overlap in the skin territories supplied by the larger arteries. Practically speaking, however, the anterior flaps of greatest value in chest wall reconstruction are the pectoralis major muscle flap based on the thoracoacromial artery and the rectus abdominis musculocutaneous flap based on the superior epigastric artery (Chapters 9 and 11). Although not a chest wall flap, the omentum is also of value for anterior defects to supplement the other flaps or for use when those flaps are unavailable (Chapter 10). The latissimus dorsi flaps, although of great use for anterior defects, belong to the posterior thoracic circulation (Chapter 8).

Other anterior flaps such as the serratus anterior, thoracoepigastric, and external oblique flaps have been described. However, the serratus, due to its small size and the location of its pedicle, has been of more value for intrathoracic defects or for coverage in the region of the axilla. This flap is limited to such special missions because of the availability of better options for external defects. The same is true for the external oblique and thoracoepigastric flaps; we have not used them in recent years for chest wall reconstruction.

The following figures illustrate these concepts. Figure 3.15 shows the deep system of large arteries that supply the structural layers of the anterior trunk. These vessels send branches through the muscular elements to supply the overlying cutaneous territories. Figure 3.16 shows the superficial system of arterioles that arborize to supply the rich subdermal vascular net of the skin. Note the anastomoses that connect the different areas to ensure collateral blood flow. Figure 3.17 depicts the general outline of the vascular territories of the anterior trunk that are most useful in chest wall reconstruction.

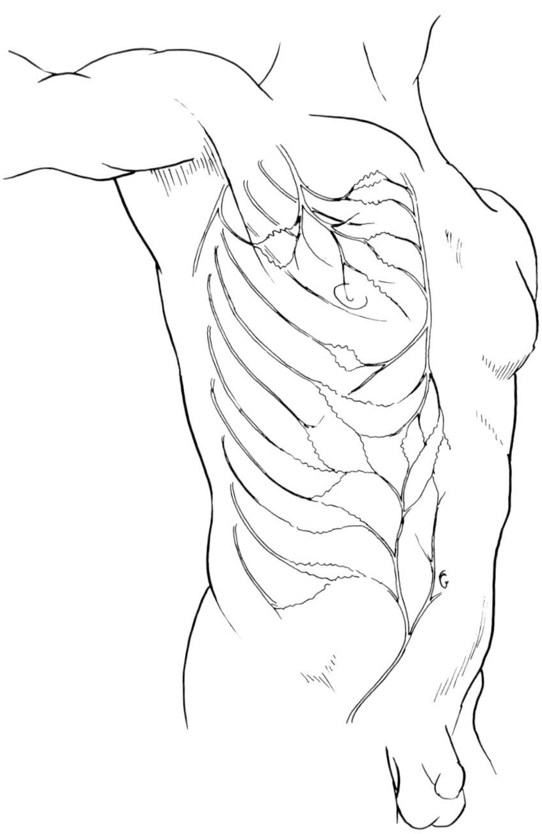

FIGURE 3.15 The deep arteries of the anterior trunk course below (and within) the musculoskeletal layer and are the source of nutrition to the skin by way of their superficial branches. Seen here are the internal thoracic, thoracoacromial, epigastric, and intercostal systems.

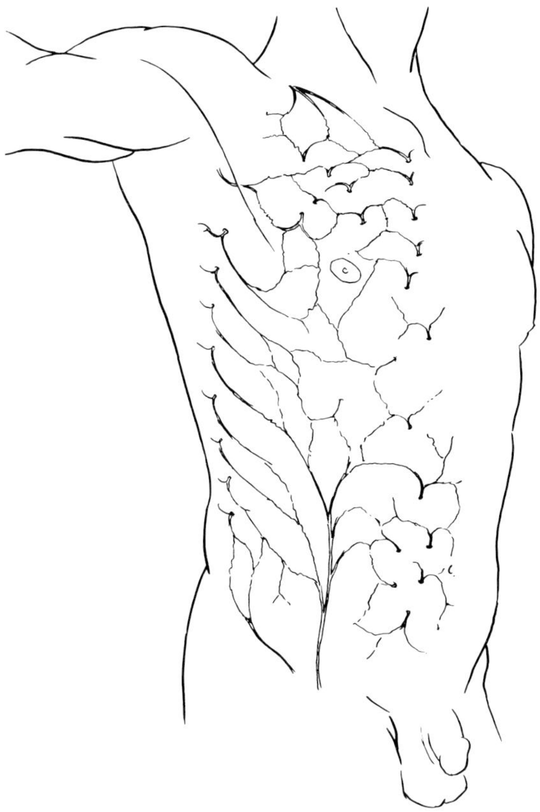

FIGURE 3.16 The all-important perforators, or perforating arterial branches, penetrate the muscular fascia to supply the skin. These represent the superficial segments of the deep system seen in Figure 3.15. In order to move large segments of skin from one area to another, these perforating vessels, as well as the larger supplying arteries, must be preserved. This can be done by moving the muscle and skin as a musculocutaneous unit, thereby incorporating the entire system into the flap. It is vitally important to ensure that the skin segment is large enough to incorporate one of these randomly emerging perforators. Otherwise, the skin undergoes ischemic necrosis, even though the muscle is viable.

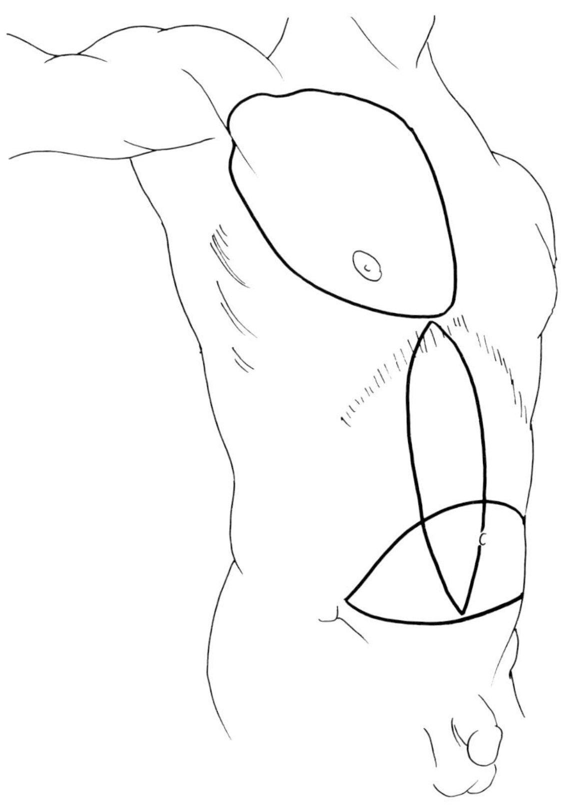

FIGURE 3.17 These are the vascular territories of the anterior abdominal and chest wall that are most useful in chest wall reconstruction. They represent general outlines of areas of the skin that can be mobilized with the underlying muscle and moved to fill full-thickness thoracic defects. Superiorly, the pectoralis major musculocutaneous territory is depicted. Inferiorly, two useful areas of the rectus abdominis musculocutaneous territory are shown (Chapters 9 and 11).

Vascular Territories of the Posterior Thorax

The skin of the posterior thorax is also supplied by transmuscular perforating arteries that exit the deep fascia in a random pattern. Less collateral circulatory flow exists in this area than over the ventral thorax since there is no corresponding ladder of vessels dorsally. However, there is overlap between the two major systems: the latissimus dorsi and the trapezius vascular territories. It is helpful to divide this area into posterolateral, posteromedial, and scapular sections of the thorax.

The largest system is the thoracodorsal/latissimus system, which supplies the entire posterolateral sector. The area corresponds to that within the borders of the latissimus dorsi muscle with a 1–2 cm margin beyond these boundaries. This extensive vascular territory can be harvested by mobilizing the latissimus dorsi muscle and overlying skin based on the thoracodorsal vascular leash. All of the skin overlying this muscle can therefore be shifted to a distant location as a musculocutaneous unit, with the muscle serving as a carrier. Conversely, the entire muscle can be harvested without jeopardizing the overlying skin due to the existence of deep perforating vessels from across the midline of the back, the scapular region, the trapezius vascular territory, and the ipsilateral paraspinous perforators. This collateral circulation can preserve the viability of the skin, in the presence of incisions, as long as at least one major source is left intact. When based on its major pedicle, the thoracodorsal artery, the latissimus is one of the most versatile of chest wall flaps since it can resurface large areas of the anterior, lateral, and posterior thorax.

Posteromedially, over the lower thorax, the skin over the latissimus muscle is supplied by the thoracodorsal system and also by a second series of vessels. This minor pedicle originates from the ninth to eleventh dorsal intercostal arteries, which perforate the deep fascia lateral to the midline. These vessels, like the thoracodorsal system, supply the latissimus and its overlying skin through transmuscular perforators. In order to harvest the latissimus based on this segmentally supplied pedicle, the major (thoracodorsal) pedicle must be divided to allow the flap to rotate into its new location. However, dividing the major pedicle in such a manner is a decision that should be carried out only by experienced surgeons and for limited indications. If used, the flap should ideally incorporate two or three of the medial perforating vessels to ensure viability. Great care must be taken to prevent torsion of the vascular pedicles when the flap is rotated into the recipient area. The threat of such torsion, in fact, severely limits the safe use of this option. This flap has been used mainly for lower midline defects since upper defects can be reconstructed with the trapezius flap.

Posteromedially, over the upper thorax, the skin is supplied by perforating vessels from the underlying trapezius muscle. These vessels originate from the superficial and descending branches of the transverse cervical artery or directly from the subclavian artery in some cases. The trapezius muscle must be incorporated in the flap if this skin is to be moved safely. Usually, the lower portion of the trapezius is employed. It is most valuable for cervicothoracic spinal defects, and the muscle is usually moved alone to fill the defect (Figure 3.18). If skin coverage is required, a split-thickness skin graft is applied directly on the muscle after it has been moved to its new location. This leaves a more natural contour at the recipient site than if an overlying skin segment is included with the trapezius as a musculocutaneous flap. In this way, a large hump on the neck or upper thorax is avoided.

The skin over the scapular region is supplied by the collateral vessels from the circumflex scapular and dorsal scapular systems. This territory is not usually applicable to chest wall reconstruction due to the presence of the bony scapula that is interposed between the chest wall and the skin. The scapular flap, however, is a reliable skin flap based on the nearby circumflex scapular vessel and can be useful for axillary defects. Its use in major chest wall resections is often limited due to the availability of other alternatives. The same is true of the upper trapezius flap (as opposed to the lower

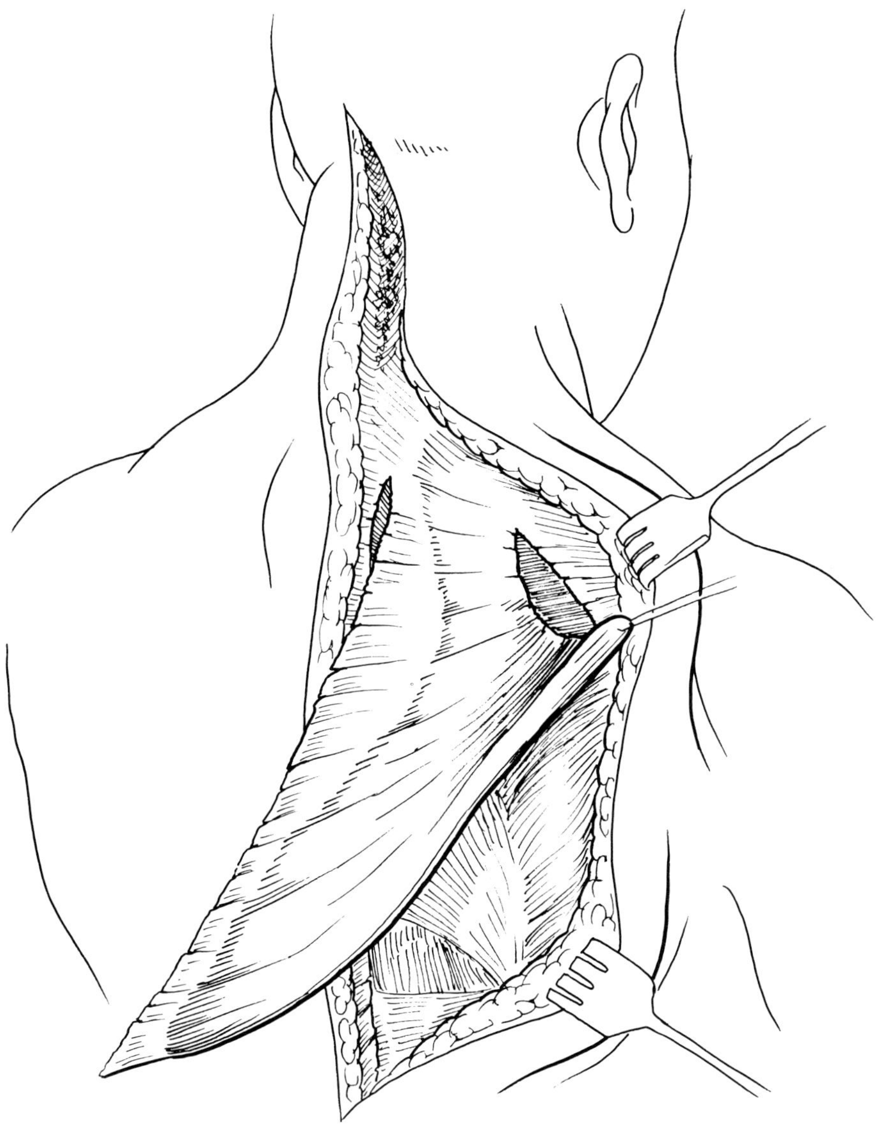

FIGURE 3.18 The lower trapezius muscle flap is useful for coverage of the cervicospinal area and can supply well-vascularized tissue to fill cavitary defects. Although the overlying skin can be carried with the muscle as a musculocutaneous flap, a skin graft is usually used instead, to avoid excessive thickness and to provide a more natural contour.

trapezius that was described), which encompasses the vascular territory about the nape of the neck, scapular spine, and acromion. This latter (upper) flap, although useful in some situations for head and neck reconstruction, carries with it the risk of neuralgias of the spinal accessory nerve. We have not used this upper flap for chest wall reconstruction.

The following figures depict the blood supply to the parietes of the posterior thorax. Figure 3.19 shows the deep system of arteries that supply the posterior muscles and their overlying cutaneous territories. Figure 3.20 shows the superficial system of perforators that arborize to supply the subdermal vascular net. Figure 3.21 outlines the general vascular territories of the posterior trunk that are of greatest use in chest wall reconstruction.

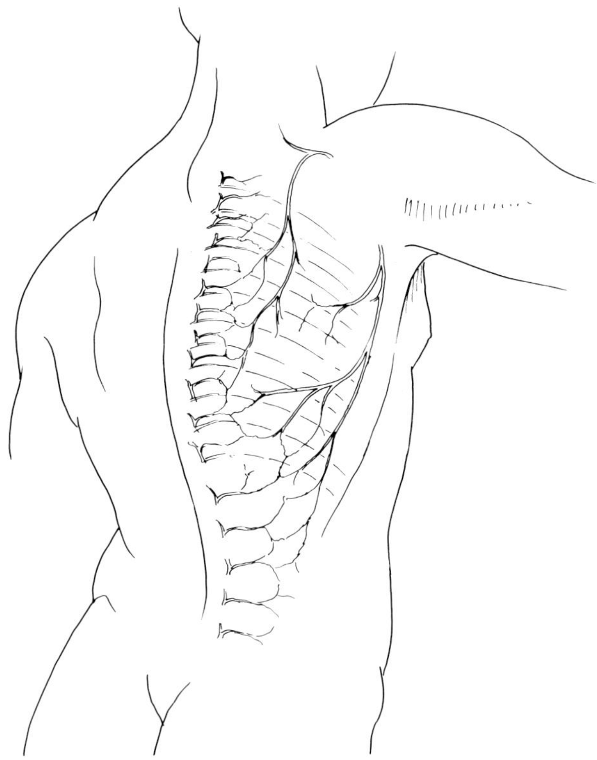

FIGURE 3.19 The deep arteries of the posterior trunk supply the muscles and their overlying cutaneous territories. Shown here are the thoracodorsal, descending transverse cervical, and lumbar arteries, whose branches perforate the muscular fascia to supply the skin. These arteries also anastomose freely with the previously shown intercostal system.

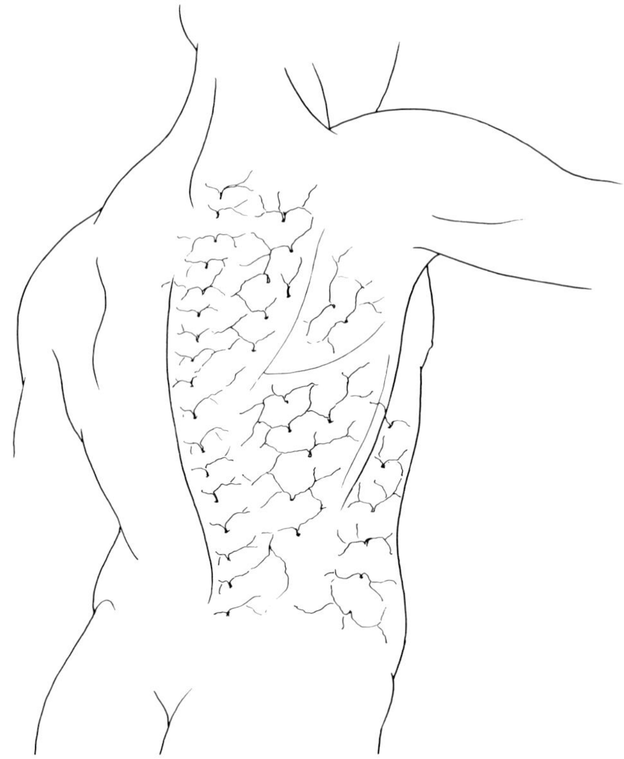

FIGURE 3.20 The superficial perforators penetrate the fascial envelope of the underlying muscle to supply the skin. These are continuations of the vessels seen in Figure 3.19. The same principles apply to these systems as to the anterior trunk.

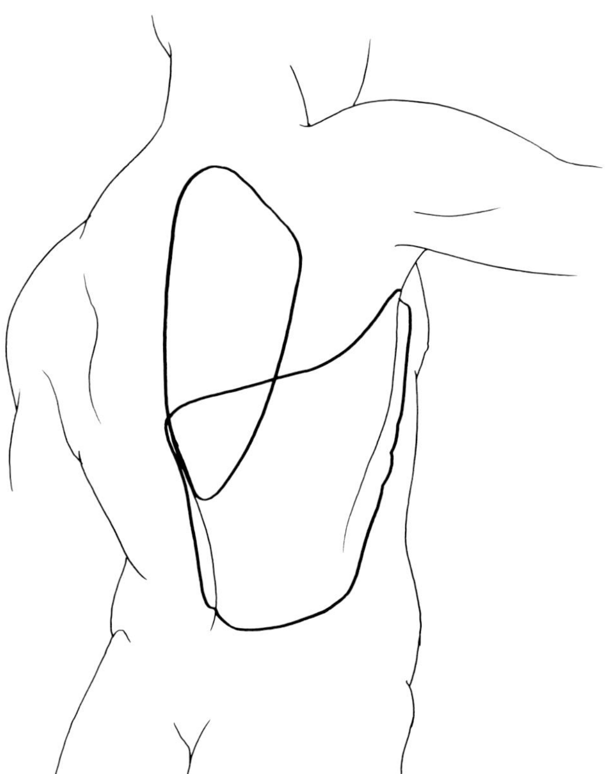

FIGURE 3.21 These are the general vascular territories of the posterior trunk. The lower trapezius flap (shown superiorly) is usually mobilized as a muscle flap, although the cutaneous territory outlined in the drawing can also be included. The latissimus dorsi musculocutaneous flap (shown inferiorly) is useful for a variety of posterior, lateral, and anterior defects. Both flaps can supply well-vascularized tissue to compromised areas.

Vascular Territories of the Lateral Thorax

The lateral thorax is an intermediate area supplied by both anterior and posterior systems. Anteriorly, the ventral ladder, formed by perforating vessels of the epigastric system, provides collateral circulation to this area. Posteriorly, the intercostal arteries contribute to the lower half of this region, extending as far as the periumbilical area (Figure 3.15). The upper half of the lateral thorax also derives flow from the thoracodorsal system through the anterior portion of the latissimus dorsi vascular territory. These systems join to enrich the watershed effect.

The most valuable flap for coverage in this area is the latissimus dorsi musculocutaneous flap from the posterior circulation. The rectus abdominis system, based superiorly, can also be of use (Figure 3.22). Figure 3.23 depicts the general vascular territories for the most commonly used flaps of the lateral thorax. An intercostal flap, based posteriorly, has been described, but we have not used it in chest wall reconstruction.

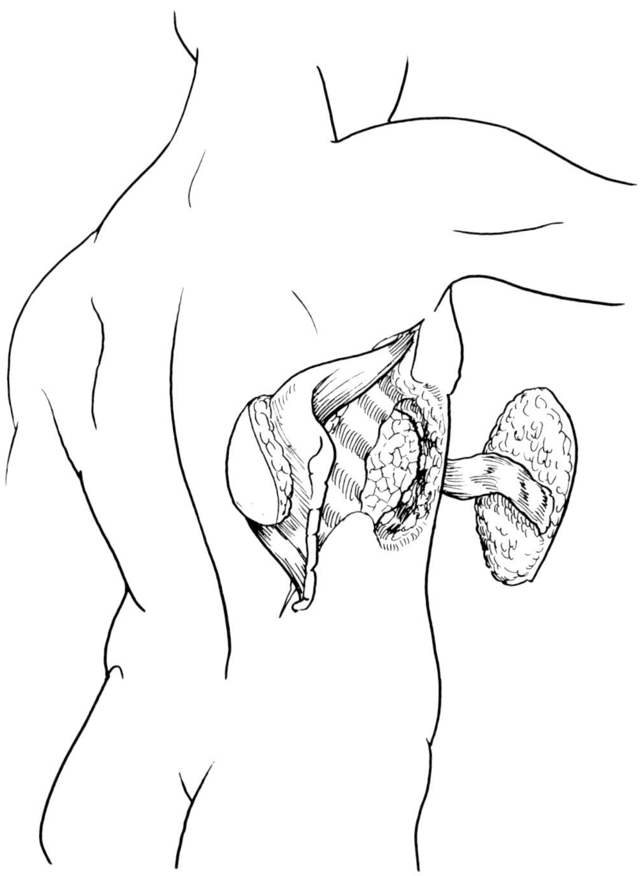

FIGURE 3.22 A full-thickness lateral thoracic defect is shown. Alternatives for a tension-free closure include the latissimus dorsi musculocutaneous flap or the superiorly based rectus abdominis musculocutaneous flap. These flaps are depicted.

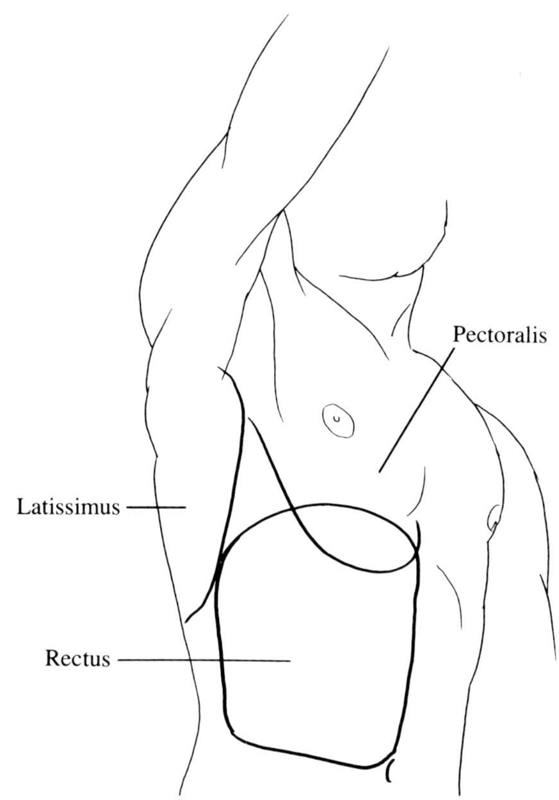

FIGURE 3.23 The general (and overlapping) vascular territories of the lateral thorax are shown. This area is also supplied, in segmental fashion, by the intercostal arteries. However, the intercostal territories are rarely used for chest wall reconstruction.

4

Preoperative Care and Considerations

A thorough evaluation before chest wall resection minimizes unexpected morbidity and contributes to a smoother operative course. The evaluation is directed at the entire patient so that any underlying or associated disease and its potential impact can be accurately assessed preoperatively. Close, early coordination with the operating room and anesthesia staffs as well as other specialists helps during this period to ensure a safe operation and to plan timely, effective management of anticipated clinical difficulties. The evaluation consists of a thorough history, careful physical examination, and selective laboratory testing.

History

Care is taken to document the chronological course (such as duration, rate of growth) and any previous treatment of the lesion on the chest wall, especially if there has been a biopsy or radiotherapy. The review of systems notes any significant diseases, particularly those requiring medication or hospitalization. Allergies to drugs or to antiseptic solutions used to prepare the patient are carefully noted, and the patient is questioned regarding any tendency toward excessive bleeding. This is particularly important since chest wall resections often require the opening of large tissue planes and the mobilization of substantial flaps to reconstruct the defect. Blood dyscrasias and associated coagulopathies could therefore result in serious hemorrhage and require excessive transfusions if not corrected before the operation. This latter problem not only increases the risk of incompatibility reactions but can also cause pulmonary insufficiency. Pertinent questions include whether the patient or family members bruise easily or have had problems with bleeding related to previous operative procedures, lacerations, or dental extractions. Conversely, familial or personal episodes of embolism or thrombosis are noted.

Particular attention is devoted to the cardiovascular and respiratory systems. The integrity of both of these systems is mandatory for safe intraoperative management and a smooth postoperative course. The patient's smoking history is important, especially the duration and extent of the habit. Past or recent respiratory infections requiring prolonged medication or hospitalization are noted. A detailed cardiac history is also taken to uncover preexisting angina pectoris or other cardiac disability. Pertinent questions include how far the patient can walk on level terrain, how many flights of stairs he can negotiate without dyspnea, what types of activities generally tire him, and what specific limitations exist. Discrete questioning concerning the patient's sexual activity can be helpful in assessing cardiovascular performance. Such activity, since it is pleasurable, can result in exertion to the limit of cardiovascular function. In males, the ability to sustain an erection is important since the absence of this capability can correlate with the presence of atherosclerotic obstruction of the iliac vessels and their branches.

The social history should uncover chronic exposure to industrial aerosols or other contaminants that could decrease pulmonary reserve. Similarly, significant ethanol intake, whether beer, wine, or hard liquor, may lead to delirium tremens and liver dysfunction in the postoperative period and should be carefully assessed.

Physical Examination

The size of the chest wall lesion is noted and its dimensions recorded. The degree of bone, skin, and muscle involvement is recorded. Tenderness, especially around radiation scars, seems to correlate well with the extent of necrosis and margins of resection. Careful notation is also made as to the possibility of involvement of major neurovascular structures by direct invasion or extrinsic compression. This is particularly true of tumors or ulcerations in the region of the clavicle that may cause compression of the axillary or subclavian vessels and the brachial plexus. Any motor or sensory disturbance of the upper extremity calls for specific muscle testing and sensory mapping. If necessary, electrical studies such as nerve conduction velocities and electromyography are obtained.

Other efforts are directed at documenting upper airway pathology, such as dental problems or undisclosed laryngeal and pharyngeal lesions, which may cause problems with intubation or require further evaluation. Indirect (mirror) laryngoscopy is performed. Certain diseases of the cervical spine can cause deformity and fixation, which can make intubation difficult if not impossible. Rheumatoid arthritis, on the other hand, can result in such spinal laxity as to cause acute cord compression when the neck is improperly flexed. These conditions must be evaluated thoroughly in consultation with the anesthesia and orthopedic surgery services before the operative date. The patient is also assessed for venous and arterial access sites. The assessment of the radial and ulnar arterial circulation of the hand (the Allen test) is prudent not only to plan for monitoring during surgery but also to assess the safety for radial arterial catheterization. Assessment of the neck veins is valuable for later placement of central venous pressure and Swan-Ganz catheters.

The condition of the skin is routinely assessed to plan for possible skin grafts. Acceptable donor areas include the thigh and buttock region. Previous incisions on the chest and abdomen are noted so that planning for alternative flaps can be initiated early and the reconstruction planned accordingly.

Laboratory Studies

Routine laboratory studies include a complete blood count, multichannel chemistry assay, urinalysis, and chest x-ray. The chest radiograph is supplemental to previous evaluations of the chest wall lesion and is done within 72 hours of the operation to assess any change in its appearance as well as to document the current status of the underlying pulmonary parenchyma. Such a film is invaluable for comparison in the immediate postoperative period.

An electrocardiogram is conducted on all individuals who have a history of cardiovascular disease as well as on individuals over 35 years of age. This test is also conducted on those individuals whose resection borders on the pericardium or may require pericardiectomy. Consultation with a cardiologist is prudent if the electrocardiogram is abnormal in any way.

If the patient has a history of blood dyscrasia, or any suggestion that the clotting mechanism is abnormal, a serum coagulation panel is obtained. In some institutions, this procedure is routine, and a platelet count and functional assay can also be conducted to complete the evaluation. If a coagulopathy is suspected, the hematologist is consulted to determine if the patient truly possesses a clotting abnormality and to plan for its successful management. If such an abnormality exists, subsequent consultation with the pathologist alerts the blood bank of the problem and arrangements can be made to preclude a shortage of transfusional components.

A routine 20-channel serum protein and chemical analysis is conducted to screen for the presence of adequate hepatic and renal function as well as for nutritional status. The nutrition evaluation, correlated with physical findings, can be augmented by other well-known tests. It is vitally important to have the patient in optimal nutritional balance before the operation. This cannot be overemphasized. If necessary, the operation must be canceled until the patient has attained anabolic goals such as weight gain and positive nitrogen balance. A mechanical bowel preparation is routinely administered, especially if the abdomen is to be entered. This also helps prevent constipation in the postoperative period. During such a preparation, an intravenous fluid is routinely administered to prevent dehydration.

Two specialized tests that are particularly valuable are pulmonary function studies and arterial blood gases. Pulmonary function studies are important because they offer an objective assessment of the patient's ventilatory capabilities. These tests, which are conducted routinely in the pulmonary function laboratory, should be available in all major hospitals. The most important of these are the forced expiratory volumes in one second (FEV_1) and the forced vital capacity (FVC).

The forced expiratory volume in 1 second permits the evaluation of any pulmonary obstructive components. Patients who have chronic obstructive pulmonary disease, for example, show a decreased FEV_1. The forced vital capacity indicates the ability of the patient to exhale a full volume of air for his body size. If the patient has a serious restrictive component, such as pulmonary fibrosis or compromise of a pleural cavity, there is usually a corresponding decrease in the forced vital capacity. Both of these parameters are obtained not only in absolute figures but also as a percentage of the predicted volume for a person of the same age and body habitus. Standard nomograms are available for comparison and evaluation of the patient's capabilities.

Comparison of the FEV_1 with the FVC should show that the FEV_1 is 80% of the FVC. This is the norm and reflects healthy pulmonary function in general. In patients with obstructive disease, the FEV_1 is decreased, and there is a prolonged expiratory phase on the spirogram. Patients with restrictive disease have a decreased vital capacity. Care must be taken in evaluating both of these parameters since mixed disease processes, that is, both obstructive and restrictive, can exist.

Another parameter is the percentage of FEV_1 and the percentage of FVC with respect to the expected values for the patient. In general terms, if the product of these two values, that is, the percentages, is greater than 2,500, then the patient will probably tolerate the resection of one pulmonary lobe. If the product is greater than 3,500, the patient will probably tolerate a pneumonectomy. If the product is less than 2,500, the patient will probably have difficulty even with a chest wall resection that doesn't remove pulmonary tissue. In other terms, the goal is to ensure that the patient will have enough functional pulmonary tissue for an FEV_1 of at least 1 liter in the postoperative period. Otherwise, he will have difficulty being weaned from the respirator and, in fact, may have a prolonged hospital course with serious respiratory complications.

The arterial blood gases are also helpful since they provide an indication of the patient's respiratory efficiency and can be somewhat predictive of later problems in weaning the patient from the respirator. They are obtained with the patient at rest, breathing room air. Determinations are expressed in millimeters of mercury for the partial pressures of oxygen (pO_2) and carbon dioxide (pCO_2) in the arterial blood. These parameters are used to determine if the oxygen saturations are in the normal range as well as if carbon dioxide levels indicate adequate ventilatory function. The pCO_2 is of value in assessing ventilatory efficiency, whereas pO_2 is more helpful in evaluating ventilation-perfusion ratios. Abnormal findings are thoroughly explored before surgery, and if questions arise concerning ventilatory capability, appropriate consultation with a specialist in pulmonary medicine is obtained.

Another helpful clinical assessment that can be included is the patient's capacity for exercise. This can be easily and personally assessed by conducting two simple tests. The first one is the patient's tolerance to level walking. The patient is allowed to walk one of the hospital floors for about 200 yards. This is done at a reasonable pace to see if there are signs of dyspnea or signs of recruitment of the accessory muscles of respiration in order to maintain adequate ventilation. The second test is conducted by walking with the patient up two flights of stairs. The surgeon notes the patient's respirations and heart rate before starting. They then walk up the stairs together at a normal pace. If the patient shows any evidence of decompensation, this test is stopped. Decompensation is reflected by abnormally increased respiratory rate, obvious recruitment of the accessory muscles of respiration, and excessively increased heart rate. If the patient can easily climb the stairs and maintain the pace with the surgeon, then he can probably tolerate the

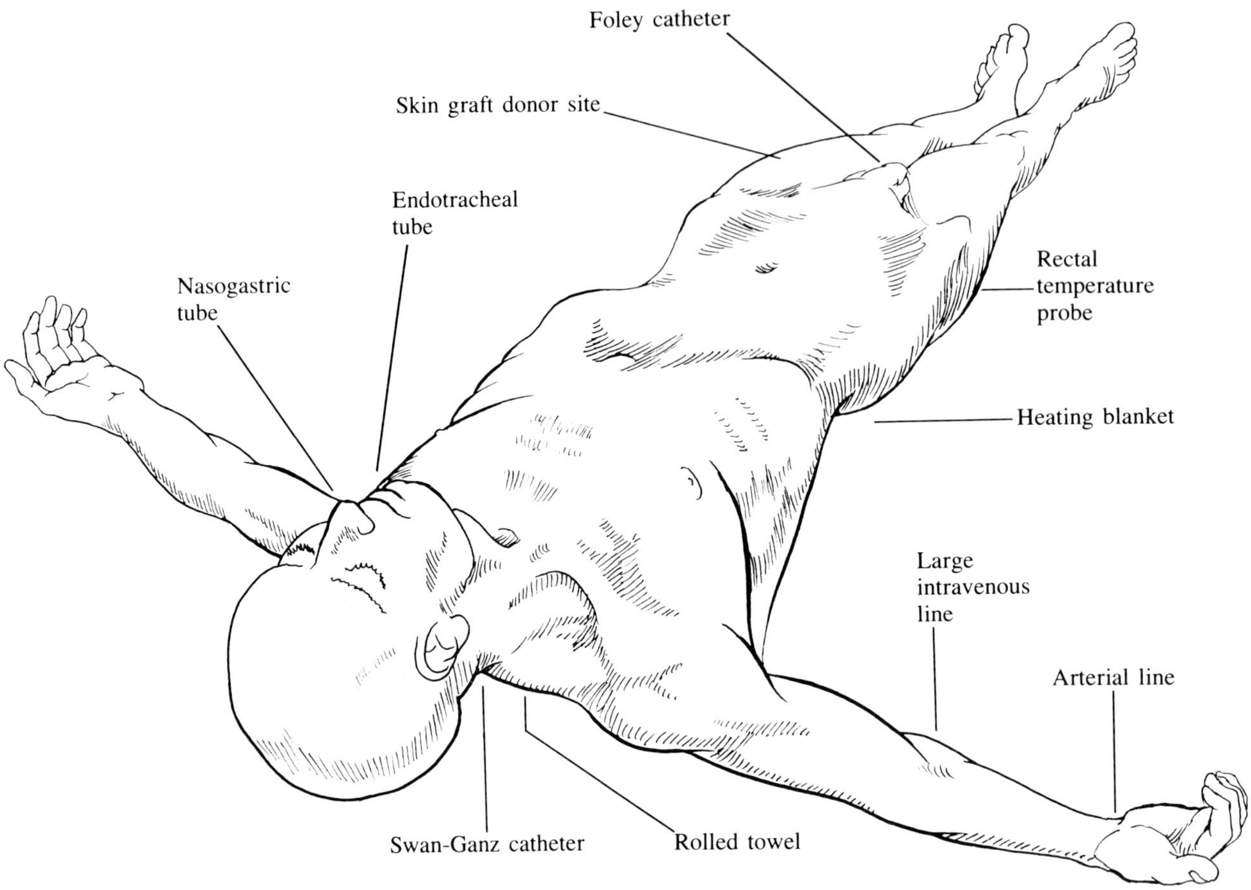

FIGURE 4.1 This illustration shows the placement of monitoring lines for a patient undergoing an anterior chest wall resection. The arterial line, large-bore intravenous lines, and Swan-Ganz catheter are placed on the side away from the lesion. If the lesion is midline, then the catheters can be placed on either side. A temperature probe is mandatory since the heat loss incurred over a long procedure can be substantial. A heating and cooling blanket is placed under the patient to assist in temperature regulation, and a Foley catheter is inserted for fluid balance monitoring. The endotracheal tube has been omitted for clarity. The anterior thigh is prepared and draped in case a skin graft is required. A rolled towel is placed longitudinally between the scapulae to elevate the anterior chest wall and sternum. The arms are extended to show the placement of the monitoring and support devices. They can be placed at the patient's sides after all the lines have been secured.

procedure well from a cardiopulmonary standpoint. If there are problems before the completion of the stairs or the 200 yards of level walking, then the patient deserves closer scrutiny or evaluation since he may not tolerate the procedure.

Any previous studies done to evaluate the lesion on the chest wall are also reviewed. These include the biopsy results as well as other information showing the extent of the lesion. Before ablative tumor surgery, it is always best to personally review the biopsy slides at the microscope with the pathologist. Arrangements can be made at that time for later frozen sections in the operating room if deemed necessary. Arteriograms, including venous phase studies, are obtained if the lesion is in close proximity to the great vessels; computerized or magnetic scans are done according to the requirements of the case. These are helpful in assessing invasion of deeper layers and thus resectional margins.

Consultation is routinely obtained with the anesthesia and operative services in order to allow them to plan for monitoring lines, positioning of the patient on the table, and ancillary procedures (such as gastrostomy or feeding jejunostomy) (Figures 4.1–4.3). For example, the arterial line should sometimes be placed so that the arm on the side of the lesion is left free and mobile during the surgery. The free arm is

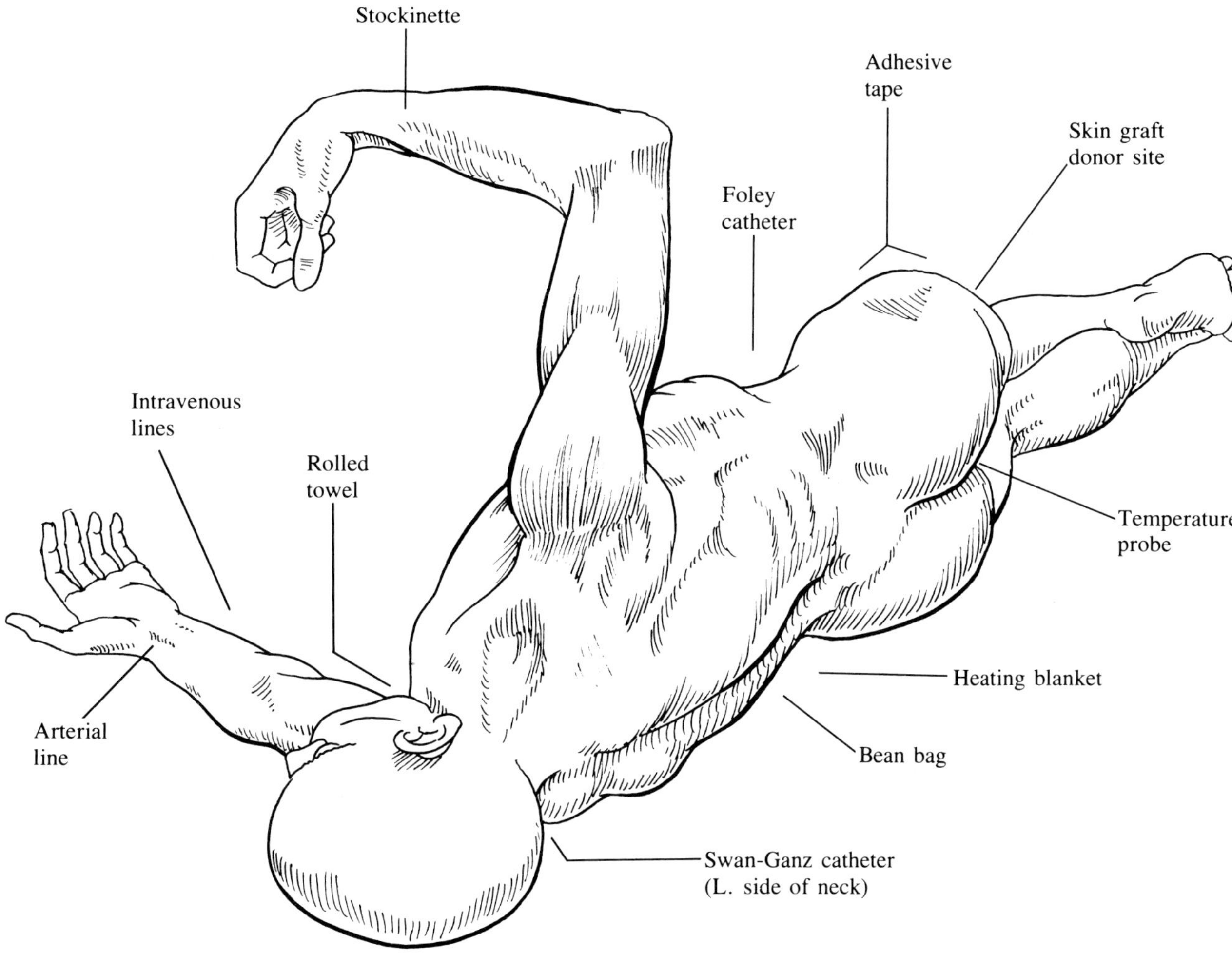

FIGURE 4.2 For lesions of the lateral chest wall and axilla, the patient is placed in the lateral thoracotomy position. The arm on the side of the dissection is prepared and left free so that its position can be changed during the case. A pillow or similar pad is placed between the legs. One leg is flexed and one leg is straight to help stabilize the patient, and all pressure points are checked for adequate padding. The arterial line, intravenous lines, and Swan-Ganz catheter are placed on the side away from the dissection and are draped out of the field. A heating and cooling blanket is placed under the patient for temperature regulation, and an orthopedic bean bag is placed under the blanket to stabilize the patient. Wide adhesive-tape bands and a safety strap are placed across the hip to complete the patient's stabilization. The buttock or lateral aspect of the upper thigh is prepared as a skin graft donor site. A rolled towel is placed in the dependent axilla to relieve pressure on the brachial plexus and vessels. The endotracheal tube has been omitted for clarity.

prepared and draped into the operative field, allowing greater liberty in approaching the resection and reconstruction. It is also suggested that Swan-Ganz or central venous pressure lines be placed on the side of the neck away from the resection. Inflatable sandbags or liberally padded restraints can be used to stabilize the patient on the operating table. Pressure points are well padded and the knee joints relaxed to preclude postoperative stiffness and venous obstruction. The neck and torso are included in the operative field to prepare for possible nodal dissection or wider excision if needed, and the shoulder area is also prepared in the event that control of the brachiocephalic vessels becomes necessary. The buttock and thigh areas are prepared for possible use as skin graft donor sites.

Other routine lines include a nasogastric tube for gastric decompression and two large intravenous pathways (including the central monitoring catheters) for fluid and blood replacement. Any blood components are administered through micropore filters to prevent microemboli to the lungs, and a Foley catheter is inserted to monitor urinary

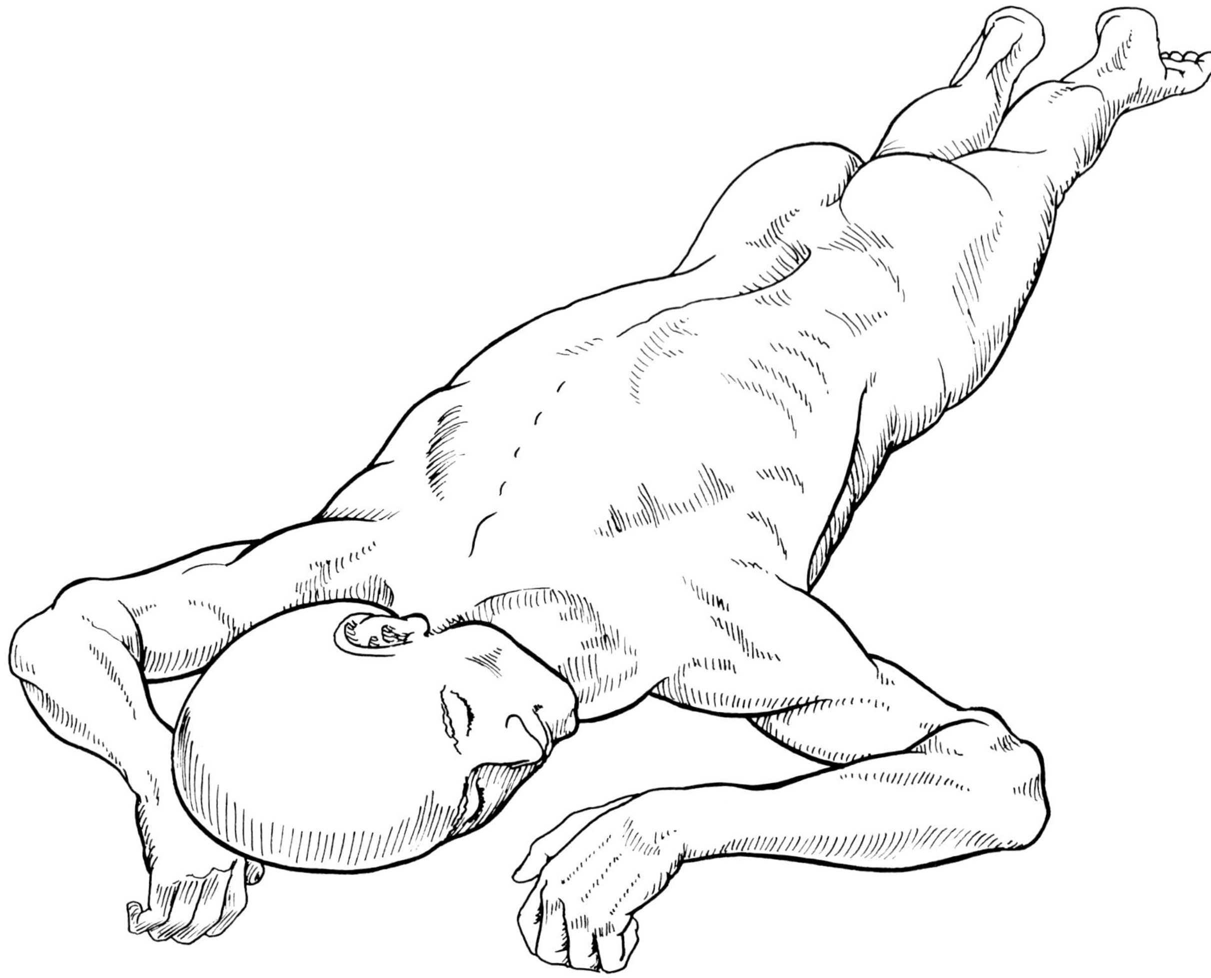

FIGURE 4.3 When the patient has a midline lesion on the posterior thorax, the monitoring devices and access lines are placed with the patient in the supine position, and the patient is then turned to the prone position. The Swan-Ganz catheter is inserted in the side of the neck to which the patient's head will be turned, and a temperature-regulating blanket is placed under the patient. Both upper extremities are supported on arm boards lowered to comfortable positions with rolled towels or other soft padding placed under the joints and in the axillae. The endotracheal tube has been omitted for clarity.

output. A temperature probe is also inserted since the procedure is sometimes lengthy and the potential heat loss substantial. A warming blanket, placed beneath the patient, is helpful for maintenance of body temperature.

In summary, a thorough evaluation of the patient's respiratory, cardiovascular, and hematologic conditions is accomplished before surgery. Preoperative consultations with the anesthesiologist and operating room staff will assure that they know how the patient will be positioned, that all monitoring equipment and lines will be placed appropriately, and that specialized instruments will be available. By anticipating problems and preventing them, it is hoped that the operative procedure and postoperative course will progress uneventfully.

Reference

American College of Surgeons, Committee on Preoperative and Postoperative Care: *Manual of Preoperative and Postoperative Care*, ed. 3. Philadelphia, WB Saunders, 1983.

5

Planning the Reconstruction

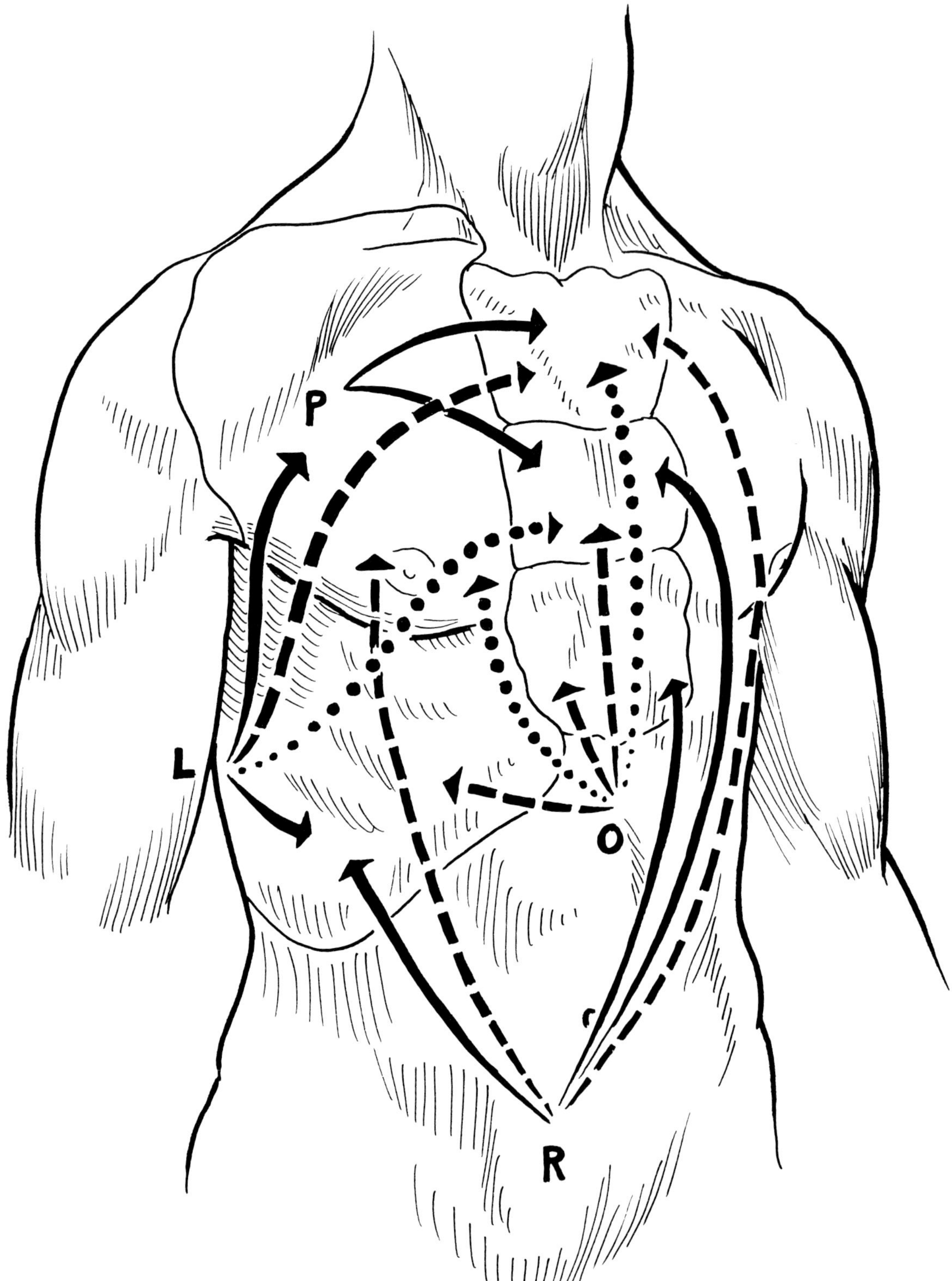

FIGURE 5 Options for closure of the anterior thorax.

Key

——→ = First choice	L = Latissimus dorsi
— — → = Second choice	P = Pectoralis major
······→ = Third choice	R = Rectus abdominus
	O = Omentum

This chapter covers the selection of the appropriate flaps and structural support for reconstruction of the chest wall defect. A discussion of the general principles is followed by a consideration of specific areas of the thorax and the decision making involved in planning the reconstruction of those areas.

General Principles

As a general rule, the goal is to provide a durable closure that seals the thorax and protects the underlying viscera. Ideally, this is done with minimum operative risk or compromise of ventilatory function. The nature of the lesion may dictate additional requirements such as eradication of infection, ability to withstand high-dose postoperative radiotherapy, local control of malignancy, or other factors covered in Chapter 6. In order to achieve such goals, it is necessary to incorporate fresh, well-vascularized tissue in the reconstruction. This is especially true when confronted with an open wound that, at the very least, is contaminated. The tissue used in the reconstruction must have a good blood supply in order to overcome such contamination and to heal successfully without an infection. If radiation injury or the fibrosis of chronic inflammation is superimposed, the need for supplying uninjured tissue is even more critical to attaining a healed and durable closure. Irradiated and fibrotic wounds have lost the ability to mount an inflammatory response sufficient for basic wound healing. In these scarred tissues, the blood vessels lack the capability to dilate and sprout new conduits to support the increased metabolic demand that accompanies protein synthesis and the phenomenon of healing. If the flaps used are poorly vascularized, the interface between the donor and recipient tissues knits poorly and a dehiscence results. Unfortunately, if this separation occurs over a full-thickness defect, it unseals the pleural space, exposes vital organs, and can quickly result in a life-threatening situation for the patient. Such complications can be avoided by proper planning and technique.

Richly vascularized muscle tissue is the first choice for supplying the nutrients and oxygen-carrying capacity required for the uneventful healing of such wounds. In addition, muscle (or musculocutaneous) flaps provide a degree of thickness that affords protection to the intrathoracic contents as well as decreases paradoxical motion during ventilation. The fascial envelope covering the muscle also offers a healthy recipient bed for the application of skin grafts. Such grafts, when applied to a thick muscle flap, heal quickly and are durable due to the thick cushion of underlying muscle.

Another important principle is the absolute avoidance of tension over the full-thickness defect in the chest wall. Flaps must be chosen so that they will reach their destination and fit loosely into the defect with no tension in any direction. If this cannot be guaranteed, then alternate or additional flaps must be recruited. The closure over the defect should literally be floppy. The paradoxical motion resulting from this mild laxity diminishes somewhat with healing and has not been a significant problem. It can, however, pose a serious problem when a total sternectomy has been performed. In such patients, instability and the paradoxical motion that ensues can cause severe ventilatory insufficiency unless the skeletal layer is also reconstructed.

If any tension exists on the chest wall, it must be shifted away from the full-thickness gap and moved to the area from which the flap was harvested. If necessary, a skin graft can be used to close this donor site. In this way, if a dehiscence occurs, it will be over an intact musculoskeletal layer of the chest or abdomen and not over the defect in the thorax (Figure 5.1).

There is controversy over the selection of different methods for chest wall reconstruction. Any one technique cannot be rigidly applied to all patients, even if the defects are quite similar. Every clinician is biased by experience or past influences, and there is no doubt that a skilled plastic surgeon can get more mileage (or reach) out of

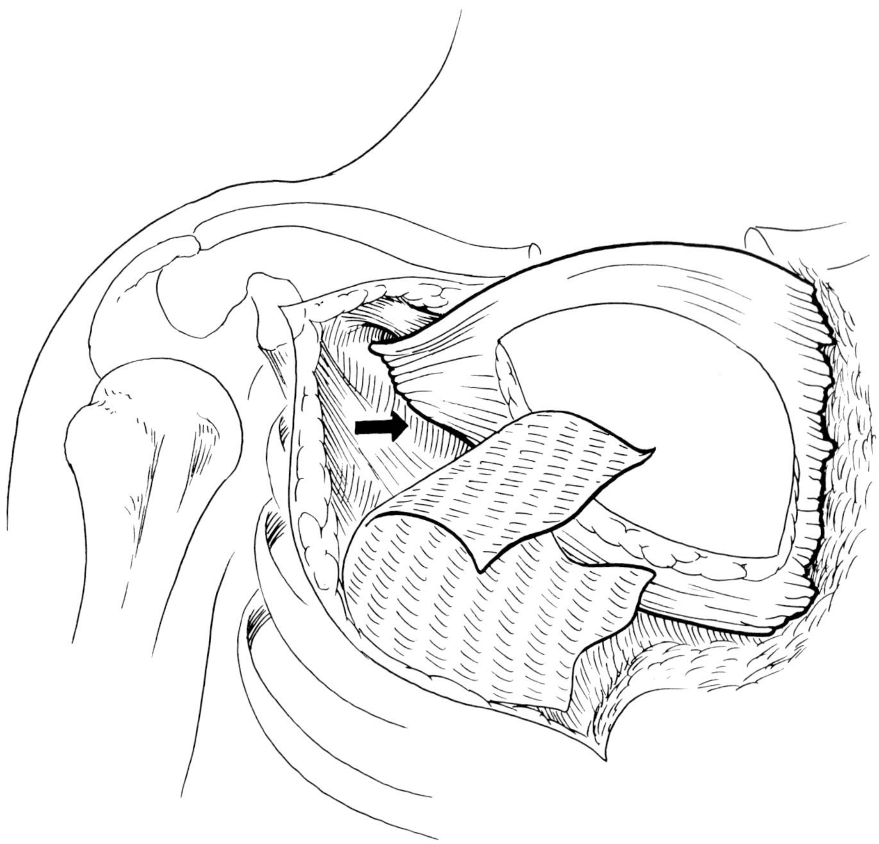

FIGURE 5.1 The principle of closure of the full-thickness defect without tension is shown. The tension is shifted to another location so that the closure of the defect is loose and floppy. If necessary, the area from which the flap was harvested is closed with a skin graft. In this example, a pectoralis major musculocutaneous flap has been shifted medially to close a manubrial defect loosely. The area from which the flap was harvested is closed with a skin graft and the tension is effectively neutralized.

certain flaps than the conservative guidelines presented in this text. However, the following considerations can provide a starting point that should be safe and clinically useful to the majority of surgeons.

Choosing the Flaps

As the surgical team examines the patient and the extent of the lesion on the chest wall, each member forms a mental picture of the anticipated defect. The thoracic surgeon considers the margins and depth of debridement or extirpation that will be required, and the plastic surgeon considers the flaps that are available to provide a durable, tension-free restoration. It is helpful to outline the proposed defect on the patient's skin with a marking pen (Figure 5.2). The distances required for each potential flap to reach the defect are then measured. More details of this technique are found later in this chapter and in Chapters 8–12. Essentially, one must know the general size and shape of the defect that is to be filled, whether the skeletal layer should be reconstructed, and which flaps are the best options to meet these requirements.

The first choice is a muscle or musculocutaneous flap because of the excellent blood supply to the muscle elements and its thickness. These factors favorably influence healing and durability. The ones most useful in chest wall reconstruction are the latissimus dorsi, the pectoralis major, the lower trapezius, and the rectus abdominis. The transverse rectus abdominis musculocutaneous flap is somewhat unusual in that it is actually a long, thin muscle that supports a sizable flap of skin and fat. This is analogous to a long, thin bridge leading to a large island (Figure 5.3). The island portion is composed of the skin and subcutaneous fat and is not as effective in chest wall reconstruction as a pure muscle flap because of its lesser blood supply. In general, skin

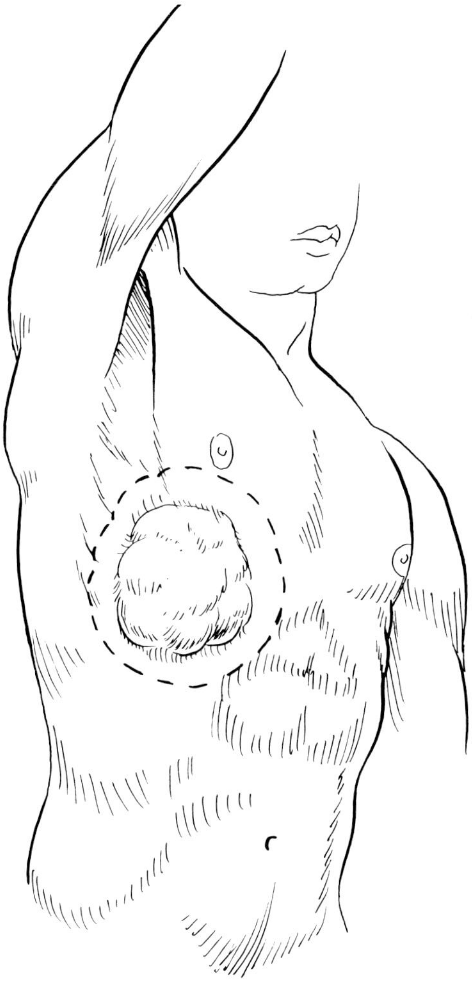

FIGURE 5.2 The proposed area of excision is outlined (dotted line) on this patient, who has a large neoplasm. This will help to plan the selection of a flap that will close the defect securely and without tension.

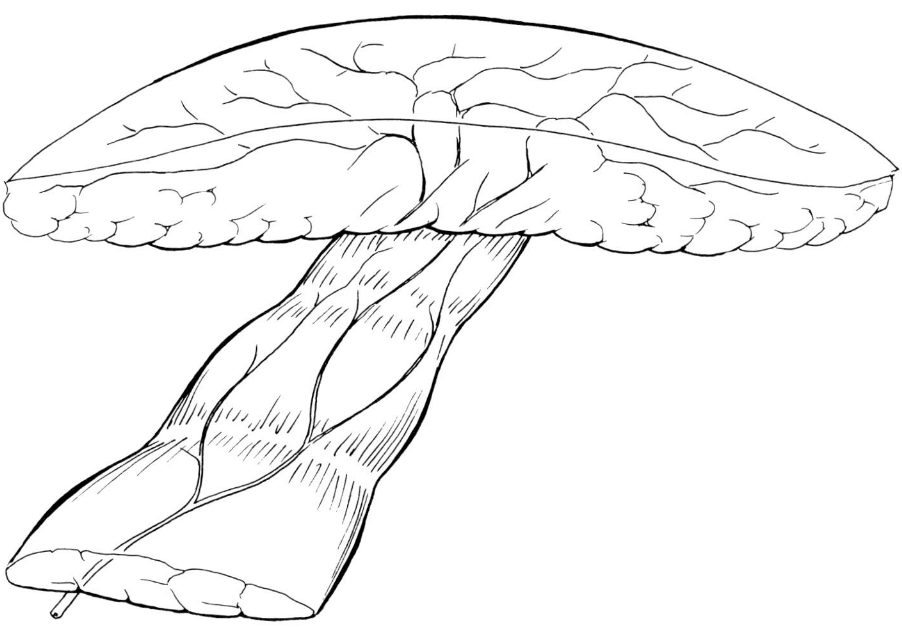

FIGURE 5.3 The transverse rectus abdominis musculocutaneous flap is different from the other musculocutaneous flaps in that it is a relatively thin strip of muscle that supports a large volume of skin and fat. These latter tissues are less favorable than muscle tissue for reconstruction. Nevertheless, this versatile flap is useful.

and fat are not as hardy or durable as a thick muscle for this type of reconstruction. Like other such flaps, it has a somewhat decreased ability to fend off infections as compared to muscle tissue. Nevertheless, the transverse rectus flap is quite useful. The omentum is a reserve choice because it lacks thickness and strength and also because it requires a laparotomy to obtain it. It is, on the other hand, richly vascularized and can support healing even in the most compromised wounds.

In considering these flaps, it is helpful to divide the thorax into anterior, lateral, and posterior sectors and discuss the alternatives available for the reconstruction of each area. The factors that limit the use of a flap and determine its range or reach are, of course, the location of the flap and length of its vascular pedicle. These are detailed in the section on the mobilization of flaps.

Anterior Chest

The Sternum The sternum can be subdivided into upper, middle, and lower portions (Figure 5.4). Upper, or manubrial, defects can be reconstructed with the pectoralis major, latissimus dorsi, rectus abdominis, or omentum flaps. The general philosophy is to consider the simplest method of reconstruction as the first option, and this usually means using the flap closest to the defect. For these upper sternal defects, the pectoralis major muscle and musculocutaneous flaps are the first choice. This flap can be separated from its origin and insertion and moved medially while still attached to its thoracoacromial vascular pedicle (Chapter 9). If no skin has been resected in establishing the defect, one or both pectoralis major muscle flaps can be mobilized to fill the defect and the presternal skin closed over the muscles primarily. If a skin deficit is present, skin grafts can be applied to the muscle surface to provide epithelial coverage.

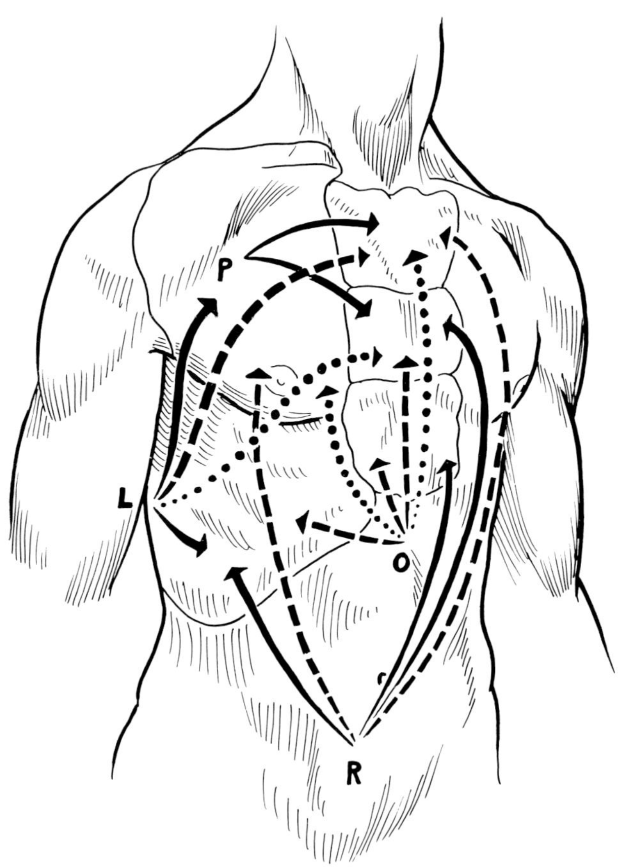

FIGURE 5.4 Options for closure of specific areas of the anterior thorax are shown. The solid arrows represent selections that are first choices; the dashed arrows, second choices; the dotted arrows, third choices. The sternum is divided into upper, middle, and lower areas. The area lateral to the sternum is divided into upper and lower regions. L—latissimus dorsi; P—pectoralis major; R—rectus abdominis; O—omentum.

The next choice is the latissimus dorsi muscle or musculocutaneous flap. It is reliable and provides excellent durability and thickness. However, it requires the patient to be on his side in order to mobilize it. It, too, can be used as either a muscle or combined muscle-skin flap, depending on the local requirements at the defect.

The next choice is the rectus abdominis, depending on its proximity to the sternal defect. One must be certain that the internal thoracic artery is intact before using the rectus since the superiorly based flap, which is used in chest wall reconstruction, depends on this pedicle for viability. Although it has been used successfully when based on lesser, intercostal arteries, such a technique is not the ideal and carries more risk.

The rectus abdominis can be used as a muscle flap alone, or as a musculocutaneous flap (tranverse or vertical), when used for sternal defects. If a muscle flap is used, the presternal skin, if intact, can be closed over the muscle, or a skin graft can be applied to the muscle surface for the closure. Alternatively, a segment of skin can be carried with the rectus abdominis as a musculocutaneous flap (see Chapter 11). If skin is needed due to the inherent tension of the presternal skin, it is not advisable to mobilize adjacent skin to close sternal defects. The use of muscle and a split-thickness skin graft or a musculocutaneous flap is preferred.

The final choice for this area is the omentum. It is reliable, has an excellent blood supply, and readily accepts skin grafts. However, it is more friable and requires a laparotomy to harvest it. The important factor in selecting these options is to understand which flaps are available and to fit the best reconstructive option to the patient's needs.

For the midsternum, the first choice is the rectus abdominis. The pectoralis major flaps can also be used for upper midsternal defects, but as one proceeds toward the xiphoid area, there is more tension on the pedicle of the pectoralis flap, and there is less muscle bulk available for use in the reconstruction. It is better to choose another flap than to stretch the vascular pedicle or close the defect under tension. After these flaps, the next choice is the omentum. It has a generous range but is subject to the limitations described earlier (i.e., friability). The next choice is the latissimus dorsi. In considering this option, one must be aware that, like the pectoralis major, its pedicle is near the shoulder, and as one proceeds caudally (toward the xiphoid), more tension is brought to bear on the vascular leash. It is therefore best for reconstructing manubrial and upper midsternal defects.

For the lower sternum (xiphoid region), the first choice is the rectus abdominis, followed by the omentum. Both of these selections are excellent for this area. Again, one must be certain that the internal thoracic artery on the flap side is intact before using the rectus abdominis. One way to ensure the patency of this vessel, in the absence of an operative flow meter or doppler, is to include a skin segment with the superiorly based flap. The fluorescein test can then be used to assess the viability of the skin and, in this way, can serve as an indirect assessment of muscle viability. This can also be of value with the other musculocutaneous flaps.

Fluorescein Test Two ampules of the dye are infused in a peripheral vein after the flap has been completely mobilized. Ten minutes later, the skin segment of the flap is gently washed with a moist sponge to clean off any stray dye. It is then closely examined in darkness with the ultraviolet lamp. If dye staining is evident within the skin, capillary flow is present and the flap is viable. Although unreliable for muscle tissue alone, this dye provides an indirect indication of muscular viability through its presence in the overlying skin. This skin segment, even if it is later removed before completing the resection, must be large enough (approximately 5 cm × 8 cm) to include at least one perforating vessel from the underlying muscle to ensure its blood supply.

Area Lateral to the Sternum This area (Figure 5.4) can be subdivided into an upper and a lower section. The upper (clavicular and subclavicular) is best covered with the latissimus dorsi muscle or musculocutaneous flap. The pectoralis cannot ordinarily

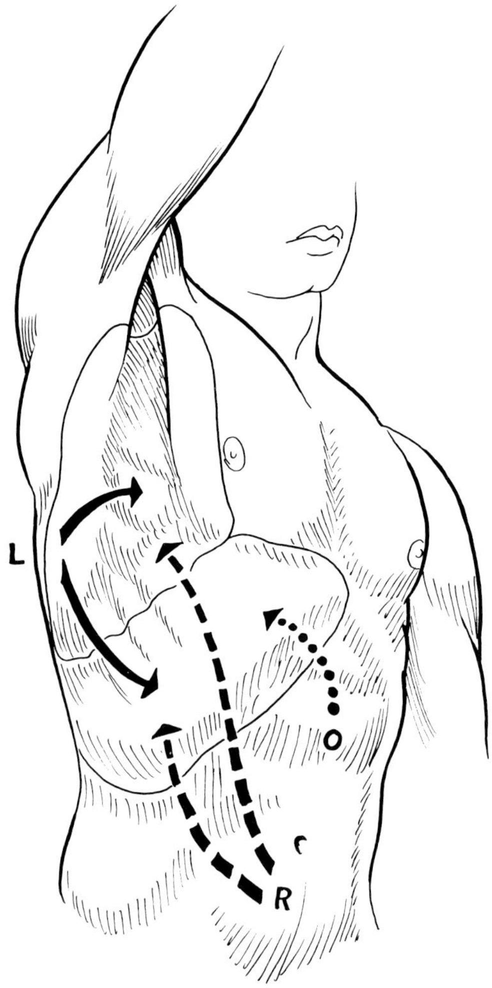

FIGURE 5.5 Options for closure of specific areas of the lateral thorax are shown. The solid arrows represent selections that are first choices; the dashed arrows, second choices; the dotted arrow, third choice. L—latissimus dorsi; R—rectus abdominis; O—omentum.

be used in this area since its pedicle has usually been ablated when the defect was established. The next choices are the rectus abdominis and omentum. If used, the rectus usually requires a fairly good-sized skin segment to reach this area. The omentum usually requires a skin graft to provide epithelial coverage.

The lower section can be reached by the rectus as the initial choice, followed by the latissimus and omental flaps. Again, the latissimus is limited by the tension on its pedicle as one proceeds anteromedially. It is better, therefore, to use the latissimus for the more posterior (or lateral) defects in this section of the thorax.

Lateral Thorax

The lateral thorax (Figure 5.5) is an in-between region but can usually be covered quite easily with the latissimus dorsi muscle or musculocutaneous flap. For upper defects that encroach on the latissimus itself, one must be certain that the vascular pedicle is intact before utilizing this option. (See Chapter 8 for the location of the vascular pedicle.) The next choice is the rectus abdominis. The omentum is the third option.

Posterior Thorax

This area (Figure 5.6) can be divided into upper midline (spinal or paraspinal) defects, scapular defects, and lower defects. For the upper midline region, the lower trapezius flap is the first choice, followed by the latissimus dorsi.

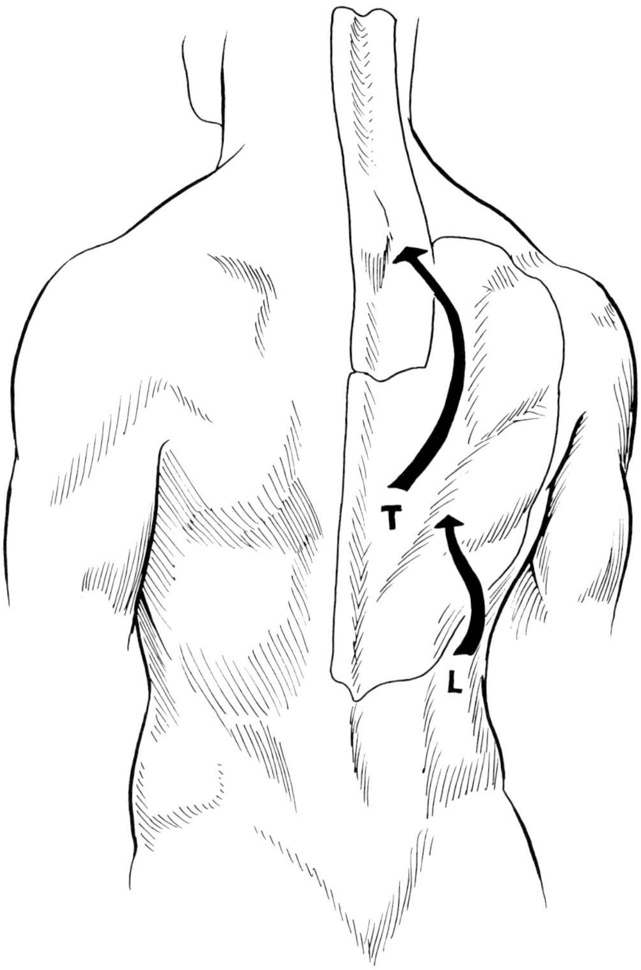

FIGURE 5.6 Options for closure of specific areas of the posterior thorax are shown. This region is divided into an upper midline area, covered best by the lower trapezius flap (T), and a lower area, covered best by the latissimus dorsi flap (L).

The scapular and lower areas can be covered in most instances by the latissimus dorsi muscle and musculocutaneous flaps. The area deep to the scapula can be covered by the latissimus flap, especially if the scapula has been removed in establishing the defect. Care must be taken, as one proceeds toward the axilla, to preserve the thoracodorsal vessels that supply the latissimus.

This section is a general outline for planning the initial steps toward reconstruction. The specific details related to each flap, as well as their limitations, are discussed in Chapters 8–12. Before selection of a particular flap, the section describing its use should be thoroughly reviewed. Table 5.1 summarizes these reconstructive options.

Structural Support

The need for providing structural support (or restoration of the skeletal layer) during reconstruction of the chest wall is modified by several factors. The first of these is the size of the defect. If the defect is small, the muscle or composite (musculocutaneous) flap alone provides sufficient stabilization. In larger defects, however, stabilization may be needed to prevent excessive paradoxical motion of the chest wall and to afford protection of the internal organs. Other factors such as the pulmonary reserve of the patient, anatomic location of the defect, and the character of the flap being used to fill the ablative gap also determine the need for further stabilization.

TABLE 5.1 Flaps Available for Reconstruction of the Chest Wall

Defects	Possible Flaps
Anterior	
I. Sternum	
A. Upper sternum (manubrium)	1. Pectoralis major muscle or musculocutaneous flap 2. Latissimus dorsi muscle or musculocutaneous flap 3. Superiorly based rectus abdominis muscle or musculocutaneous flap 4. Omentum
B. Midsternum	1. Superiorly based rectus abdominis muscle or musculocutaneous flap 2. Omentum 3. Pectoralis major or latissimus dorsi
C. Lower sternum (xiphoid)	1. Superiorly based rectus abdominis muscle or musculocutaneous flap 2. Omentum
II. Lateral to Sternum	
A. Upper (clavicular and subclavicular)	1. Latissimus dorsi muscle or musculocutaneous flap 2. Superiorly based rectus abdominis musculocutaneous flap 3. Omentum
B. Lower	1. Superiorly based rectus abdominis musculocutaneous flap 2. Latissimus dorsi muscle and musculocutaneous flap 3. Omentum
Lateral	
	1. Latissimus dorsi muscle and musculocutaneous flap 2. Superiorly based rectus abdominis musculocutaneous flap 3. Omentum
Posterior	
I. Upper Midline	1. Trapezius muscle flap with split-thickness skin graft 2. Latissimus dorsi muscle or musculocutaneous flap
II. Scapular and Lower	1. Latissimus dorsi muscle and musculocutaneous flap

Obviously, patients who have good pulmonary function will tolerate a larger defect and its attendant paradoxical motion better than an individual who exhibits poor pulmonary reserve. In older patients with chronic restrictive or obstructive changes, stabilization of even small defects may be required to allow the patient to be effectively weaned from the ventilator postoperatively. The anatomic location of the defect also plays an important role since certain portions of the chest cage are partially supported by the structures already present. This is particularly true on the upper posterior aspect of the chest, where the scapula and adjoining musculature provide sufficient support. Finally, the need for stabilization is also dictated by the character of the flap used in the reconstruction. If the flap is thick and robust and includes muscle tissue, then the need for additional stability beneath the flap is less. For example, the omentum may require underlying structural support because it is friable and thin and may be further attenuated by the surgical dissection. If stabilization is required, two categories of material can be considered: (1) autogenous tissue and (2) alloplastic devices.

Autogenous Tissues

Autogenous materials involve the use of free tissue transplantation (grafts) or the interposition of nearby living structures. The most durable grafts are bone grafts. These

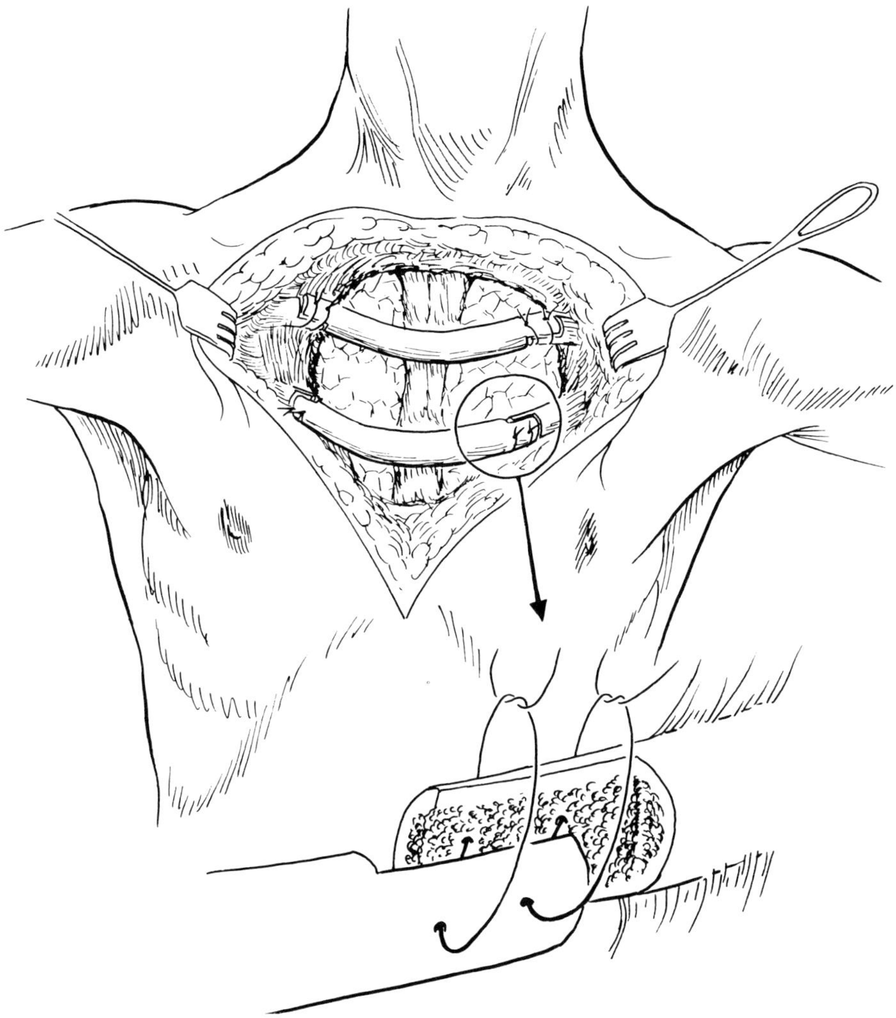

FIGURE 5.7 For greater stability, rib grafts are notched so that they can be secured with transfixing wire sutures. This technique also allows for a greater area of contact between the cancellous portions of donor and recipient bone. This increases the likelihood for survival of the bone graft.

free pieces of bone are secured into the defect and form a matrix for gradual replacement by new bone. Such grafts are most successful when placed in contact with a large surface area of intact trabecular bone at the margins of the defect and into a richly vascularized recipient bed (Figure 5.7). In such an environment, the osteocytes within the graft have a greater chance for survival, and osteoblasts can be recruited to gradually replace the grafted tissues with new bone. Otherwise, the graft is absorbed, leaving only a fibrous remnant. Even this, however, can provide an element of support or stabilization even though the original bone graft has failed. In considering bone grafts, the ribs offer the best option. The iliac crest and the tibial donor sites are mentioned only for completeness and are rarely used. Iliac crest bone could be used if ribs are unavailable, but because of the curvature of the crest, it doesn't easily conform to the recipient area. Removing sections of the proximal tibia for use as bone grafts dangerously weakens the tibia from loss of bone and can result in fracture upon weightbearing.

Segmental rib grafts may be used intact or may be fabricated into split grafts. When the rib is used as a split graft, a portion of the rib can be returned to its normal anatomic position and half of the rib (the external half) is removed and transferred to the site where stabilization is necessary. An easier and more popular option is to employ the intact rib segment or to split the rib longitudinally and use both halves in the reconstruction. Removal of multiple ribs can be self-defeating if loss of stability in the previously healthy part of the chest wall results. Fortunately, this is rare if only one or two ribs from each side are used. To avoid this, the ribs at the margins of the defect are left intact and ribs that are one or two spaces away are removed as the grafts. This technique maintains overall stability.

The disadvantages of rib grafting are donor site pain and possible instability in a previously healthy area of the chest wall. Composite grafts consisting of fascia lata combined with bone grafts or bone chips are not used extensively due to resorption of the graft and lack of stability. Perhaps the least desirable of the autogenous tissues is fascia lata. It is a soft membrane, transferred without its blood supply, which has a tendency to stretch and become flaccid after it has been sewn into the defect. Multiple strips are usually required and must be fixed in parallel to achieve closure. Such grafts handle contamination poorly and can become a nidus of necrotic, infected tissue. It can therefore result in serious local infection or mediastinitis.

The interposition of autogenous tissues involves the movement of adjacent ribs and muscle into the defect from the margins. A rib (or portion of the rib) and intercostal muscles above or below the defect are freed anteriorly and positioned diagonally across the defect while still attached posteriorly. Such interpositions are often unsatisfactory since they expand the area of instability and contribute little support.

Alloplastic Materials

A number of synthetic materials have been tried. Solid plates made of metal, lucite, and fiberglass have been used for stabilization of the chest wall but are not popular. They are immobile, unyielding slabs of foreign material that are situated in an elastic and constantly moving chest wall. In this situation, they have a tendency to erode through the surrounding tissues, which are less durable, and serious hemorrhage or exposure through the skin has been reported following their use. They have been replaced in recent years by the more flexible variety of synthetic monofilament meshes.

Certain types of clothlike materials are commonly employed in chest wall reconstruction. The metallic meshes have generally lost favor since tantalum, a material that initially enjoyed popularity, was shown to fragment due to the incessant motion of the chest wall. Stainless steel, which has less of a tendency to fragment, is difficult to handle. For these reasons, as well as a general lack of elasticity, and the fact that they are radioopaque, the metal products are not frequently used. Other metal materials such as long, thin metal struts still find occasional use in reinforcing the synthetic meshes.

Newer synthetic materials such as Teflon™, nylon, polypropylene, and Gortex™ screens have found increasing use in the repair of chest wall defects. The most commonly used of these is polypropylene screening. It is relatively easy to handle, pliable, and somewhat tolerant of contamination due to its large weave and monofilament construction. It can also be trimmed to fit any defect.

Technically, the material is sewn in place with a number of interrupted polypropylene sutures. The sutures are placed so that they come through both the screen material and the periosteum. They are tied on the superficial side, and the synthetic screen is affixed to the inner (deep) aspect of the defect (Figure 5.8). This is done in such a way that the material is tight and devoid of folding or kinking. The other meshed materials are used in much the same way.

Disadvantages incurred with these materials have included chronic infection, relaxation of tension (flaccidity), and failure along the suture line (dehiscence of the mesh). When infection or chronic drainage occurs, a trial at local wound care is warranted; such treatment sometimes succeeds. This is especially true if muscle flaps or omental flaps have been used to provide the coverage. Such success seems to be related to the vascularity of the flaps. With skin flaps, or the skin portion of rectus abdominis flaps, success is less likely, and the contaminated mesh usually must be removed in order for healing to occur. Flaccidity is normally well tolerated and requires no intervention. Dehiscence or suture line failure, on the other hand, can usually be repaired with a good chance of success.

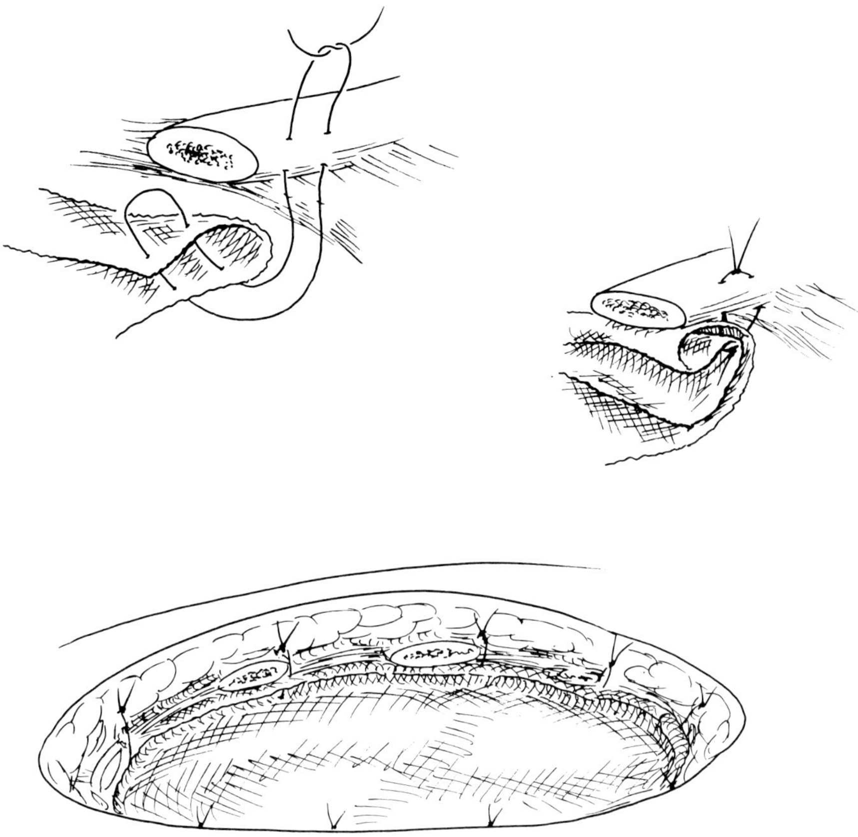

FIGURE 5.8 A technique for securing the alloplastic mesh to the edges of the defect is illustrated. The suture is placed on the cephalad side of the rib to avoid the neurovascular bundle. It is attached to the deep side and stretched to preclude folding or kinking. It forms a tray for the flap.

These problems have led many surgeons to abandon attempts at providing structural support and to employ muscle or musculocutaneous flaps alone. This is certainly an alternative with small and moderately sized defects.

Composite units of synthetic material, such as the methyl methacrylate sandwich, have been used in chest wall reconstruction. This technique allows the methacrylate cement to harden between two layers of synthetic mesh. If this sandwich is used in a flat portion of the thorax, it is molded on a flat surface such as the back table of the operating room. If it is to be shaped in conformity with the lateral chest wall, it is molded over a curved retractor. It is best fabricated away from the patient since the reaction is markedly exothermic and can burn the flesh. This technique is rarely recommended due to problems associated with erosion, exposure, and hemorrhage.

In summary, both synthetic materials and autogenous tissues can be used to achieve stabilization of the chest wall. Each has its assets and its liabilities. One should consider using the flaps alone wherever possible. In doing so, disadvantages such as donor site pain and instability (rib grafts), infected prostheses, and other morbidity can be avoided. This, of course, may be inadvisable in dealing with certain defects, especially the larger ones. If prosthetic material is deemed necessary, the first choice is the prolene or nylon mesh. It usually affords reasonable protection, stabilization, ease of handling, and toleration of some degree of contamination.

Multiple Flaps

The indication for the use of multiple flaps is simply the presence of tension. Such tension is usually caused by a shortage of available tissue when employing a single flap to achieve closure. It can also be occasioned by the inadequate reach of a flap that was expected to easily fill the farthest corner of the defect. When such problems occur in the operating room, alternate flaps must be hastily recruited to achieve a tension-free seal of the thorax. It is therefore best to prepare for such a situation so that recruitment of the extra flaps will be a natural and planned extension of the operation rather than a hasty and ill-prepared expediency. In assessing the anticipated defect preoperatively, one must choose not only a primary option but also a secondary set of plans. With the patient standing, the defect is measured with the measuring tape (see details of specific flaps in the section on mobilization of flaps). With each flap, particular attention is devoted to measuring the distance from the root of the pedicle to the most distant portion of the flap. With one end of the tape still at the root of the vascular pedicle, the working end of the tape is lifted up off the in situ flap and swung around to the defect. If the flap is a good option, the tape should easily fit into the portion of the defect that is to be filled. This simple maneuver is repeated for other flaps in the area until a clear choice of flaps emerges. Some flaps are ruled out with just one measurement.

In this way, a plan is formulated to deal with the unexpectedly large defects that inevitably occur. They may result from extension of a malignancy into adjacent structures that requires a wider excision to obtain clear margins. Or the defect may be enlarged by removal of more infected or necrotic tissue (as in posttraumatic or postradiation debridements). Whatever the cause, one must position and drape the patient so that access to the alternate or additional flaps is assured. This is discussed in more detail in Chapter 13.

For example, if a large upper midsternal defect is anticipated, and one is considering the rectus abdominis and latissimus dorsi flaps for the closure, the distances are

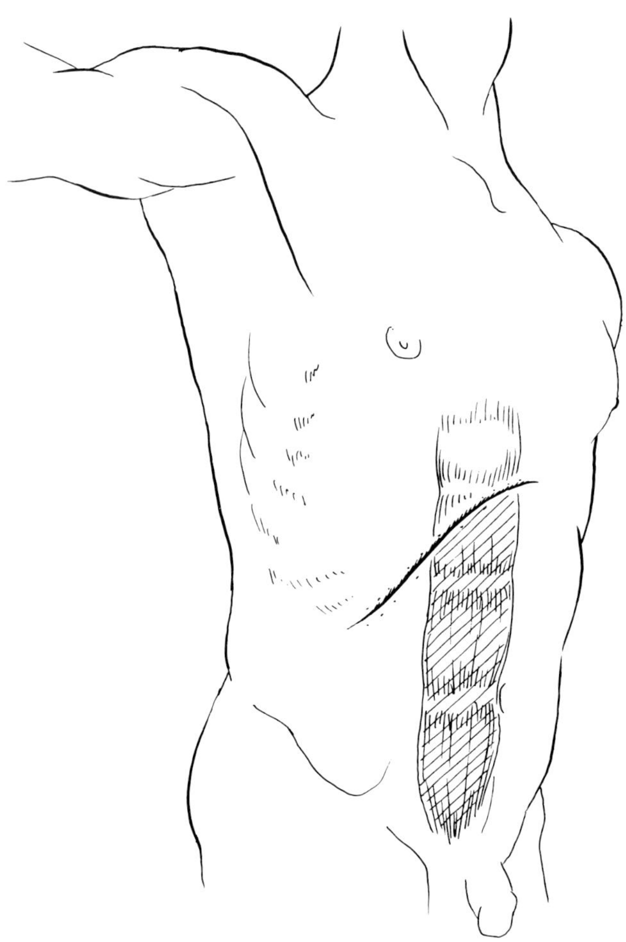

FIGURE 5.9 This healed right subcostal incision from a previous abdominal procedure contraindicates the use of a superiorly based rectus abdominis flap on that side. Such a flap would not survive since the epigastric vessel was ligated and does not reconstitute with time.

measured as shown in the sections on these flaps. If the flaps are found to be adequate, the patient is prepared and draped so that both flaps can be easily mobilized during the operation. This same process is done when preparing to use alternate flaps in other sectors of the thorax: measure the critical distances and available options for coverage; prepare for multiple flaps; and ensure a tension-free closure.

Precautions

The presence of surgical scars in the area of the flap or crossing the vascular pedicle may contraindicate the use of that flap. Once an incision has divided the blood supply on which the flap depends, the vessels never reconstitute and the flap distal to the scar fails. This is of critical importance in planning the reconstruction since previous incisions may rule out certain reconstructive options.

The common incisions of importance are a right subcostal incision (e.g., from previous cholecystectomy) that divides the pedicle to the superiorly based rectus abdominis flap and a previous posterolateral thoracotomy incision that divides the pedicle to the latissimus dorsi flap (Figures 5.9 and 5.10). Any such scar must be studied before selecting nearby flaps.

In summary, it is desirable to plan the extirpative and reconstructive phases of the operation meticulously and well in advance. Details such as flap selection, the need for stabilization, and preparation for the use of multiple flaps are considered for each patient so that the procedure will be completed efficiently and with minimum risk.

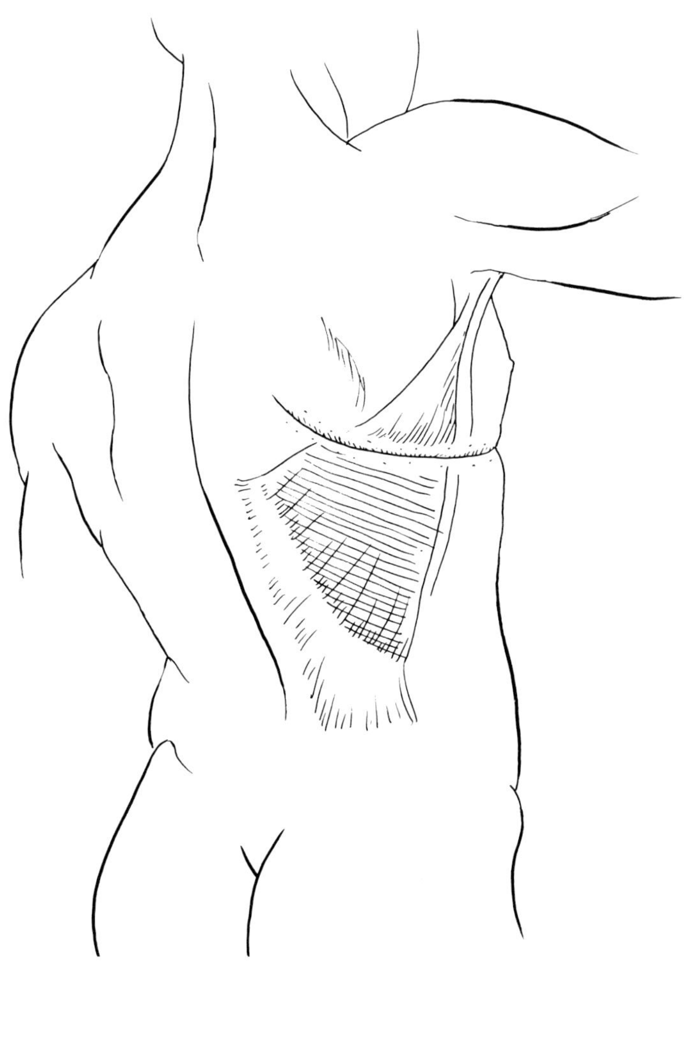

FIGURE 5.10 This posterolateral thoracotomy scar contraindicates the use of the latissimus dorsi flap since the vascular pedicle was interrupted during the procedure. The flap distal to the old incision would fail.

6

Resection and Debridement of the Chest Wall

The most common indications for removing portions of the chest wall are related to the extirpation and local control of tumors and to the removal of devitalized tissues secondary to infection, radiation, or trauma. These entities may be present alone or in various combinations. For example, a radionecrotic ulcer may contain residual malignant tissue and nonviable bone and cartilage and be even further compromised by a fistula or infection. Certain principles should be considered before extensive resectional or debridement operations. These are discussed in this chapter. The treatment, of course, should be tailored to fit the patient's needs, medical condition, and realistic goals for cure or palliation.

Neoplasms

Tumors may arise from the primary layers of the chest wall, as blood-borne metastatic deposits or as an extension from a source within (or external to) the thoracic laminae. Neoplasms that invade the deeper layers occasionally arise from tissues superficial to the fascia, such as recurrent mammary carcinomas or neglected skin cancers. Benign or malignant growths may also originate from within the thoracic cavity as tumors of the mediastinal structures, nerves, lung, or pleura. In evaluating a mass on the chest wall, it should be remembered that approximately 50% of all chest wall neoplasms are benign in nature.

Preoperative Evaluation

A tumor of the chest wall may have certain characteristics that suggest malignancy. These characteristics include anterior location (especially sternum), rapid growth, rest pain, radiographic evidence of bony erosion or destruction, and invasion of contiguous organs. This latter finding (visceral invasion) carries a poor prognosis. A malignancy is also more likely to exhibit overlying skin fixation, show central degeneration on scanning studies, and have satellite lesions. In contrast, benign lesions are more likely to have a less rapid growth pattern, be located posteriorly or laterally on the chest wall, and exhibit no truly invasive properties. Special attention should be devoted to a history of trauma involving the ribs. Old rib fractures can mimic neoplastic lesions. These are, of course, generalizations, and the definitive study is a histological analysis of the mass itself.

The routine preoperative evaluation is discussed in Chapter 4, but the assessment for a tumor should include plain radiographs and computerized tomography in addition to the general workup. Magnetic resonance scanning is being evaluated as an additional diagnostic tool. Computerized scanning has been the most helpful modality in assessing the extent and invasive properties of any given lesion.

The Biopsy

After the appropriate studies have been obtained and evaluated, the definitive histological picture must be considered. This means a diagnostic sampling of the tumor. There is controversy as to the indications for and the type of biopsy that should be performed. In general, an excisional biopsy (one that totally removes the lesion) is preferred whenever possible. This method results in the most accurate histological analysis and is therapeutic as well. However, it should be accomplished only if the surgical team is fully prepared to ablate the lesion locally and to proceed with the reconstruction of the resulting defect. Certainly, situations may arise when this is not possible or practical, and yet a tissue sampling must be obtained to find out what one is dealing with. In these instances, an incisional biopsy or needle biopsy is undertaken, depending on the pathologist's ability to analyze the small sample accurately.

Whichever of these latter two methods is prescribed, it is best when it is accomplished by the same surgical team that will later excise the lesion. If a malignancy is suspected, the patient should also be evaluated by the chemotherapist and radiation oncologist who may later be called on to treat the patient. This is done before any biopsy so that all members have the opportunity to examine and stage the tumor clinically. This examination is much easier and reliable when accomplished without the swelling, inflammatory changes, or scarring that inevitably occurs after any biopsy. Unfortunately, some patients are referred for definitive treatment after these important steps have already been done, and the receiving team is somewhat at a disadvantage.

The philosophy to perform excisional biopsy as a first choice at our institution has evolved in part through recommendations by the Armed Forces Institute of Pathology, whose different branches routinely analyze our specimens. Incisional (or partial) biopsy samples have failed to include malignant cell populations that were later discovered when the entire specimen was submitted. This, of course, has important implications for treatment and prognosis. Thus, there is a risk that an initial sample, obtained by incisional biopsy, may be designated incorrectly as a benign lesion. This is due to the fact that chest wall tumors sometimes have both benign and malignant cell lines interspersed randomly within the confines of the lesion. This is especially true of larger lesions and of chondrosarcomas, which are among the most common of chest wall malignancies. The smaller the sample (e.g., needle biopsy), the more likely it is that an important area will be missed in the biopsy.

In addition, incisional biopsies do not always heal properly and can give rise to an indolent ulcer that is compromised by contamination or infection. This is more common with fast-growing malignancies, previous irradiation, or when the skin is stretched over large lesions and becomes attenuated. If a biopsy site fails to heal, the resulting open and contaminated wound increases the risk of infection when the tumor is later resected and the defect reconstructed. Another problem is that although some tumorous growths do in fact exhibit healing after incisional biopsy, the resulting pleomorphism in the healing area can mimic malignant degeneration. These metaplastic changes can later cause diagnostic confusion when the mass is studied after the definitive resection.

Despite these risks, incisional biopsy is admittedly easier. It is sometimes championed since chemotherapy and radiation therapy are considered to be the first-line treatment for certain tumors, such as plasmacytomas. On the other hand, even with these tumors it is possible to increase diagnostic accuracy as well as to reduce the tumor burden (in preparation for chemotherapy or radiation therapy) by removing the entire lesion (i.e., excisional biopsy). Histological patterns of borderline malignancy within the tumor can then be subjected to special studies such as electron microscopy, so that the growth can be classified before subjecting the patient to anticancer medications or radiation treatments.

Resectional Margins for Benign Growths

For suspected benign lesions, a 1- or 2-cm margin of clinically normal tissue around the lesion usually suffices for the excisional biopsy. If the final diagnosis is confirmed to be of a benign nature, the margin of normal tissue decreases the risk of recurrence and does not significantly increase the size of the resulting defect.

If incisional biopsy is chosen, one should attempt to obtain a large and representative portion of the tumor and close the incision without tension. There should be no undermining or opening of additional tissue planes since this increases the risk of spreading the tumor.

All consultations with the oncology specialists should be accomplished before any biopsy, and the pathologist should have input as well. The pathologist may desire 1-mm glutaraldehyde-preserved pieces of tissue for electron microscopic study.

If a suspected benign lesion is found to be malignant after histological analysis, then a more aggressive resection is accomplished as outlined next. This can be done during the same hospitalization.

Resectional Margins for Malignant Neoplasms

There is controversy as to what procedure constitutes an adequate resection for cancer of the chest wall. Some authors have advocated removing a segment that includes one rib cephalad and one rib caudal to the margin of the neoplasm. Total excision of the involved rib has also been recommended. This has been interpreted to mean the full anteroposterior length of the rib. We prefer to perform the initial full-thickness incision at a distance (approximately 5 cm) from the lesion. Through this thoracotomy, the extent of the tumor is assessed bimanually. This examination within the pleural space notes adherence to lung or any visceral involvement that would contraindicate total removal.

The en bloc resection (including resectable viscera) includes 5 cm of clinically normal tissue in the plane of the chest wall as measured from all borders of the neoplasm. This is determined by palpation and inspection and includes 5 cm of normal rib, both anterior and posterior to the tumor (clinical margins). Frozen sections are done on the tissues at the periphery, with the knowledge that some tissues (such as bone) are not amenable to such analysis. The goal is to secure local control by obtaining histologically uninvolved tissue for at least 1–2 cm from the resectional margin (histological margins). The 5-cm clinical margins, incorporating at least one rib above and one rib below the lesion, seem to attain this goal (histological margins) in the majority of cases. In our experience, wider resections do not improve the prognosis. Once a lesion has developed satellite areas within a rib or within other areas of the chest wall, the prognosis is very poor. Extended resections, encompassing large portions of the chest wall in order to chase such lesions, do not improve the prognosis but do increase morbidity. It also does not rule out hematogenous metastases, which may have already occurred.

Invasive lesions from superficial organs (such as the skin or breast) and tumors invading the chest wall from within the pleural space are treated as indicated by the primary disease process as well as its chest wall extension. One of the most frequent superficial cancers has been recurrent breast carcinoma following mastectomy and radiation therapy. Such disease generally presents as a nonhealing ulcer and involves not only the skin and subcutaneous fat but the deeper layers as well. Biopsy of the ulcer often confirms recurrent malignancy. Treatment is directed at full-thickness resection of the diseased, radionecrotic tissue and immediate restoration with healthy flaps. Staged reconstruction is done only in truly septic wounds.

Extension of a tumor into the chest wall from within the thorax (e.g., a Pancoast tumor) may require a partial chest wall resection. The same principles of resection (i.e., 5 cm of clinically normal tissue plus the adjacent ribs) apply to these lesions. They are usually removed from within the thorax and the skin can sometimes be spared. The following general discussion is limited to some of the more common malignancies of the chest wall.

Malignant Tumors

Primary chest wall malignancies generally fall into one of five major types, with a sixth classification containing all of the other types. The five most frequently encountered tumors are (1) chondrosarcoma, (2) fibrosarcoma, (3) osteogenic sarcoma, (4) solitary plasmacytoma, and (5) Ewing's sarcoma. Each of these neoplasms has certain characteristics that may suggest the diagnosis. Some of these are outlined next for each of the tissue types.

Chondrosarcomas may arise at any age but are more frequently seen in young and middle-aged adults. These relatively common lesions are usually slow-growing tumors that are locally persistent and invade contiguous structures. Chondromas and chondrosarcomas seem to be at different points along a spectrum of growth potential, and chondrosarcomas often have benign chondromatous elements within them. Hence, an incisional biopsy of such a lesion may yield benign tissue. Radiographically, these tumors are lobulated masses, of variable density, which are at or near the costochondral junction or within the costal cartilages. They are more likely to be anterior on the thoracic wall. Local resection generally provides good control with 5-year survival of 85–90% reported. Recurrence is usually local and related to inadequate extirpation. The keystone of successful therapy is wide excision of the primary tumor. When the disease has recurred locally or is particularly aggressive, synchronous areas within the chest wall may be seen, and the prognosis is much poorer. Pulmonary lesions, which signal advanced disease, may also become apparent at this time. Unfortunately, chemotherapeutic agents and radiation therapy are relatively ineffective against these growths.

The next most common malignancies have been fibrosarcomas, which range from insidious and slow-growing to exceedingly aggressive. These, too, are more frequently seen in young and middle-aged adults, with occasional occurrences in the older population. They often present as a mass that invades the muscular tissue and portions of the thoracic skeleton and may even follow previous radiation therapy for other lesions (these are particularly aggressive). Adequate excision is the primary mode of therapy for these lesions since chemotherapy and radiation therapy have little effect on them. As with chondrosarcoma, these lesions are best treated by the first radical excision since recurrent lesions are generally refractory to subsequent therapy. Advanced disease may not only present as a local recurrence but frequently shows up as pulmonary metastases as well. Survival rates for the adequately excised primary lesion are generally in the 40–60% range at 5 years. Survival diminishes precipitously with recurrence and pulmonary metastases.

Osteogenic sarcomas are relatively uncommon on the chest wall. They generally occur in younger individuals, with the highest frequency in the second or third decades of life. These lesions sometimes exhibit a characteristic sunburst pattern on the plain x-ray, along with variable components of rib destruction. The sunburst appearance is related to raylike projections of calcium within the neoplasm. Although chemotherapy and radiation have resulted in variable success over short intervals, radical extirpation is the mainstay of treatment. Recurrent tumors usually present with pulmonary metastases rather than local lesions. In its advanced stages, the disease has an exceedingly poor prognosis. Although long-term survival has been recorded with osteogenic sarcoma, the expected cure rate is less than 50%.

Solitary plasma cell sarcomas or plasmacytomas are usually found in older individuals. Although they are sensitive to radiation, we have generally resected the chest wall mass as an excisional biopsy. Most patients who have been treated for this entity subsequently develop multiple myeloma. After the excisional biopsy, these patients must be closely followed by the oncology services, and chemotherapy or radiation treatment administered as indicated. Unfortunately, this tumor does not have a reliable radiographic presentation when it involves the chest wall. It may mimic a healing rib fracture, a metastasis, or one of the other primary chest wall tumors. When the patient develops systemic myeloma, it is usually responsive to chemotherapy for a variable time. In some patients, this progression of the disease has occurred many months after resection of the tumor, and extended survival is not unusual with the newer modes of combined therapy.

The final type of tumor is Ewing's sarcoma. It is generally seen in childhood or adolescence and can exhibit a characteristic radiographic pattern. This finding, described as onion skinning, relates to rapid growth and elevation of the periosteum at the tumor margins. The computerized tomographic scan can be helpful, but a histological specimen is needed to confirm the diagnosis. Chemotherapy and radiation have offered only limited success, and wide excisional surgery should be a part of any treatment plan.

TABLE 6.1 Common Chest Wall Malignancies

Tumor	Age Group	Location	Prognosis	Chemotherapy	Radiation Therapy
Chondrosarcoma	Young to middle-aged adults	Often anterior (near costochondral junctions)	Good with adequate excision	Poor	Poor
Fibrosarcoma	Young to middle-aged adults	Any region	Fair with adequate excision	Poor	Poor
Osteogenic sarcoma	Young adults	Any region	Fair with adequate excision	Variable	Variable
Plasmacytoma	Older adults	Often anterior	Fair (multiple myeloma)	Good	Good
Ewing's sarcoma	Adolescents	Often anterior	Poor (less than 20%)	Poor	Poor

Satellite lesions or pulmonary metastases can occur early in the course of the illness and make survival unlikely, although occasional survivors are recorded. The average 5-year survival is less than 30%.

All other tumors can be grouped in the final category. They may include such diverse lesions as rhabdomyosarcoma, malignant desmoids, and other infrequent neoplasms. Few of them exhibit a characteristic radiographic appearance. Diagnostic biopsy should be carried out, and our preference is wide excision with primary reconstruction. Close cooperation with the oncologists and pathologists furnishes the best approach (see Table 6.1).

Infection

Infection of the chest wall is usually secondary to ulceration of a tumor, trauma, breakdown of skin after high-dose radiation therapy or, more commonly, following a thoracic operative procedure. It may also occur as a result of bacterial seeding from within the thorax or as hematogenous dissemination from a distant source. The treatment of these latter two entities is directed at the source of infection, while treating any abscess on the thorax by means of incision and drainage. Antibiotic therapy is also employed in a regimen directed at the specific organism.

Infections related to malignant ulceration are usually in the nature of contamination of a nonhealing area. Although a cellulitis may occasionally supervene, the therapy is directed at a palliative (or curative) resection of the ulcerative lesion. This effectively removes the nidus of infection as well as the tumor. Due to the contamination of the operative site, broad-spectrum antibiotics are administered during the perioperative period. Surface cultures are of limited value since these open wounds, like any such skin disruption, grow a confusing array of bacteria. After the excision, the chest wall is restored primarily (if at all possible) with a healthy, well-vascularized flap. Such closure with thick, robust flaps allows the area to successfully withstand any residual contamination as well as tolerate additional postoperative radiotherapy. (See the following section on radiation ulcers.)

Posttraumatic infections are usually due to residual necrotic tissue or foreign bodies within the injured area. Therapy is directed at incision, drainage of purulent material, and thorough debridement of any remaining debris. In contrast to radiation ulcers, the posttraumatic wound is usually left open for an early delayed closure. Occasionally, flap coverage is required. The general treatment of traumatic chest wounds is discussed later in this chapter.

As indicated, infections related to radionecrotic ulceration respond poorly to anything short of wide excision and replacement with a healthy, well-vascularized flap. Serial debridement serves only to enlarge and deepen the nonhealing cavity, and a skin graft virtually always fails to heal properly due to the poor recipient bed that is irreversibly damaged by the radiation. The principle is a one-stage excision and immediate restoration of the defect with uninjured tissues (see following section).

The most common infection is postoperative. It usually involves the sternum and follows a median sternotomy that was used for an elective cardiac operation. A frank dehiscence may occur with exposure of the heart. More commonly, there is gradual onset of sternal tenderness, instability, and a low-grade fever. Spontaneous drainage of pus at a point along the midline incision frequently results in a chronic sinus that intermittently discharges purulent material. After appropriate evaluation to determine the extent of the infection (there is a good correlation between the area of tenderness and the eventual extent of the debridement), the incision is reopened and a thorough debridement is accomplished. Resection of the infected tissue is taken back to normal bone, and any deep sutures are removed. Pledgets that are grossly involved are removed if this can be done safely. The wound is then packed open with moist, sterile sponges for delayed closure within a few days. Wet-to-dry dressings are changed once per shift on the ward and the wound evaluated daily.

When considered appropriate, the next debridement is accomplished in the operating room, and if the wound is clean, it is closed. The closure usually involves the use of a unilateral rectus abdominis muscle flap, a pectoralis flap, or an omental flap, which is used to fill the cavitary defect with healthy tissue. The skin can usually be easily closed over this flap. Such staged debridement and the use of a well-vascularized flap give a high rate of successful closure. A word of caution is in order before selecting the rectus abdominis muscle flap. If the internal mammary artery has been used to revascularize the heart or if it is not patent on arteriography, the rectus muscle cannot be used since it depends on this artery for its blood supply.

Radiation Ulcers

Measures that fall short of wide excision and immediate closure with fresh, uninjured flap tissue often fail. The blood supply is so poor to these radiation-damaged areas that they have no capacity to mount an adequate healing process. They, in fact, worsen unless treated.

The staged debridement phases are usually bypassed since the ulcer enlarges if allowed to desiccate or remain open for lengthy periods of time. When the patient is deemed to be medically prepared for the operation, a wide resection and primary reconstruction are undertaken. The ultimate extent of the resection correlates well with the extent of preoperative tenderness. The ulcer is removed, along with the necrotic skeletal elements, until normal, uninjured tissue is reached. The error is in being too conservative in the removal of questionable tissue.

As indicated, in contrast to trauma or other infections, an attempt is made to close the defect at the same operation. If the defect is left open, there is risk that more necrosis will supervene in this damaged, irradiated bed of tissue. However, if the wound is deemed too contaminated, it must be packed open, and a delayed closure is performed as soon as it is safe to do so, preferably within a few days of the initial debridement. The closure, in any case, must incorporate well-vascularized muscle or omental tissue so that uneventful healing will take place. Since the damaged skin has been removed, it, too, must be replaced. This is usually done by applying a meshed, unexpanded skin graft directly onto the fresh muscle flap or omentum. Meshed grafts tolerate contamination well, yet heal as a sheet if applied unexpanded and kept moist for several days until the interstitial areas epithelialize.

This approach results in a secure, reliable closure in the majority of patients. However, as indicated, the surgeon must be prepared to excise the skeletal elements widely to ensure such success. Any necrotic cartilage must be looked on as a foreign body. Failure to remove it radically results in recurrent infection and fistulization, often with multiple sinus tracts.

Resection and Debridement of the Chest Wall for Trauma

Penetrating trauma of the chest wall requires special considerations due to the unique physiology of the thoracic bellows as well as the important structures contained within the chest. In dealing with severe injuries, serial debridement may be necessary to remove residual foreign bodies, devitalized bone, and necrotic tissue. Once these materials are eradicated (and, preferably, when healthy granulation tissue is apparent), reconstruction can be safely considered.

Such posttraumatic debridement requires careful assessment and individualization of treatment. The patient with extensive injury may require intubation and ventilatory support due to instability of the thoracic skeleton or to underlying parenchymal injury. This is particularly true if the wound is extensive enough to compromise the function of a major portion of the lung.

In the acute situation, if the patient has poor ventilatory function due to gross instability or air leakage, a unilateral or double-lumen endotracheal tube may be used to temporarily secure adequate ventilation to the healthy lung. The use of such a tube allows the good lung to be ventilated, yet excludes the air leak on the injured side until the injury can be repaired. After stabilizing the patient's ventilatory and cardiovascular status and dealing with other immediate life-threatening problems, the thoracic wound can then be carefully evaluated. This is done in the operating room after the fluid resuscitation is well underway. Once the patient is under general endotracheal anesthesia, the lung and chest wall can be methodically evaluated. Debridement is started by excising the wound edges and any exposed areas that are obviously devitalized. Muscle viability may be tested by applying a brief electrical current to see if the muscle will contract. A muscle stimulator or low coagulation current may be used for this purpose. If the muscle bundles twitch, they are most likely viable and have a reasonable chance of recovery. Muscle tissue that is obviously devoid of blood supply or vitality may be conservatively trimmed from the wound edge. Once the debridement at the margins has been extended back to healthy tissue, attention is turned to the deeper structures.

The lung is assessed for hemorrhage and devitalized parenchyma. Such tissue and any foreign bodies are removed and the injured area irrigated. Once the bleeding is controlled and debridement completed, the lung is expanded by opening the second lumen of the double-lumen tube. In cases of irreversible damage, resection of segment, lobe, or lung may be required. This is particularly true in patients who have been injured by high-velocity projectiles in military (or urban) battles. The loss of a lobe or segment in a young, healthy individual does not result in significant respiratory disability. Removal of the badly injured lobe can provide better control of hemorrhage, decrease the potential for prolonged air leak, and significantly lower the risk of postoperative empyema.

As the lung is reexpanded, any air leakage is noted. The use of absorbable, figure-of-eight sutures may help to contain hemorrhage or to seal small bronchioles that remain open on the debrided surface of the lung. Once hemostasis is obtained and all major air leaks are sealed, the lung is inflated and inspected again to ensure that no further foreign material is present. The lung is then deflated by disconnecting the second lumen on the endotracheal tube and allowing the lung to collapse. The entire pleural space is copiously irrigated to eradicate all residual clots and to remove any substances such as clothing, shards of bone, pieces of shrapnel, and other material from the environs. After the pleural cavity and chest wall have been thoroughly examined, the lung is once again reexpanded.

Chest tubes are situated to withdraw air and any residual fluid that may accumulate. One tube goes to the apex of the chest to withdraw air. It is inserted through a

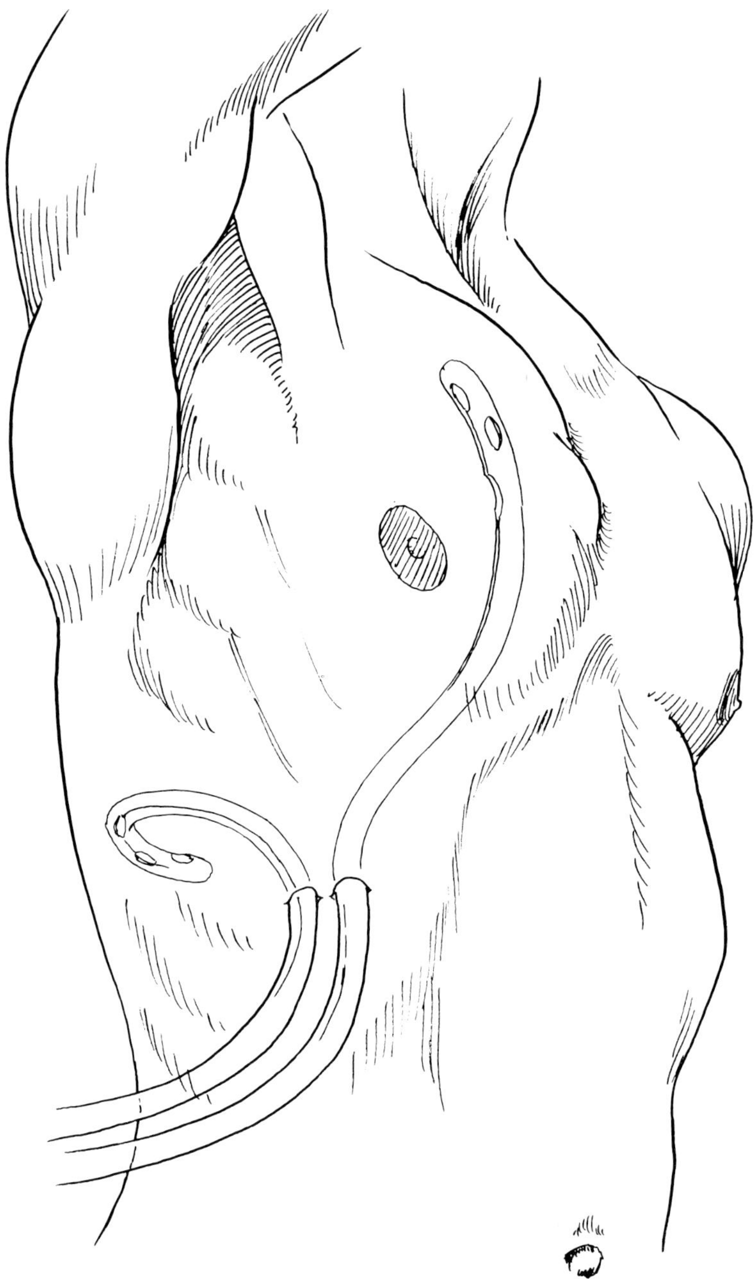

FIGURE 6.1 Chest tube placement after debridement for severe trauma is shown. In general, at least two large tubes are situated to withdraw air and postoperative fluid accumulations. One is positioned at the apex of the pleural space, and the other near the diaphragm, posteriorly in the costophrenic recess.

separate low incision and is directed upward toward the second interspace in the midaxillary or midclavicular line. Two additional tubes may be situated near the diaphragm. One of these, a number 40 right-angled tube, is oriented to lie in the costophrenic sinus posteriorly against the diaphragm. In some situations, the second tube along the anterior costophrenic sinus may or may not be necessary to achieve adequate drainage of the pleural space (Figure 6.1).

After the chest tubes have been secured, a large, sterile, occlusive dressing is placed in the defect so that it provides a protective seal. A copious, vaseline-impregnated gauze dressing is used and layered into the base of the wound and at the margins until a large, firm pack is in place. The chest tubes are then hooked up to high suction (between 40 and 100 mm of mercury pressure) to expand the lung fully and to allow it to fill the hemithorax.

The wound is closely inspected on a daily basis as the occlusive dressing is changed and the chest tubes are kept to high suction to encourage adherence of the lung to the margins of the defect. During the inspection, a careful search is made for residual foreign bodies or nonviable tissues. If further debridement is necessary, it is done under the controlled conditions of the operating room and under general anesthesia. The sharp debridement required in these wounds is exceedingly painful and should not be conducted in the intensive care unit.

Once the wound is clean (and, preferably, has developed a surface of healthy granulation tissue) and the exposed lung has become adherent to the chest wall, then reconstruction may be safely attempted. All air leaks should be completely eliminated. Once the wound is prepared, the appropriate stabilization and flap coverage can complete the restoration of the chest wall. The use of synthetic materials in such wounds is discouraged except when a massive section of the chest wall has been lost. Such injuries can cause an extreme ventilatory paradox that renders the patient totally dependent on the respirator. In such instances, it may be necessary to use a synthetic mesh to restore the skeletal layer at the initial reconstructive operation. Another alternative is to seal the wound with healthy flaps, wait a few days to rule out any local suppurative process, then perform a stabilization operation as a final stage. The patient can then be extubated safely. This is an extreme case but is offered to help in dealing with the patient who cannot come off the ventilator because of the loss of a large portion of the chest wall.

Loss of Major Portions of the Chest Wall

The loss of a large section of the chest wall is usually related to trauma, the ablation of tumors, or excision of radionecrotic ulcers. If there is no contamination to be dealt with (e.g., large tumors without ulceration), immediate stabilization of the musculoskeletal layer (usually via synthetic mesh material) followed by primary closure with composite (musculocutaneous) flaps is the method of choice. With such stabilization and coverage, the patient can usually be weaned from the respirator within the first few days. In some instances, rib struts may be required to afford even more stability. These cases must be individualized and contingency plans developed by the team preoperatively to cover any anticipated problem (see Chapter 5).

Another situation in which extensive resection is necessary is the large radionecrotic ulcer, which is compromised by a supervening infection and an extensive area of chondritis. Such involved costal cartilage must also be resected since, once infected, the cartilage acts as a foreign body—especially when further compromised by radiation. Any debridement that falls short of complete excision of the involved cartilage results in recurrent abscess, fistulization from underneath the flaps, and failure to heal. The radiated tissues must be radically resected and the chest wall restored with healthy, well-vascularized flaps. Secondary closure should be avoided if at all possible since granulations form poorly on the irradiated tissue, and leaving such injured tissues open can actually extend the area of necrosis. Of course, one is occasionally forced to perform a delayed closure if the radionecrotic ulcer is grossly infected. In such an instance, the closure is performed as soon as the wound is clean.

It is vitally important that the closure of these large defects be accomplished without any tension whatsoever. The closure is loose and floppy over the defect and any tension is moved to another area of the chest wall. This usually means the use of multiple flaps (Chapter 5).

7

Postoperative Care

The postoperative care of a patient who has had a major chest wall resection and reconstruction can be challenging, depending on the extent of the ablative defect, the amount of paradoxical motion that follows, and the patient's overall condition. A considerable volume of intravenous fluid has usually been administered during the operation, and the patient may well have received blood component replacement as well. Such variables, along with other specific requirements due to preexisting medical conditions, have an additive effect that must be considered in caring for these individuals. In general, three areas require special attention: (1) the cardiovascular system, (2) respiratory function, and (3) nutritional requirements.

Cardiovascular System

Particular care is exercised in evaluating and supporting the cardiovascular system after a chest wall operation. The requirements are similar to those seen after a major thoracotomy or cardiac procedure. This is particularly true if there is a history of preexisting cardiovascular disease, such as myocardial infarction. The surgeon must carefully balance intravenous fluid requirements and blood component therapy to maintain homeostasis without precipitating pulmonary edema or excessive tissue swelling. Certain techniques used to monitor cardiovascular status after surgery are extensions of those effectively used during the operative procedure. The arterial line is maintained until the patient is off the respirator and arterial blood gases have returned to acceptable levels. The Swan-Ganz catheter is ideally maintained until the patient is off the respirator and the postoperative mobilization of third-space fluid is complete. The area dissected during the operation is relatively wide, and the edema generated by these tissues can be substantial. This fluid returns to the vascular compartment 48 to 72 hours after the surgery, and this is attended by a noticeable diuresis. During this time, the Swan-Ganz catheter can effectively monitor cardiac status through pulmonary capillary wedge pressure measurements and provide insight into left-sided cardiac function.

As indicated, mobilization of third-space fluid usually results in a brisk diuresis. Some patients, however, may require cautious administration of a diuretic to enhance urinary flow. Such therapy is indicated when the left atrial pressure begins to rise without evidence of increased urinary output. If this occurs, therapy is initiated with small (5–10 mg) intravenous doses of furosemide to prompt the diuresis. Occasionally, larger doses (up to 40 mg at a given time) may be required to achieve this effect. Again, caution is warranted to ensure that renal function is unimpaired before the administration of additional medication. The serum electrolytes, especially potassium, are monitored. Potassium concentrations, depending on preoperative levels, the extent of muscle trauma during the operation, and renal function, can fluctuate widely during this diuresis and increase the risk of cardiac arrhythmias.

Judicious fluid replacement may minimize the edema generated in the third space. It is prudent to balance the fluid replacement such that the urinary output is 20–50 cc per square meter of body surface area per hour. Efforts are made to maintain the intraoperative and postoperative hematocrit in the range of 30–35%, with a hemoglobin of 10–12 g. This allows good oxygen transport capability and capillary flow, yet does not require excessive fluid replacement. Preoperative correction of low hematocrit and hemoglobin concentrations, either by nutritional support with postponement of operation or transfusion, is indicated so that the patient starts the operative procedure at optimal levels. Transfusions are usually given as packed cells in accordance with modern concepts of blood component therapy. All blood products are filtered through a micropore system to decrease microembolic phenomena, which can cause injury directly to the capillary endothelium and indirectly to the alveolar membranes of the lungs. Such trauma evokes edema in the pulmonary interstitium, which can decrease compliance as well as the capability of the lung for gas exchange.

If the patient is more than 65 years of age, has a history of cardiac disability, or has any findings of underlying cardiac dysfunction, prophylactic digitalization is strongly considered. Such therapy is started immediately after the operation in anticipation of the mobilization of third-space fluid. Digoxin is administered intravenously in divided doses such that 1.5 to 1.75 mg is given during the first 48 hours after surgery. Such therapy increases the inotropic response of the heart and works to suppress certain cardiac arrhythmias. The most common arrhythmia is atrial fibrillation with a rapid ventricular response. In this event, the goal of digitalization is to modulate the ventricular response to a more natural rate. Atrial fibrillation should be anticipated in these patients when there is mobilization or manipulation in the vicinity of the pericardium or the root of the lungs.

Another arrhythmia seen after manipulations close to the pericardium or adjacent to the ventricles is premature ventricular contraction. This condition is usually associated with ventricular irritability and is facilitated by hypokalemia. If premature ventricular contractions appear postoperatively, serum electrolytes should be drawn and the potassium concentration confirmed. After this has been slowly corrected, and if the arrhythmia persists, lidocaine is administered by the intravenous route as a 100-mg bolus. A lidocaine drip is instituted at any time if the premature ventricular beats are multifocal, are coupled, appear close to the T wave, or show a frequency such that cardiac output or blood pressure have diminished.

The Swan-Ganz catheter is helpful in evaluating cardiac performance during this critical period since it can give an estimate of cardiac output through the thermal dilution technique. Baseline values for cardiac output are obtained in the operating room as soon as the thermodilution catheter is inserted. This is particularly true for patients who may have cardiac dysfunction. Cardiac output determinations are repeated during the operation as necessary to assess cardiac performance and peripheral perfusion.

These assessments continue in the immediate postoperative period to compare current values with previous determinations. A decreasing cardiac output may call for early digitalization. Such timely therapy may enable the heart to deal with the increased fluid mobilized during the second to fourth postoperative day. Rarely, positive inotropic support is required, usually in the form of intravenous dopamine, in those patients who demonstrate decreased cardiac output with a rising left atrial pressure. Pulmonary capillary wedge pressures in excess of 18 mm of mercury suggest decreasing left ventricular performance. It is possible to maintain the left atrial pressure by appropriate administration of small volumes of fluid coupled with intravenous dopamine by way of constant, slow infusion. Such an infusion is generally associated with increased cardiac output, slightly decreasing left atrial pressure, and increased peripheral arterial pressure. A diuresis is also noted, due mainly to increased renal perfusion. Such support for patients who have had major chest wall resections has been required infrequently in our experience.

Respiratory System

The initial goal is a gradual decrease in ventilatory support and timely extubation. The patient is moved from the operating room to the intensive care unit with the endotracheal tube in place under ventilatory support. The anesthesiologist regulates the ventilator during the operation and works closely with the surgeon during the immediate postoperative period. Initially, the patient can be maintained on a tidal volume of 10 cc/kg with approximately 10 to 12 breaths per minute. (See Chapter 2 for a review of ventilatory physiology.) Arterial blood gases are drawn as soon as the patient is stabilized on this regimen (about 15 minutes). The inspired oxygen concentration is initially set at 100% and rapidly tapered according to the patient's response. For example, if the initial blood gases show a pO_2 greater than 100 and a saturation in excess of 95%, the inspired oxygen concentration is cut back to 70% and the process repeated. Adequate ventilation is also assessed, and is reflected by a pCO_2 which is ideally in the vicinity of 35–45 mm of mercury. If the oxygen concentration is less than 100 mm of mercury and the saturation is less than 95%, the normal 5 mm of positive end-expiratory pressure (PEEP) is increased, and both sides of the chest are again auscultated to assure that the lungs are expanded and ventilation is occurring on both sides. An immediate chest x-ray is always taken in the intensive care unit so that adequate expansion of both lungs and appropriate position of tubes and monitoring lines are confirmed. This latter assessment applies to chest tubes, nasogastric tube, monitoring lines, and endotracheal tube.

After acceptable values are attained for both pO_2 and pCO_2, intermittent mandatory ventilation (IMV) is instituted, starting at 10 breaths per minute. Blood gases are again determined, and if they are well maintained, the inspired oxygen concentration is gradually decreased to 40% and the IMV decreased until the patient is breathing without support. For example, the blood gases are obtained on 70% oxygen, then on 50% oxygen, then on 40% oxygen, while maintaining ventilation (pCO_2 in the range of 35–45 mm Hg). If the pO_2 remains above 100 mm of mercury and saturation stays above 95%, the inspired oxygen concentration can be decreased to 40% with a sufficient number of breaths per minute to assure that the pCO_2 remains between 35 and 40 mm Hg.

Lactic acidosis at this time is corrected by first assuring adequate perfusion so that renal regulatory mechanisms are able to correct the acidosis. If the metabolic acidosis is particularly severe or prolonged, sodium bicarbonate can be cautiously administered intravenously in single ampules of 44 mEq each. After each ampule is given, the arterial blood gases are checked to ascertain any persistent negative base excess.

Once adequate blood gases are achieved on 40% oxygen, the IMV mode is decreased. With each decrease in mandatory ventilation, arterial blood gases are again obtained. When the patient has achieved 2–4 breaths per minute on 40% oxygenation, is awake, and has regained muscular strength and control, the spirometer is used to further assess the capabilities of the patient. Quiet respirations are measured, and tidal volumes should be greater than 10 cc per kg of body weight (i.e., the 70 kg person should be able to move at least 700 cc per breath at rest). The maximal inspiratory effort should generate 30 cm of water (negative pressure), and the forced expiratory volume should attain 15 cc/kg (i.e., 1,050 cc for the 70-kg person). Another staged approach is to place the patient on a blow-by tube (T tube) with 40% inspired oxygen, check the blood gases again, and extubate the patient if the arterial gases have reached the prescribed goals. Much of this relates to individual preference by the surgeon. Most patients who can easily maintain themselves on an IMV of 2 breaths per minute, are alert, and responding appropriately can be extubated safely. Greater caution must obviously be exercised in those individuals who have respiratory disability or who are lethargic. It is wise to provide ventilatory assistance overnight and plan on extubation early the next day. This prevents exhaustion of the patient and permits unhurried extubation under optimum conditions for both patient and staff.

Suctioning

While the patient is on the respirator, mist humidification and frequent intratracheal suctioning are needed to clear mucus secretions. Small aliquots of saline, injected directly into the endotracheal tube, can loosen inspissated mucus and are aspirated with the suction tube immediately following the injection. On limited occasions, patients may require bronchoscopy to remove a mucus plug successfully. Clinically, the obstruction is heralded by lobar atelectasis evident on physical examination and confirmed by chest x-ray. These tenacious secretions are difficult to remove by the usual catheters but can be withdrawn through the bronchoscope while the patient is still on the respirator. This usually requires a side arm on a number 9 or 10 endotracheal tube to accommodate the fiberoptic scope. The patient is placed on 100% oxygen during bronchoscopic examination and the IMV is increased to 10. If the patient is reactive, paralyzing agents may be required to accomplish the task efficiently and safely. Rarely, the mucus plugs may not be amenable to removal by the fiberoptic instrument. In these instances, rigid bronchoscopy, performed by a skilled endoscopist, is required since the intratracheal tube must be removed and a ventilating bronchoscope introduced into the trachea. After this procedure, the patient is returned to the respirator with a larger endotracheal tube in place if possible (size 9 or greater) so that suctioning is easier and fiberoptic bronchoscopy may be conducted if necessary.

After extubation, active pulmonary toilet is continued. Blow bottles may be considered, but the newer incentive spirometric devices requiring the elevation of colored plastic balls through suction on the mouthpiece are most helpful in decreasing atelectasis. These are used throughout the early postoperative period, combined with good respiratory therapy and physical therapy. These may be discontinued when the patient is fully ambulatory, is coughing well, and shows no evidence of chest wall discomfort on deep inspiration.

Chest tubes are used when the pleural space has been violated during the operation. They are placed in an area away from the chest wall repair and inspected frequently. The tube placement is confirmed radiographically in the immediate postoperative period and also at any time the patient exhibits a problem related to ventilation. A daily chest x-ray is obtained as long as the tube is in the patient and immediately following its termination. The tube is stripped frequently to ensure that it is not occluded by clots, and the drainage chamber is kept in the most dependent position. The drainage system is maintained at 20-mm Hg negative pressure since this is usually adequate not only to drain fluid accumulation but also to keep the lung expanded even if there is an air leak. The use of rubber tubing between the chest tube itself and the collecting system facilitates stripping either manually or with roller devices.

Another modality that may be used to augment pulmonary toilet and postoperative analgesia is the intercostal nerve block. Such therapy is customarily employed in consultation with the anesthesiologist and, on the ward, is usually done with the chest tubes in place to preclude pneumothorax. Bupivicaine is employed as a half percent solution and injected along the intercostal nerve routes on the operative side. In the operating room, this can be done at the conclusion of the resection and before the reconstruction is started. Three intercostal nerves above and below the incision as well as the involved segment are targeted. When properly used, this technique can decrease postoperative pain for up to 48 hours and thereby increase the ability of the patient to cough effectively. Care must be taken not to enter the dural sheath near the nerve root since vasodilatation and a subsequent fall in blood pressure can sometimes occur if the local agent is introduced into the dural sac. Severe vasodilatation of the vasculature in the lower extremities can ensue, resulting in significant systemic hypotension. Intercostal nerve blocks can be repeated as necessary in patients who have poor respiratory function and who have had a large resection.

The Gastrointestinal Tract

The gastrointestinal tract requires monitoring and attention both for the handling of normal secretions and the use of its absorptive capacity to maintain nutrition. This aspect of postoperative care is vitally important and cannot be overemphasized. The patient must be provided with excellent nutritional support in order to recover without complication. Such support is planned and initiated preoperatively. If the peritoneal cavity has been entered (e.g., if the omentum has been recruited for the reconstruction) and particularly if the patient requires long-term ventilatory support, a jejunostomy of the Witzel type should be considered. This technique is particularly useful in keeping abreast of the caloric demand occasioned by the healing of such a large wound since feedings may be started with an elemental diet almost immediately after surgery. A number 18 red rubber catheter (which has extra holes cut in it) is introduced into the jejunum at a convenient location distal to the ligament of Treitz (Figure 10.15). The jejunum is secured to the abdominal wall lateral to the rectus abdominis muscle and away from the blood supply of any other flaps that may be needed.

The usual seromuscular tunnel is fabricated with Lembert sutures, and efforts are made to prevent internal herniation. Initially, the tube is connected to gravity drainage only. During the first postoperative day, an elemental diet is started at half-strength, using approximately 50 cc per hour with careful monitoring of the abdomen and visual assessment of the flow. This is gradually increased to full flow (100–150 cc per hour). With such efforts, long-term caloric support may be maintained without the necessity of parenteral nutrition or uncomfortable nasogastric irritation. It is rare that the caloric requirements of the healing wounds are in excess of what can be introduced in the jejunostomy. If this occurs, supplemental parenteral nutrition can be employed. The access pathway for such therapy should be away from the chest wall reconstruction because of possible local complications secondary to infection or manipulation around the suture lines.

A gastrostomy is used in addition to the jejunostomy in those patients who have had repair of a tracheoesophageal fistula and any other type of reconstruction in which long-term gastric decompression is required. This is particularly useful in decreasing gastric reflux over the suture lines of the repair and also in decreasing the risk of aspiration. A standard Stamm-type gastrostomy is joined to the anterior abdominal wall and brought out through a stab incision lateral to the rectus abdominis muscle (to prevent any injury to the pedicle of the rectus abdominis flap). Both the jejunostomy and gastrostomy may be well maintained for long periods. In fact, some patients can be discharged with gastrostomies and jejunostomies if they require late postoperative nutritional support and decompression. These tubes are easily removed but must be in place long enough for a secure tract to form before removal. This ensures that leakage of viscus contents does not occur into the peritoneal cavity upon removal. Stomal drainage decreases within 24 hours and usually seals within 5 to 7 days after removal of the tube.

The patient may require a mild laxative or colonic stimulation to encourage the first bowel movement after surgery. A mild suppository or Fleet's enema can be useful in this regard.

Additional Postoperative Considerations

The patient is carefully monitored for thromboembolism as any patient should be after major surgery. The usual care is given as required with the Foley catheter. A closed system is maintained and proper meatal care is administered. The Foley is discontinued as soon as the patient is capable of voiding on his own. The core body temperature is frequently reduced due to operative heat losses. Consequently, temperature monitoring devices should remain until core heat is stabilized in the normal range. Warming blankets are used only if the temperature is severely reduced. The indwelling rectal probe or other means of continuous temperature monitoring is usually continued until the patient is able to sit in a chair.

Care of the Flaps

The flaps used in reconstruction are frequently inspected to look for evidence of ischemia. The most common reason for failure of musculocutaneous flaps is venous obstruction. This is usually caused by technical error during the operation and is due to tension and the absence of a truly loose closure. It is manifested by a mottled, bluish discoloration and areas of coolness to the touch. There may also be a sluggish capillary refill. Temperature monitors can help in this assessment, but early and frequent postoperative examination is required regardless of the presence of such devices. Such venous engorgement is due to torsion, pressure, or tension on the vascular pedicle of the flap and requires immediate decompression if the flap is to survive. Removal of sutures at the bedside is the first measure. If unrelieved in a few minutes, the flap is totally mobilized in the operating room. Provisions are made for closure by other flaps at this time.

The suture lines around the flap are lubricated with an antibacterial ointment to prevent crusting and secondary infection, and no dressing is applied unless meshed skin grafts are used. The donor site of the flap and the skin grafts are treated in standard fashion, and the drainage is recorded from the suction catheters from beneath the flaps. Meshed grafts are kept moist with saline-soaked sponges to prevent desiccation of the uncovered interstitial areas. These are usually epithelialized from the graft in 3 to 4 days, and the moist dressings can be discontinued at this time. The graft is then lubricated daily with an antibacterial ointment to prevent scaling. This, too, can be discontinued after several weeks, but the patient should be counseled as to the tendency of the grafted skin to peel. This is due to the absence of sebaceous activity in grafted skin and can be permanent, depending on the thickness of the skin graft and inclusion of sebaceous glands with the graft.

Summary

As with the resection and reconstruction, the postoperative care must be individualized for each patient. Both services are intimately involved with the patient even though one is responsible for orders and initiation of care. With proper management in the operative and postoperative period, excellent results can be obtained. In the last 18 years at our institution, approximately 170 major chest wall resections have been conducted in patients of all ages for a variety of reasons. Only two postoperative deaths have ensued: one from a late myocardial infarction in an elderly man and one in a young woman who died of rampantly aggressive generalized breast cancer. The postoperative morbidity has been comparable. With fastidious operative and postoperative care, comparable results can be obtained at most institutions equipped to handle a patient with a major operative procedure.

References

American College of Surgeons, Committee on Preoperative and Postoperative Care: *Manual of Preoperative and Postoperative Care*, ed. 3. Philadelphia, WB Saunders, 1983.

Graeber GM, Snyder RJ, Fleming AW, et al: Initial and long-term results in the management of patients with primary chest-wall neoplasms. *Ann of Thor Surg*, 1982;34:664.

Graeber GM: Discussion of paper by McKenna RJ, McMurtrey MJ, Larson DL, Mountain CF: A perspective on chest wall resection in patients with breast cancer. *Ann of Thor Surg*, 1984;38:482.

SECTION II

Mobilization of Flaps

8

The Latissimus Dorsi Muscle and Musculocutaneous Flaps

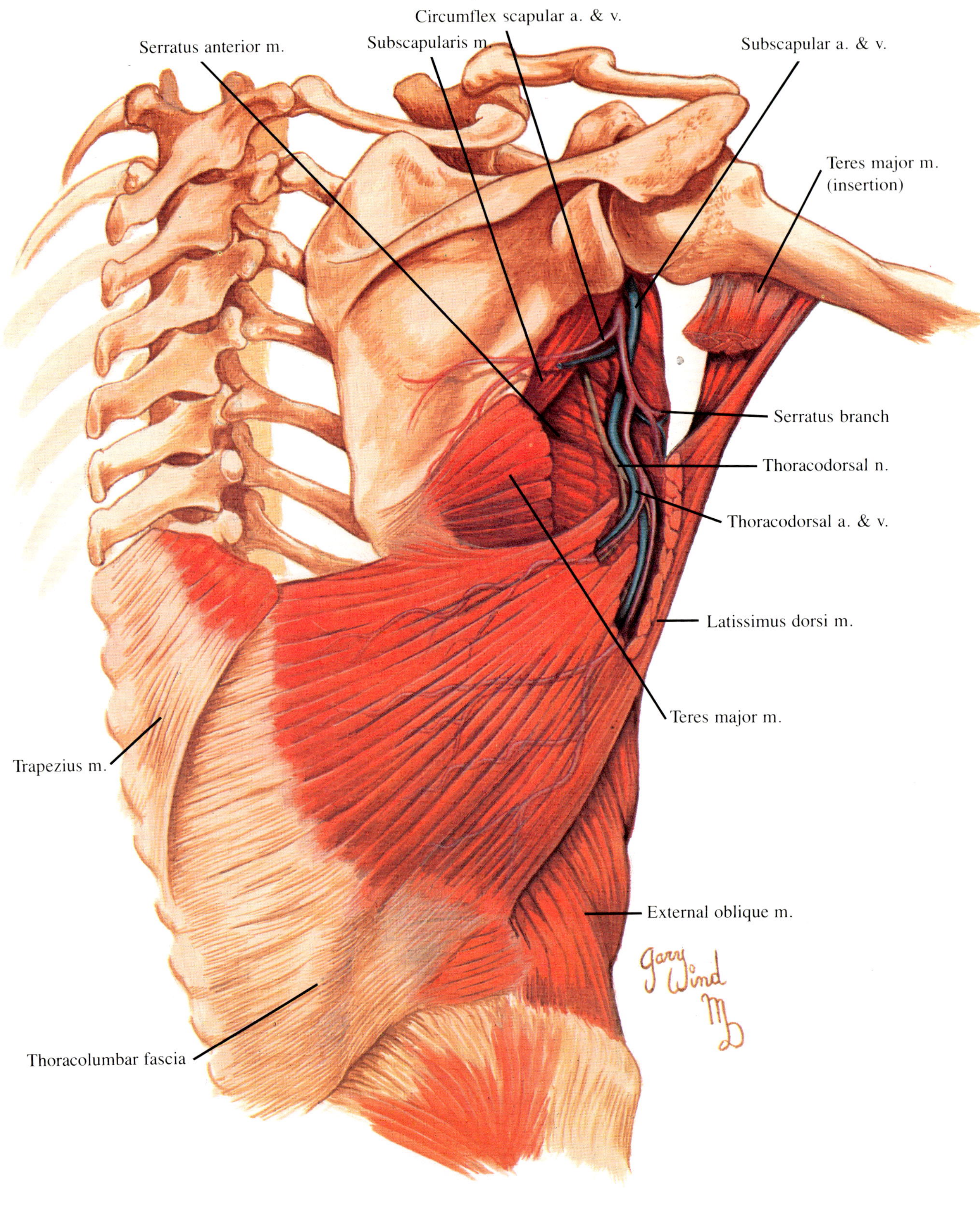

The latissimus dorsi muscle and its immediate neighbors are shown in cutaway fashion to demonstrate the dominant thoracodorsal neurovascular pedicle and relationships at the origin and insertion of the muscle.

Anatomy

The latissimus dorsi muscle covers a roughly triangular area of the lower back from the sacrum up to the level of the seventh thoracic vertebra (Plate 8.1 and key drawing). The muscle originates from a broad aponeurosis which attaches to all of the spinous processes caudal to T6 and which fuses inferiorly with the posterior layer of lumbodorsal fascia. The aponeurosis attaches laterally along the posterior crest of the ilium and may contain muscle fibers at its free margin. A small triangular area at the cephalad end of this origin is deep to the trapezius muscle, whose aponeurosis begins at the spinous process of T12. The rest of the latissimus is superficially located, just beneath the subcutaneous fat. Additional fibers of the latissimus originate from the lower three or four ribs, between digitations of the external oblique, and join the deep aspect of the muscle. The cephalad margin of the muscle is joined to the inferior angle of the scapula by muscular fasciculi. The muscle fibers converge and spiral 180° around the teres major, to insert into the crest of the lesser tubercle of the humerus and into the floor of the intertubercular groove. There are rarely any significant variations in the muscular configuration.

The skin of the back is thick and bound to the deep layers by dense septa of the fibrous dorsal superficial fascia. The deep investing layer of fascia splits to enclose the fleshy part of the latissimus and fuses with the lumbar aponeurosis (the union of latissimus aponeurosis and the posterior leaf of the lumbodorsal fascia).

The predominant blood supply to the latissimus comes from the thoracodorsal artery, which is the continuation of the subscapular branch of the axillary artery after the subscapular gives rise to the circumflex scapular artery. The thoracodorsal artery and accompanying thoracodorsal vein run between the subscapularis and the serratus anterior and give off one or two sizable branches to the latter. The vessels then pass anterior to the teres major to reach the deep surface of the latissimus along its cephalad border approximately 2 cm from the lateral muscular edge and 8–10 cm from its humeral insertion. There is some variation in the origin of the circumflex scapular, but the thoracodorsal artery is constant. After reaching the deep surface of the muscle, the thoracodorsal vessels bifurcate in about 90% of individuals into two major branches. The lateral branch follows the direction of the muscle fibers about 2 cm from the lateral border. The other branch passes medially approximately 4 cm from the cephalad edge. When this major transverse branch is absent, there are three or four branches of the lateral vessel that parallel the upper muscular fibers. Both arrangements permit the division of the latissimus into two or more viable flaps. Dye injection studies demonstrate the perforating branches of these vessels supplying the overlying cutaneous territories.

The thoracodorsal nerve arises from the posterior cord of the brachial plexus about 3 cm proximal to the subscapular vessels and joins the thoracodorsal vessels to supply the latissimus with innervation from C6, C7, and C8. The nerve branches in the same pattern as its accompanying vessels.

The latissimus extends, adducts, and internally rotates the arm. It also pulls the shoulder caudally and posteriorly.

General Characteristics

With proper technique, the latissimus dorsi flap is eminently reliable and can provide thick, durable coverage to large defects in practically all sectors of the chest wall. It can be used as a combined muscle-skin flap or as muscle alone to fill cavitary defects. The exposed muscle is an excellent recipient bed for skin grafts, and because of the thickness of the muscle, the healed grafts are well padded for increased durability.

The entire muscle (Figure 8.1) may be mobilized on its vascular pedicle and transposed to the defect. Since it belongs to that category of muscles that provide

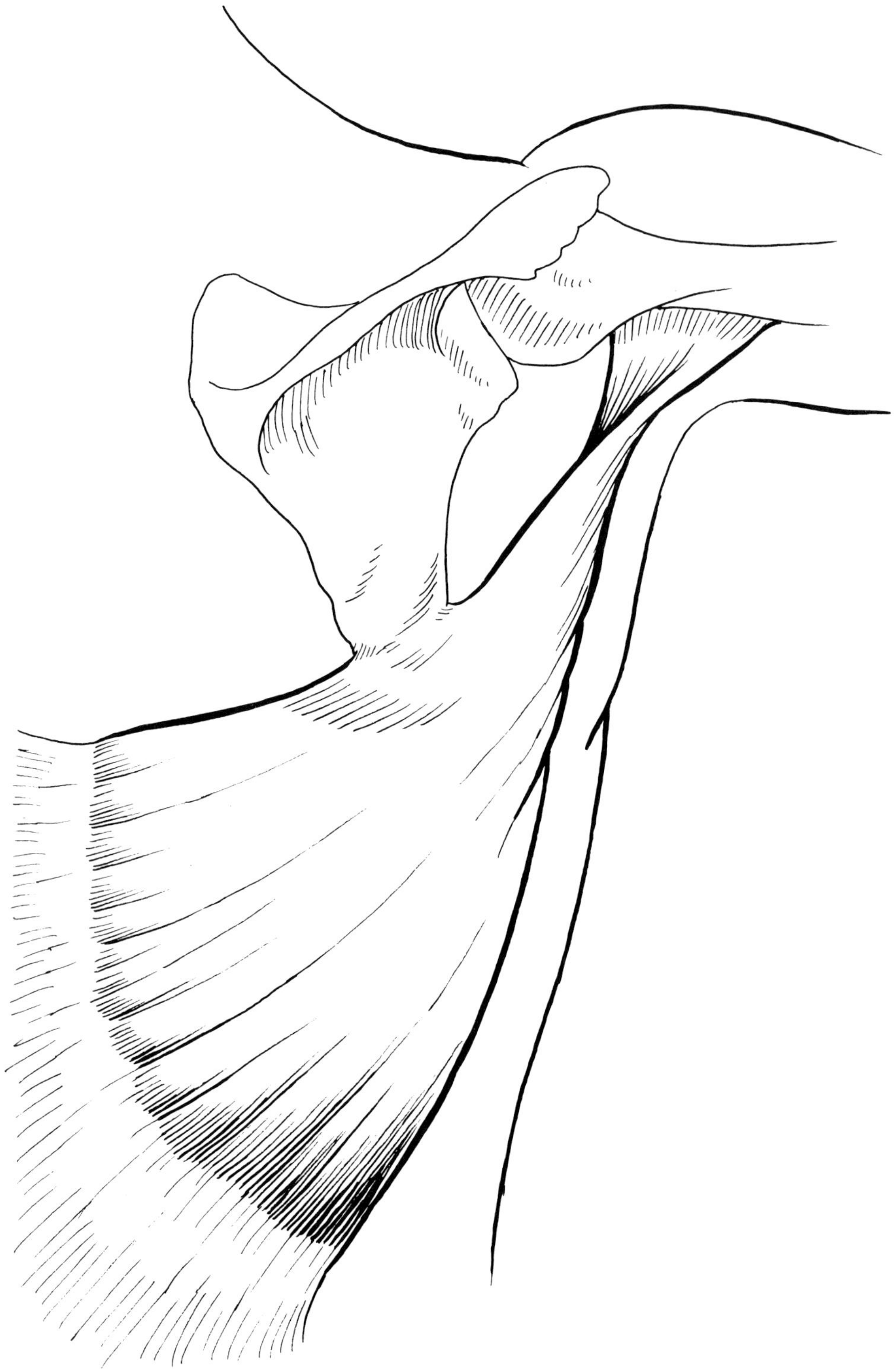

FIGURE 8.1 The entire latissimus muscle may be mobilized on its vascular pedicle, giving durable, thick coverage to many areas on the chest wall.

nutrition to the overlying skin by way of perforating arteries, it can also be used as a combined musculocutaneous flap. The muscle then acts as a carrier for the skin and subcutaneous tissue needed at the defect. Virtually the entire territory of skin overlying the latissimus can be safely carried by the muscle (Figure 8.2). However, the skin defect left by total removal of the muscle-skin unit will require grafting of the donor site. The donor site can be closed primarily if the skin defect is less than 10 cm wide in the adult patient. Although large skin segments are very reliable, small ones are less so because

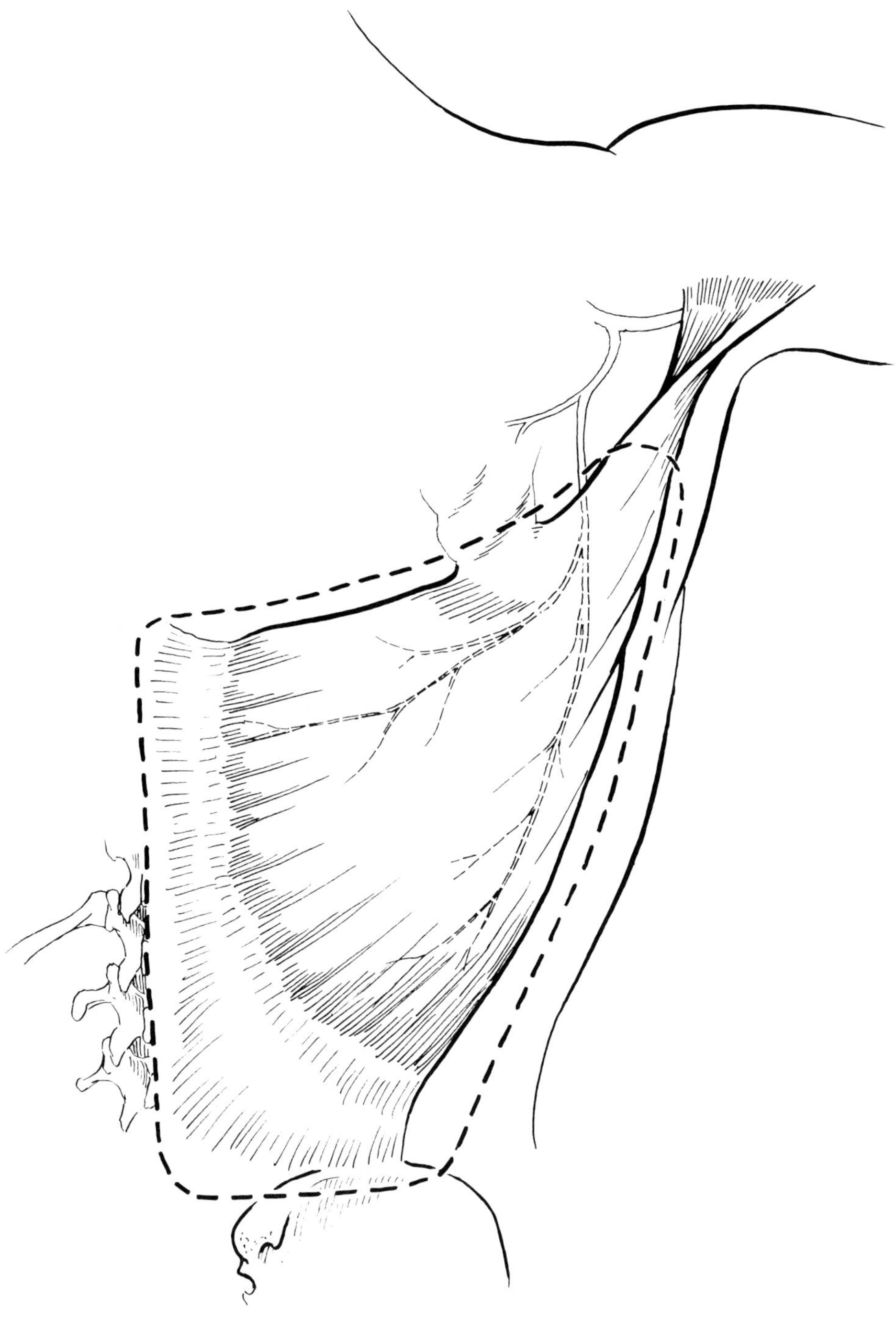

FIGURE 8.2 Virtually the entire territory of skin overlying the latissimus can be safely carried by the muscle. Usually, however, only a portion of the skin is used, and the donor area can be closed primarily.

they may not include a perforating vessel from the muscle. These numerous vessels enter the skin from the muscle several centimeters apart in a somewhat random fashion. If the skin does not incorporate such a vessel, it will undergo necrosis even though the muscle will be viable. Thus, the skin portion of the flap should be at least 6–8 cm in its shortest dimension. Although the vascular territory of the latissimus extends a few centimeters beyond its borders, the most reliable area of skin is that which directly overlies the muscle.

It is possible to use the muscle without including its dominant blood supply, the thoracodorsal vessels. This ''reverse'' latissimus, which is based on the perforating arteries about the lower paraspinous musculature, has been used for midline spinal defects (see Chapter 3, Figure 3.8). Its range and arc of rotation are more limited, however. To date, we have not found common use of this alternative. The same is true concerning the use of the latissimus flap based on reverse flow through the artery to the serratus musculature. This latter design has been used in postmastectomy cases where the thoracodorsal artery had been previously divided proximal to this branch.

Preoperative Planning

The decision to use the latissimus dorsi muscle flap or combined muscle-skin flap to cover a chest wall defect is based on the reconstructive requirements of the defect, the condition of the latissimus itself, the size of the muscle and available skin relative to the defect, and the useful range of the mobilized flap.

The condition of the muscle is important since one of the goals is to supply healthy, durable, and richly vascularized tissue to enhance primary healing of the defect. Muscle that has been denervated (for example, by injury during a previous mastectomy) is best avoided since the atrophic changes render it thin, pale, and sometimes unreliable from a vascular standpoint. Likewise, a previous thoracotomy that has transected the muscle makes it relatively useless as a reconstructive option, since the muscle and skin distal to the old incision will undergo necrosis if mobilized again. This distal portion is the most useful part of the unit for most reconstructions.

The latissimus may be tested by having the patient place the hands on the hips and push inward toward the midline while the surgeon palpates the anterior edge of the muscle (Figure 8.3). If it contracts, the neurovascular pedicle is intact and the muscle can be safely used for the reconstruction.

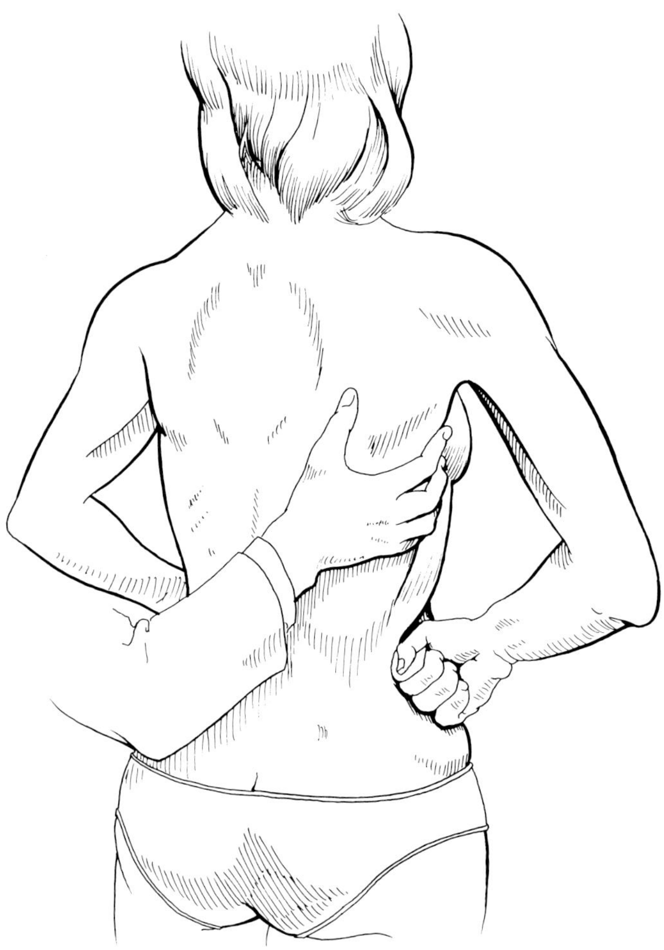

FIGURE 8.3 The latissimus may be tested by having the patient place the hands on the hips and push inward toward the midline while the surgeon palpates the anterior edge of the muscle.

Next the size of the muscle is compared to the size of the defect for which it will be used. The principle is to ensure a tension-free closure of the defect or, if tension should exist, to shift it to a point well away from the gap in the chest wall. This is particularly critical for full-thickness defects. In this way, if a dehiscence occurs, it will not occur over the critical area but rather over intact parietes. If there is any question as to size or tension at the defect, the use of one or more additional flaps must be considered in the planning phase (see Chapter 5 for selection of additional flaps).

As stated earlier, the larger the cutaneous island carried with the muscle, the more reliable is its viability since it will be more likely to incorporate a large feeding artery from the muscle to the skin. In some cases, it may be deemed more appropriate to use the muscle alone and then apply a split-thickness skin graft for epithelial coverage. Such grafts heal readily on this well-vascularized muscle.

The range or ''reach'' of the flap is the most distant extent for which it can provide reliable coverage. This range is limited by the vascular pedicle, which forms the stationary ''pivot'' point of the flap. There must be no tension on this lifeline.

To get a quick, general appraisal of the range of the latissimus, a tape measure is applied to the thorax from the posterior axillary fold down to the distal limit of its origin (Figure 8.4). This latter point corresponds to the junction of the latissimus with the paraspinous muscle group near the lumbar spine, just even with the highest point on the iliac crest. The tape at the axillary fold represents the stationary pivot point of the flap, which is the vascular pedicle. The lower point on the tape represents the farthest reach of the flap.

Posteriorly, the flap will cover upper thoracic, midline spinal, and scapular defects as well as those about the upper shoulder (Figure 8.5). The intact scapula and its musculature present an obstacle to its use in the upper regions, however.

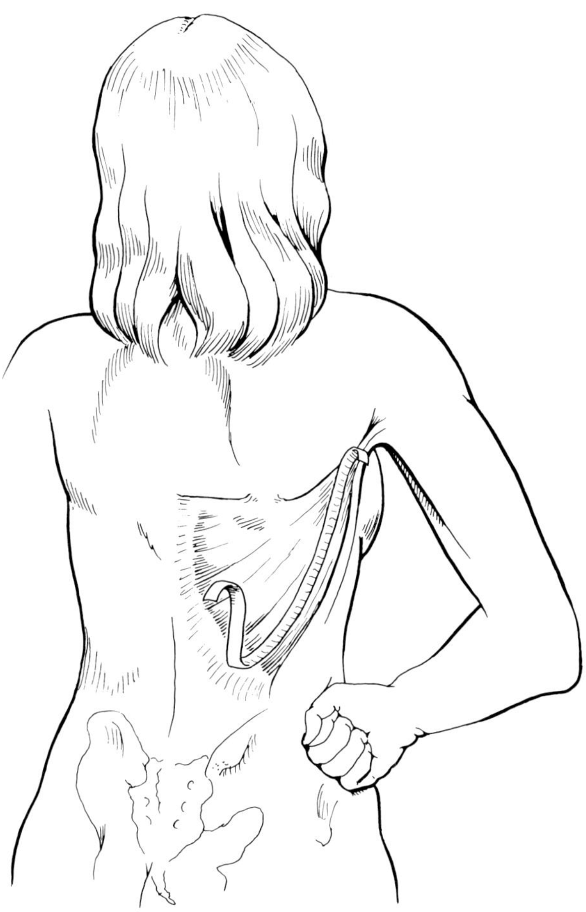

FIGURE 8.4 A tape measure is applied from the posterior axillary fold down to the distal limit of the latissimus origin.

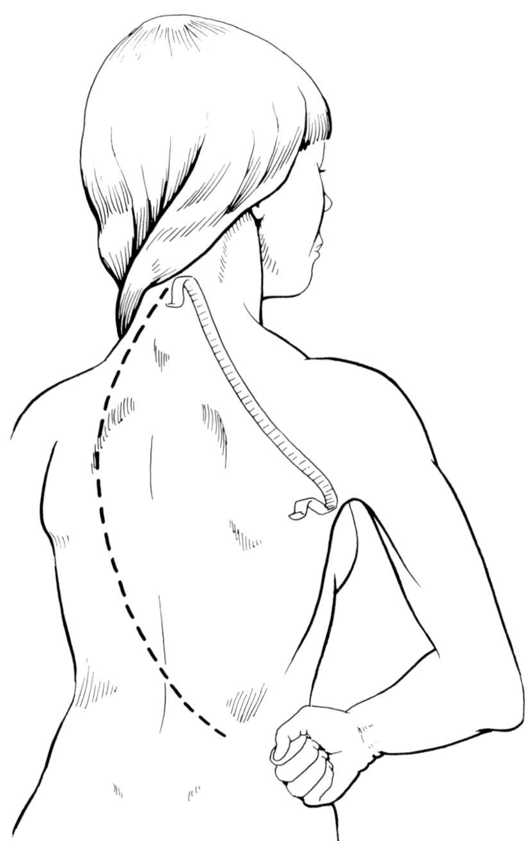

FIGURE 8.5 Posteriorly the flap will cover upper thoracic, midline spinal, and scapular defects as well as those about the upper shoulder.

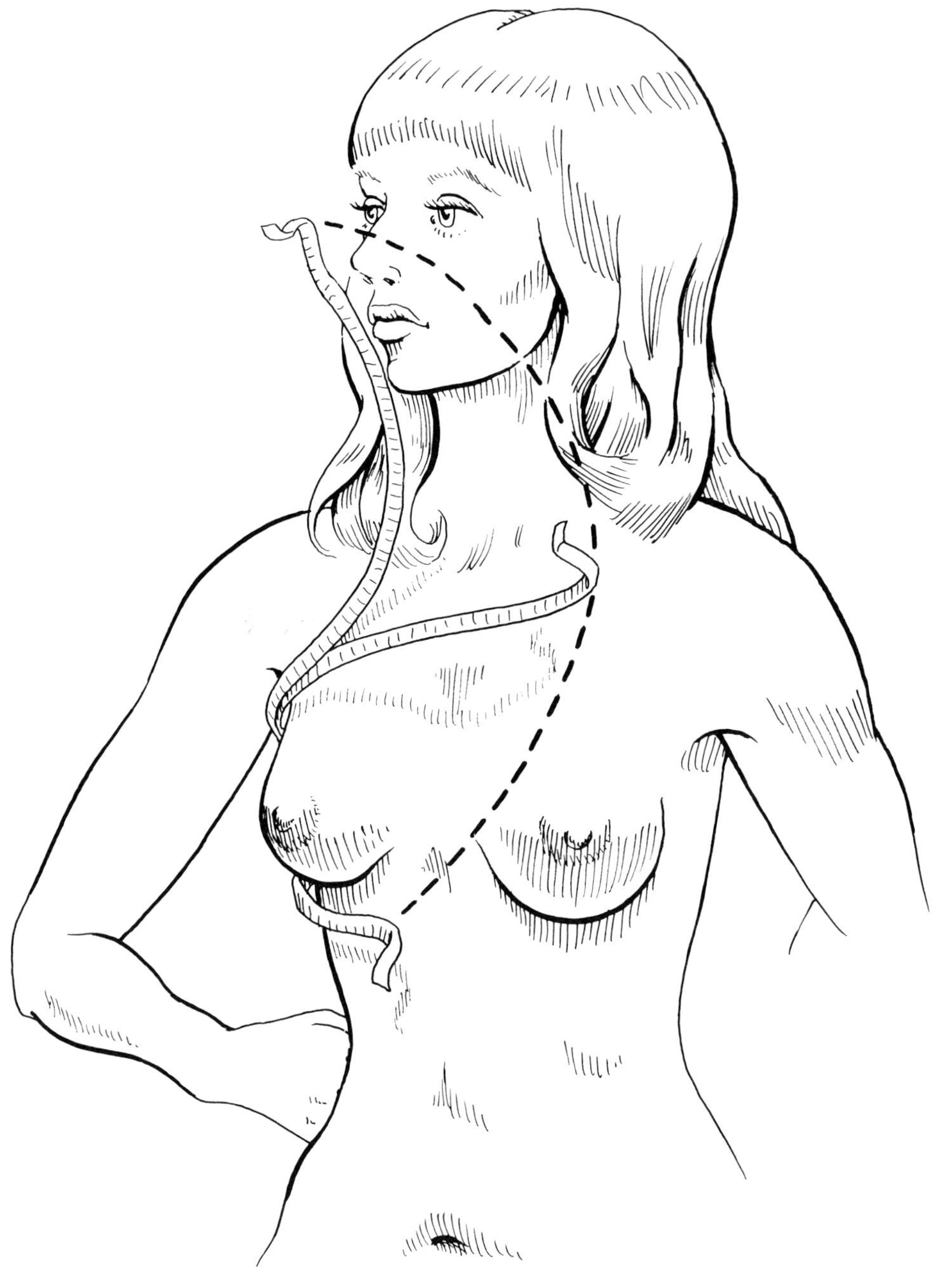

FIGURE 8.6 Anteriorly the latissimus will reach the parietal area of the skull, the ipsilateral supraorbital ridge, the pharynx, and the intraoral regions. It can reach as far as the contralateral mid-clavicular line and is most useful for upper sternal, ipsilateral clavicular, and upper chest wall defects.

Anteriorly, after the latissimus is brought through the axilla, it will reach the parietal area of the skull, the ipsilateral supraorbital ridge, the pharynx, and the intraoral regions (Figure 8.6). It will cross the midline of the neck as far as the opposite midclavicular line and easily cover defects of the upper three-quarters of the sternum. As the xiphoid region is approached, the more distal limits of the flap are pressed into service and tension can be a problem. Laterally, the flap will reach all areas from the axilla down to the costal margins.

Returning to the planning phase, the lower point on the tape is now moved to the distal limit of the existing or planned surgical defect in the chest wall (Figure 8.7). It should easily cover the defect.

If this first measurement is good, a hand towel or other nonelastic cloth can be helpful in specific planning. The cloth is placed on the patient and cut or folded to correspond to the patient's actual latissimus (Figure 8.8). The proposed skin island is

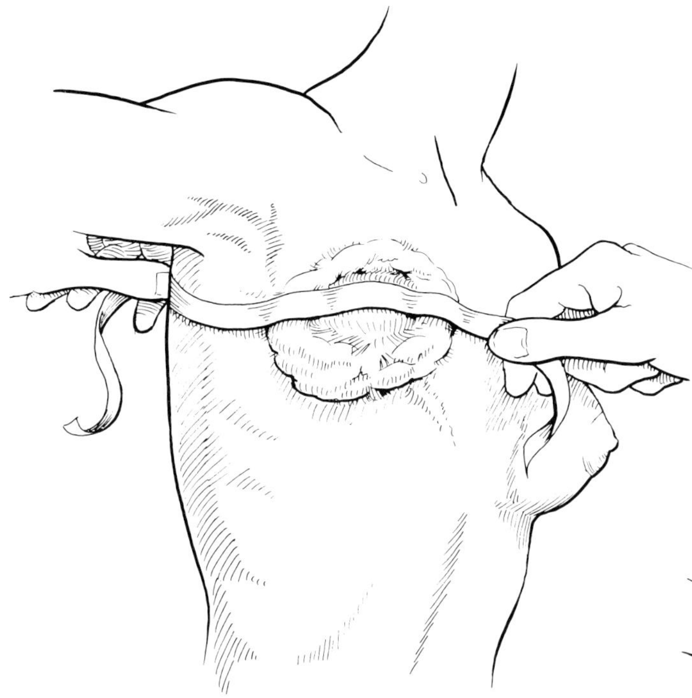

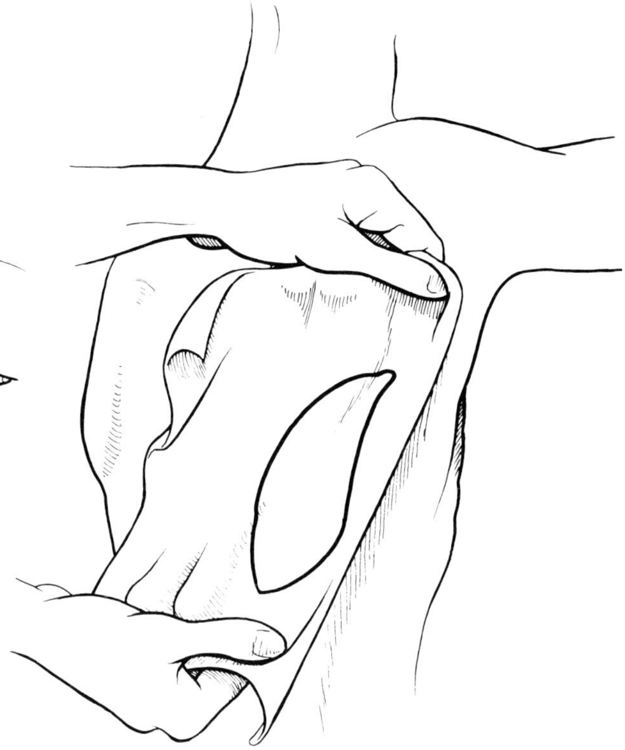

drawn on the cloth, and the mobile end of the cloth ''flap'' is rotated over the planned operative defect, keeping its ''pedicle'' on the posterior axillary fold (Figure 8.9). This will give an idea as to the ultimate reach of the flap as well as to how the skin island will conform to the anticipated defect in the chest wall. After making any adjustments in the cloth flap and the skin island, and if the latissimus is found to be suitable for the task, the incision can be outlined.

FIGURE 8.7 The lower point on the tape is moved to the distal limit of the chest wall defect.

FIGURE 8.8 A nonelastic cloth is cut or folded to correspond to the patient's latissimus, and a proposed skin island is drawn on the cloth.

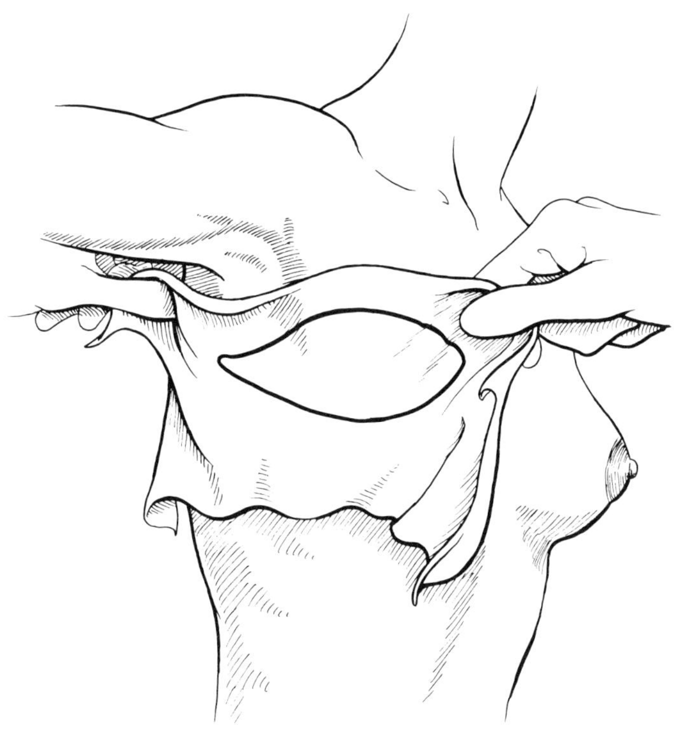

FIGURE 8.9 The mobile end of the cloth ''flap'' is rotated over the planned operative defect, keeping the pedicle end at the posterior axillary fold.

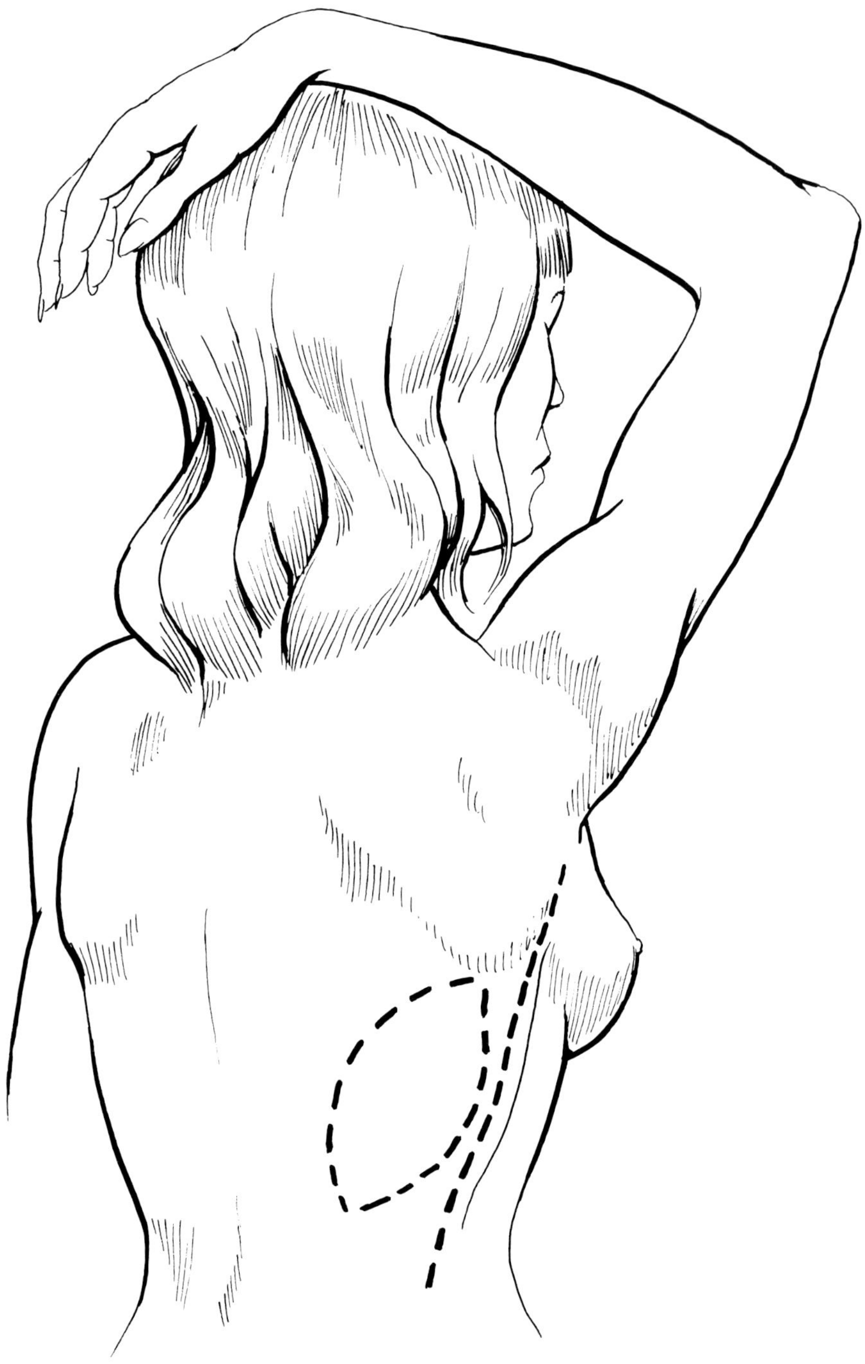

FIGURE 8.10 The incision site is marked. The straight line is used when only the muscle is to be mobilized. The ellipse is used when a segment of skin is to be used with the muscle.

The patient's hand is placed again on the head so that the muscle is tightened. This will allow the anterior edge to be more readily palpable. The surgeon's fingers are moved over the ribs until the muscle is rolled under the fingers. This anterior margin is then marked. If the latissimus muscle alone is to be used, the incision will be along this margin (Figure 8.10). If a combined muscle-skin flap is to be used, the skin island is marked as determined before on the cloth "flap." In mobilizing this combined flap, enough access to the muscle will be available after the skin island has been incised so that additional incisions are usually not needed.

If required, these measurements can also be made or adjusted with the patient on the operating table. This is particularly true if the defect turns out to be a different size than anticipated.

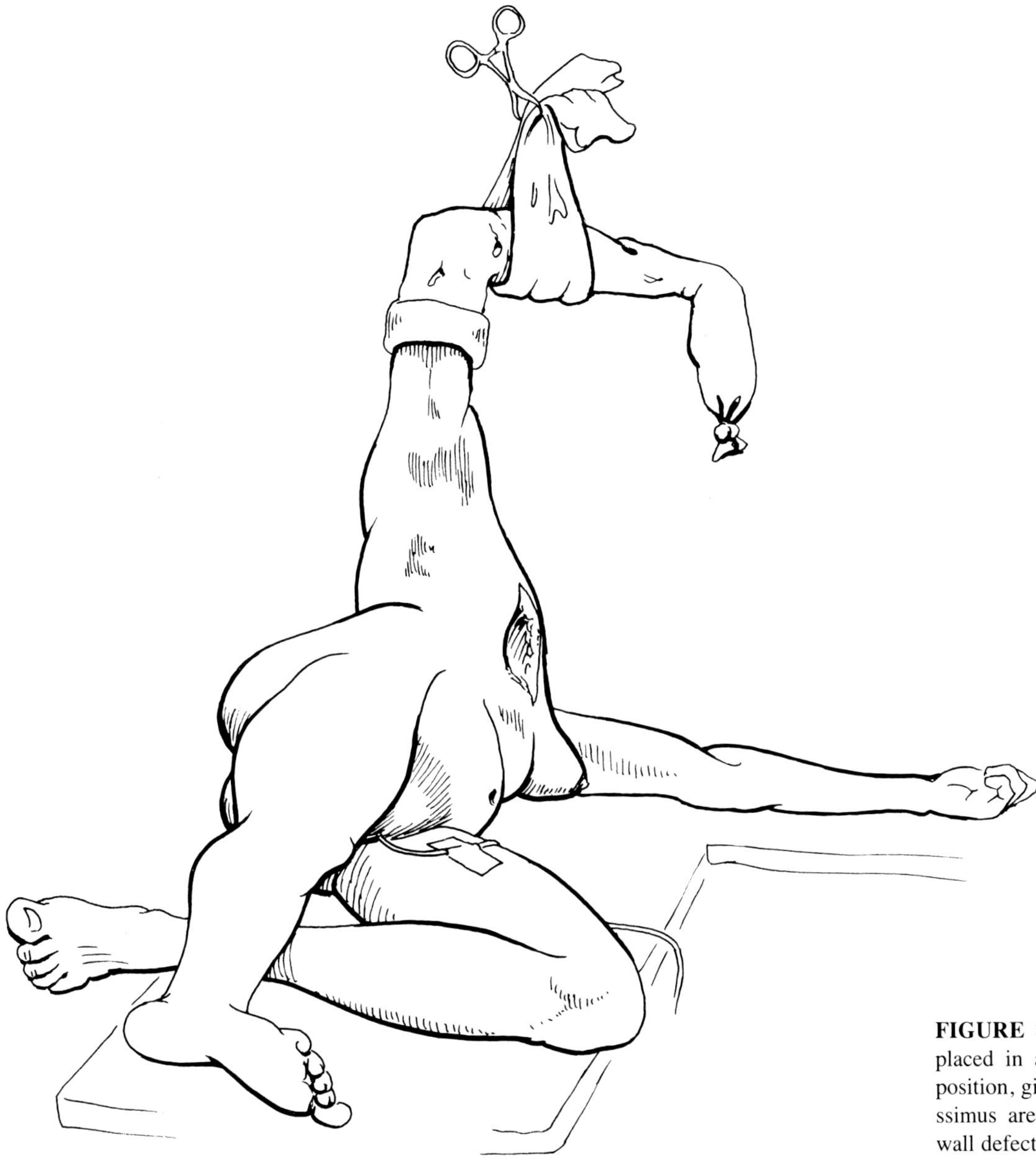

FIGURE 8.11 The patient is placed in a lateral thoracotomy position, giving access to the latissimus area. The anterior chest wall defect is also shown.

Mobilization of the Musculocutaneous Flap

The best position for access to the muscle is with the patient on his side as for a lateral thoracotomy (Figure 8.11). For posterior and lateral defects, the patient will usually remain in the lateral position throughout the operation. For anterior defects, however, the patient will usually be supine for the surgery related to the defect, then turned to the lateral position for mobilization of the latissimus flap. For this procedure, the patient is prepared and draped as follows: After endotracheal anesthesia, the patient is placed on his side and the exposed upper extremity, thorax, neck, hip, and abdomen are prepared. The lateral buttock and thigh are also prepared and draped in anticipation of possible skin grafting of the muscle or flap donor site. Drapes are stapled to the skin, a double stockinette is placed on the arm, and the patient is turned to the supine position. The anterior field is then prepared and draped.

After the ablative portion of the operation has been completed, the patient is turned to the lateral position. The margins of the previously marked skin island are incised to the

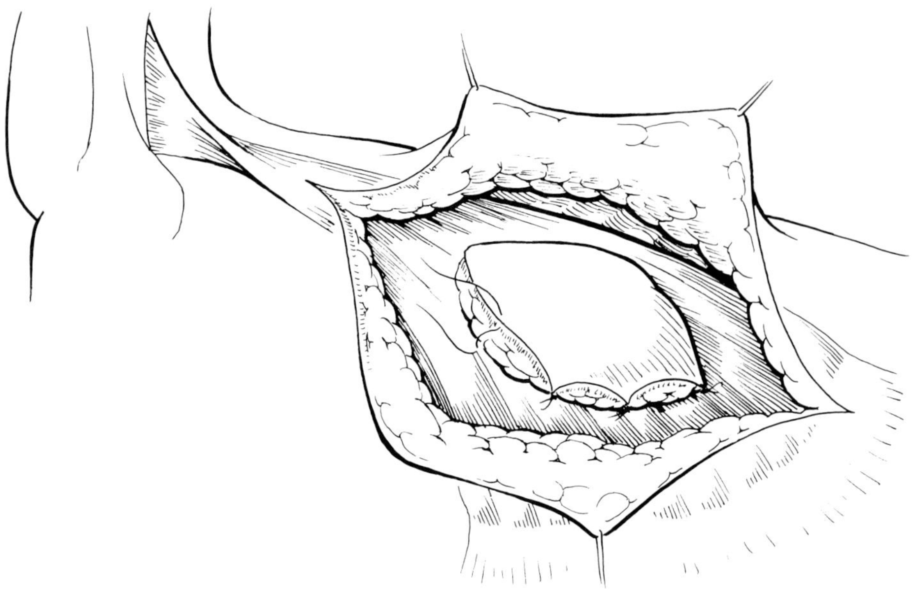

FIGURE 8.12 The skin is incised down to latissimus fascia, the skin island is tacked down, and the anterior edge of the muscle is identified.

latissimus fascia (Figure 8.12). Several tacking sutures are placed from the fascia to the dermis of the skin island. These temporary sutures will prevent the skin segment from separating from the muscle and shearing the perforating vessels upon which it depends for survival. The skin and subcutaneous fat along the lateral margin are retracted away from the muscle, and the anterior edge of the muscle is located. The dissection proceeds along the anterior edge, which is defined by the longitudinal direction of its fibers. This fiber direction is helpful in differentiating the latissimus from the underlying serratus anterior muscle, whose fibers run obliquely and inferiorly from posterior to anterior. The skin and fat are sharply elevated from the latissimus in all directions, in effect uncovering the entire superficial aspect of the muscle except for the skin island. Since the fat is more adherent to the fascia as one approaches the iliolumbar area, sharp dissection is usually necessary (Figure 8.13). In this area, a lighted mammary retractor may assist in visualizing the numerous perforators as they exit the muscle on their way to the skin. In this way, they can be grasped with fine forceps and cauterized prior to transection.

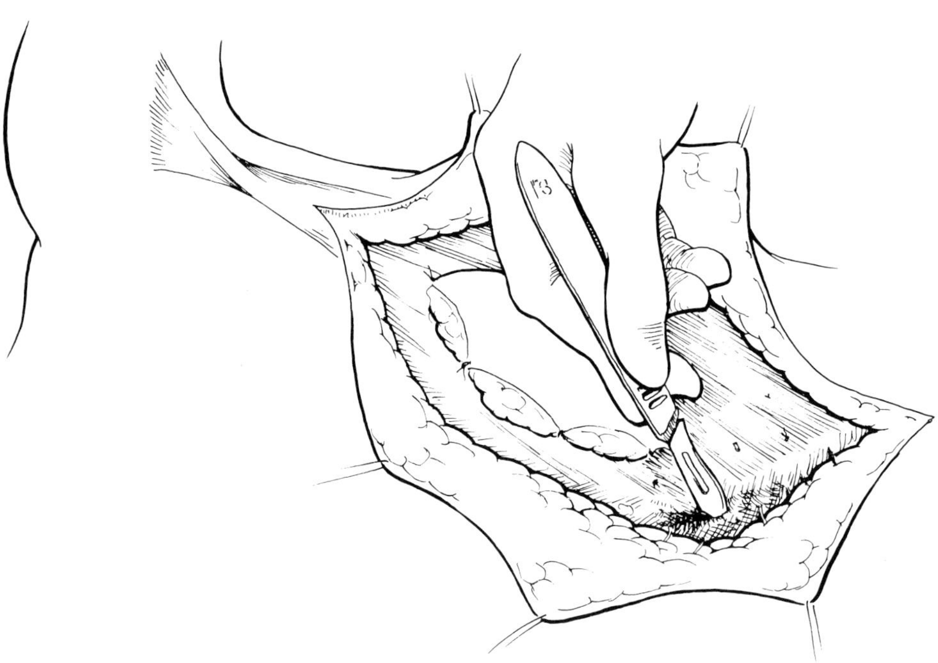

FIGURE 8.13 Sharp dissection is necessary to elevate the skin in the iliolumbar area.

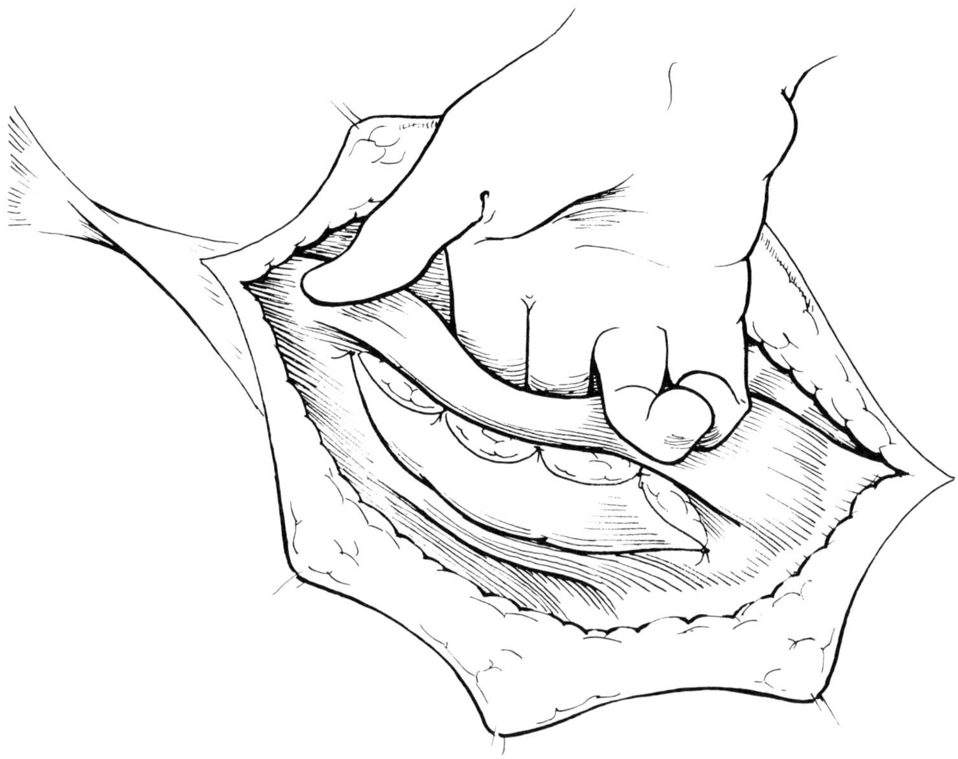

FIGURE 8.14 The submuscular dissection is begun at the anterior edge of the latissimus. Care is taken not to injure the muscle during its elevation.

Next, the submuscular dissection begins, starting at the midpoint of the anterior edge (Figure 8.14). The dissection proceeds caudally to the iliolumbar region as far as possible toward the iliac crest. The dissection is carried medially to the paraspinous muscles, which are identifiable by the longitudinal direction of their fibers. The latissimus is freed until it can be grasped between the thumb and fingers as far caudally as possible (Figure 8.15). The caudal border is then transected with the scalpel or cutting

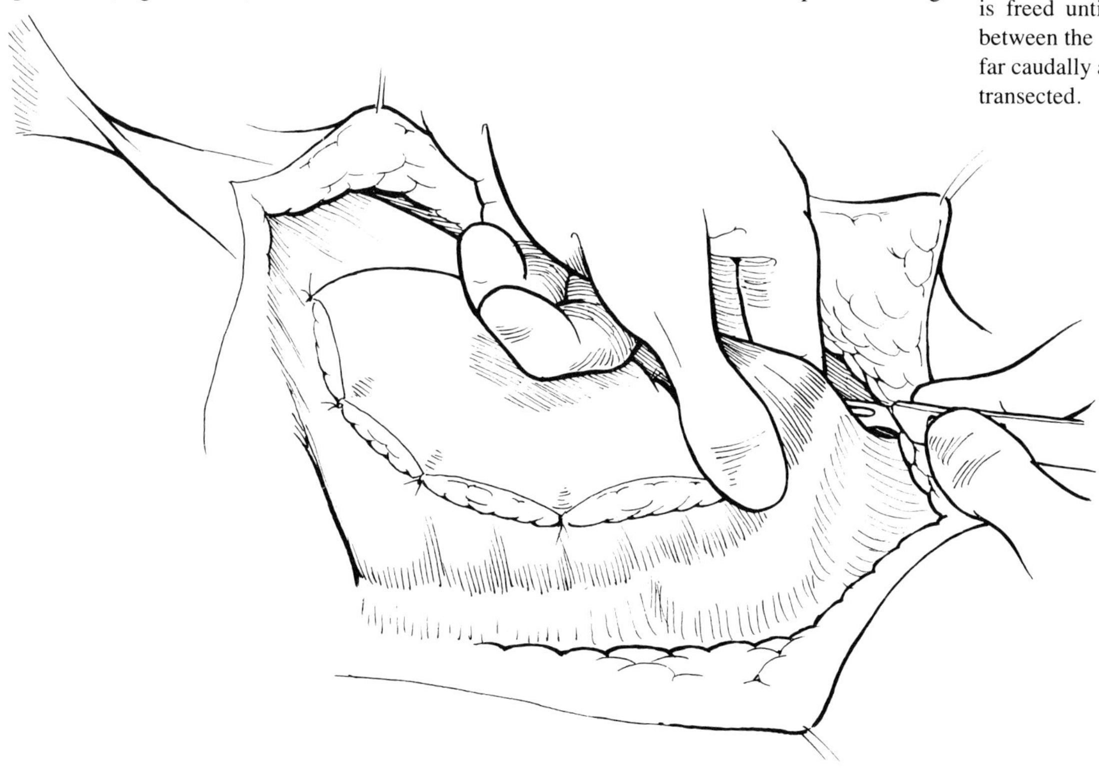

FIGURE 8.15 The latissimus is freed until it can be grasped between the thumb and fingers as far caudally as possible. It is then transected.

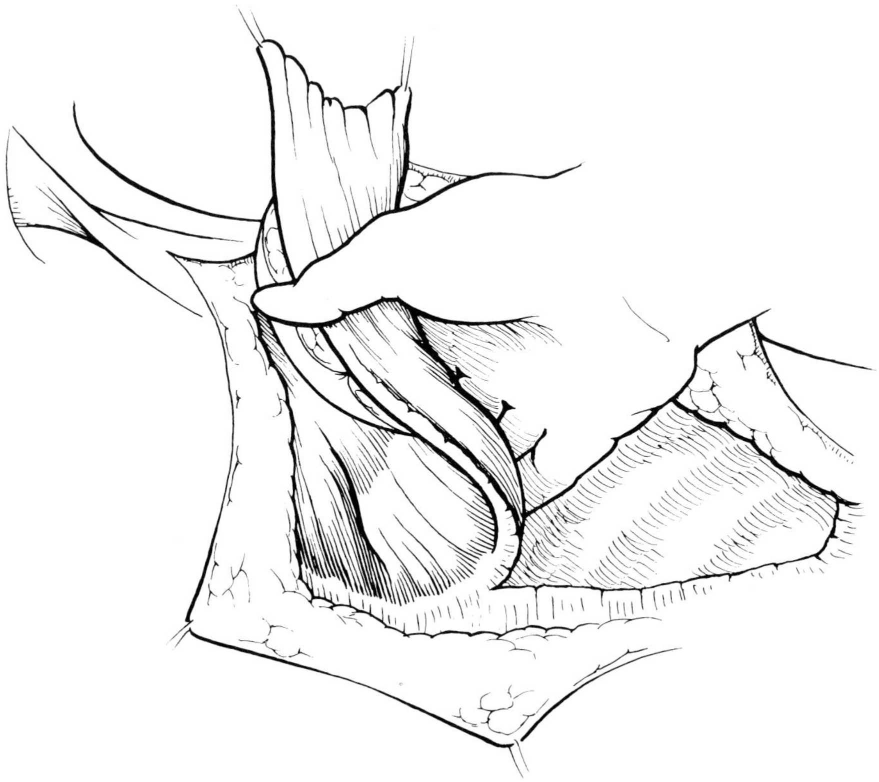

FIGURE 8.16 The submuscular plane is dissected with the fingers. This separates the muscle from the ribs and serratus fascia.

current of the electrocautery. After hemostasis is achieved, the origin of the muscle is serially divided from its spinal attachments, working cephalad near the midline of the back. As the muscle is released, it is gently elevated and retracted with silk sutures to prevent injury, and the filmy submuscular plane over the ribs of the midthorax is opened with the fingers (Figure 8.16). After detachment of the spinous origins is completed, the cephalad border of the muscle is sharply freed from any attachments over the inferior angle of the scapula, working carefully toward the axilla (Figure 8.17).

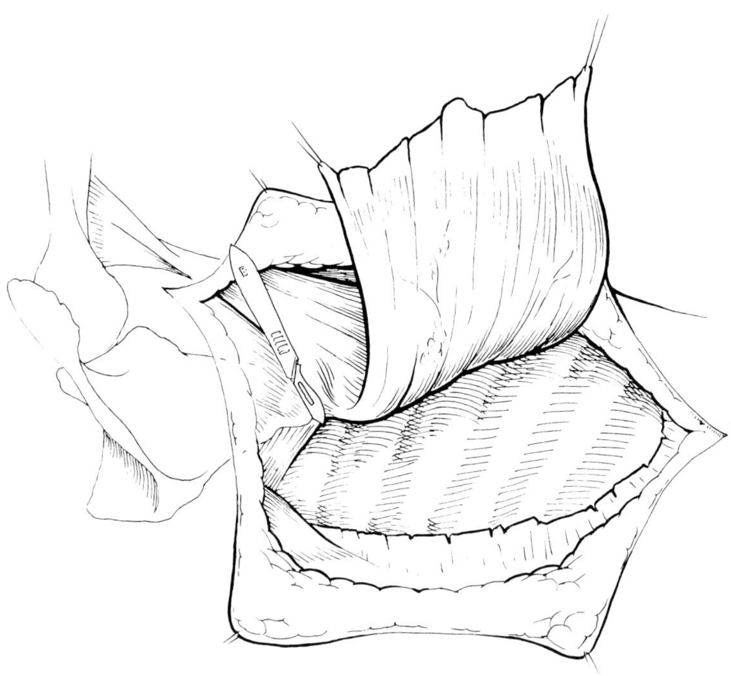

FIGURE 8.17 The muscle is sharply freed from the inferior angle of the scapula, and the thoracodorsal pedicle is carefully located.

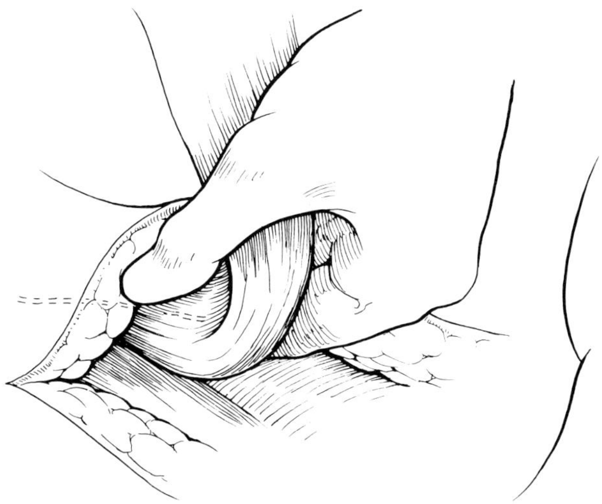

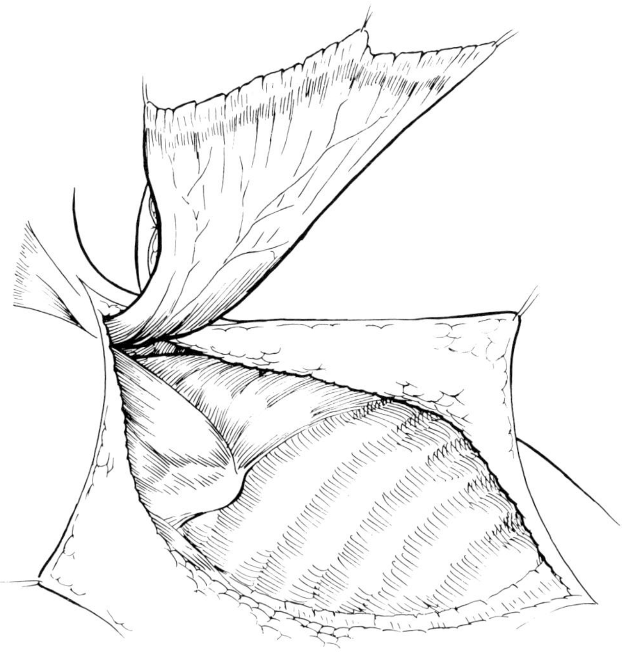

At this point the muscle is lifted up and a search is made for the thoracodorsal vascular pedicle. The index finger gently feels along the deep aspect of the muscle as the fibers begin to thicken and coalesce toward their humeral insertion (Figure 8.18). A few inches below the actual insertion, the arterial pulse will be felt and the muscle may be lifted in order to visualize the pedicle directly. As the muscle is freed from its posterior and parascapular attachments near the axilla, it will gain more range for coverage of the defect (Figure 8.19). However, this should be done with an eye toward protecting the pedicle at all times. The pedicle is on the deep aspect of the muscle, so that *superficial dissection is safe*. Any dissection deep to the muscle or near the insertion must be done millimeter by millimeter with the pedicle *under direct visualization*. Although a few centimeters can be added by transecting the insertion of the muscle (Figure 8.20) and/or mobilizing the pedicle up to the subscapular artery and its origin from the axillary artery, this must be done cautiously. The circumflex scapular and serratus branches are ligated

FIGURE 8.18 The arterial pulse is palpated near the insertion of the muscle.

FIGURE 8.19 The muscle is fully mobilized with the pedicle under direct vision.

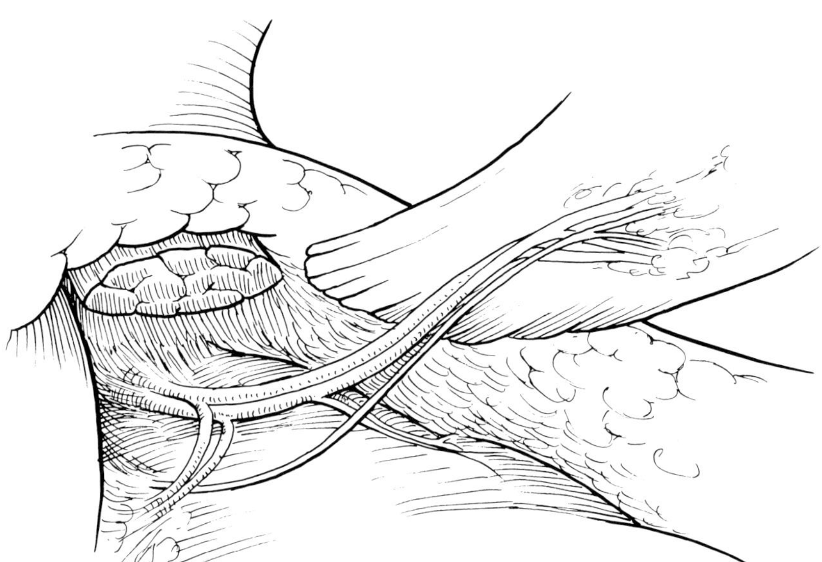

FIGURE 8.20 Transection of the muscle origin may add a few centimeters to the range of coverage.

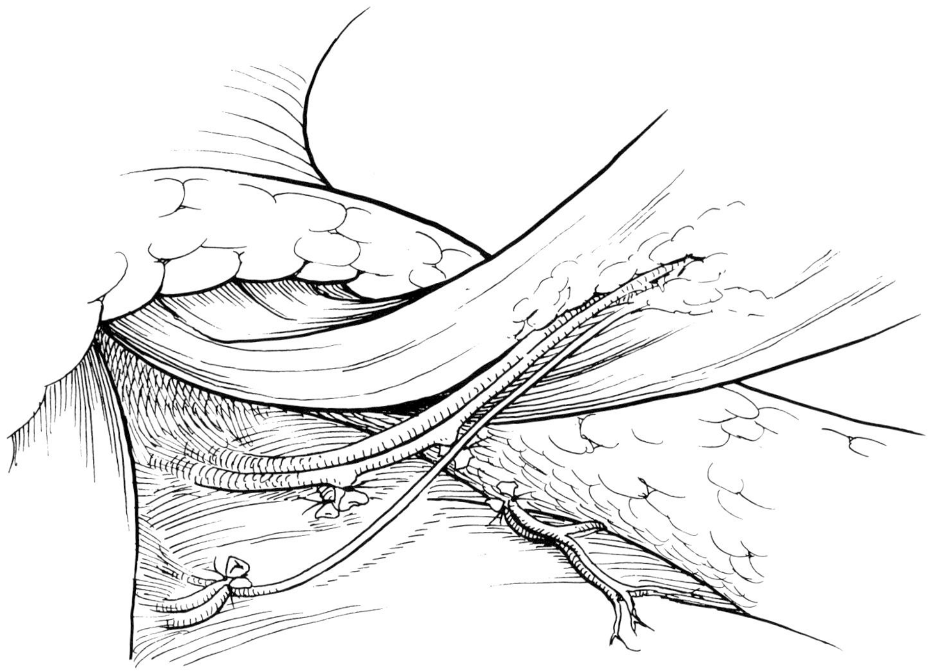

FIGURE 8.21 The pedicle may be mobilized up to the origin of the subscapular artery by dividing the circumflex scapular and serratus branches. The nerve is left intact.

and divided during this latter maneuver (Figure 8.21), and it is best not to rely on this additional reach if the original measurement is short. If this is the case or if there is any tension on the pedicle, additional flaps will be necessary to close the defect safely.

When covering an anterior defect, the flap is protected with moist pads momentarily and attention turned to transferring the flap to the defect. The subcutaneous fat is dissected off the deep fascia of the axilla so that a transaxillary tunnel is opened through which the muscle can be transferred. Anteriorly, the tunnel is dissected back toward the axilla in a similar fashion. It should be large enough so that the surgeon's open hand can easily pass through it (Figure 8.22). If there is any tightness, the skin and fat comprising

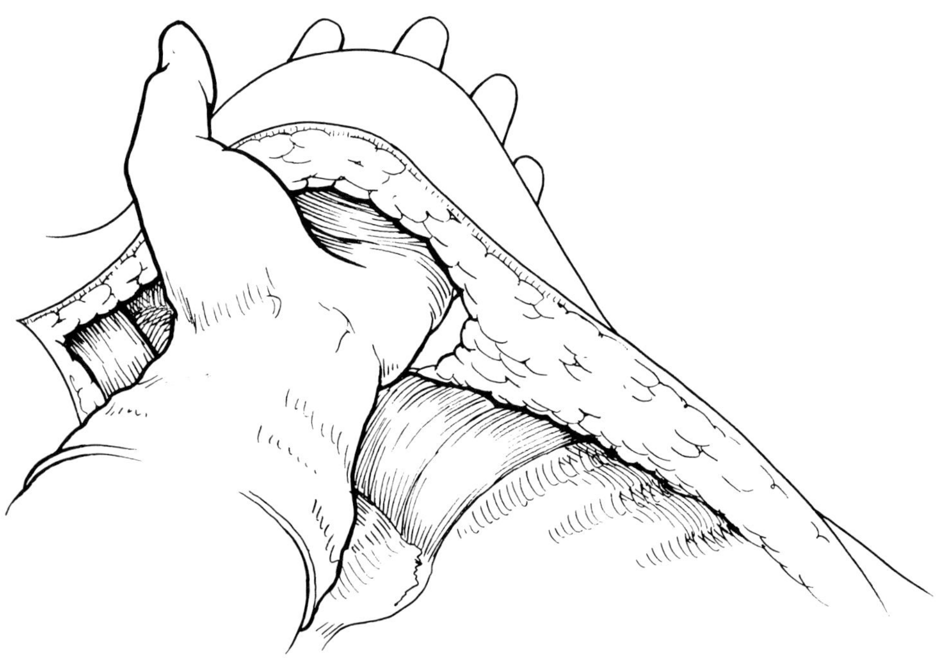

FIGURE 8.22 The tunnel should be large enough so that the surgeon's open hand can easily pass through it.

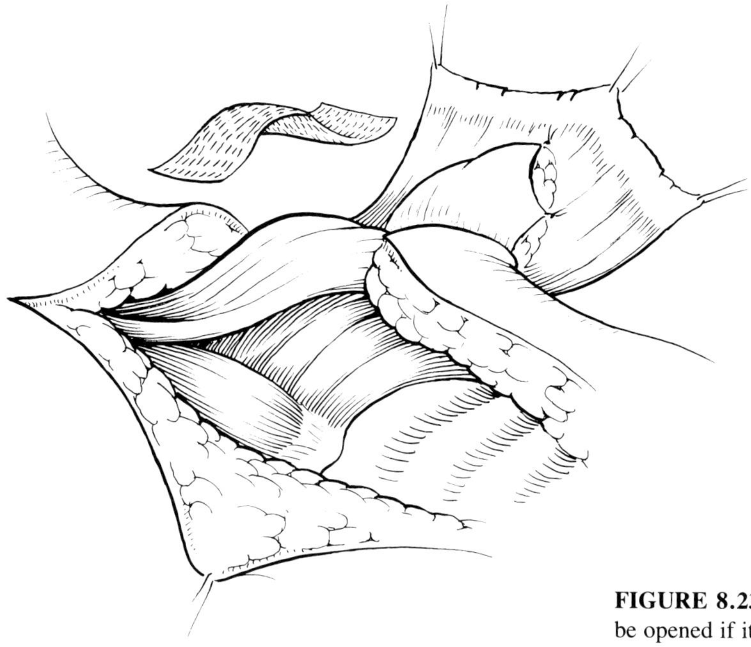

FIGURE 8.23 The tunnel may be opened if it is too tight.

the roof of the tunnel are completely opened so that the flap has a direct, open route to the defect (Figure 8.23). The exposed latissimus muscle in the resulting "trough" can be covered with a split-thickness skin graft if necessary.

The flap is transposed to the defect and brought back for further mobilization if there is any tension (Figure 8.24). As stated earlier, the insertion may be transected for

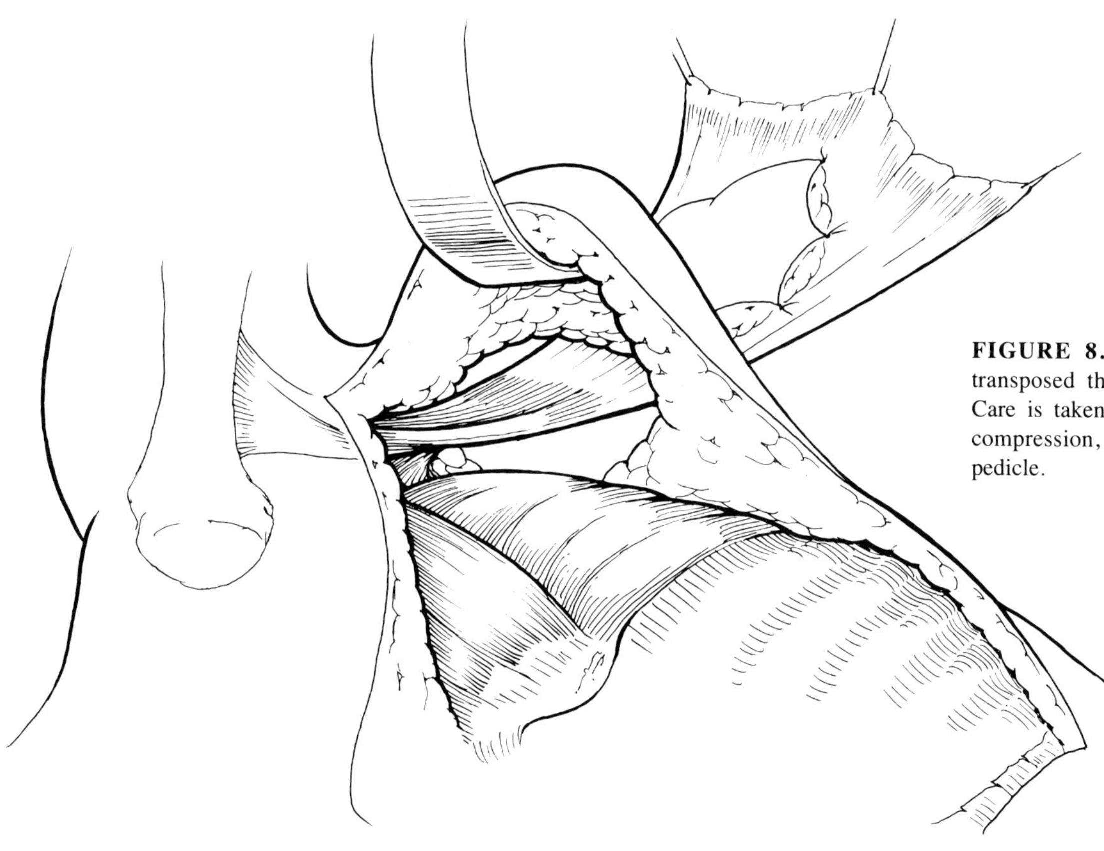

FIGURE 8.24 The flap is transposed through the tunnel. Care is taken to avoid tension, compression, or torsion on the pedicle.

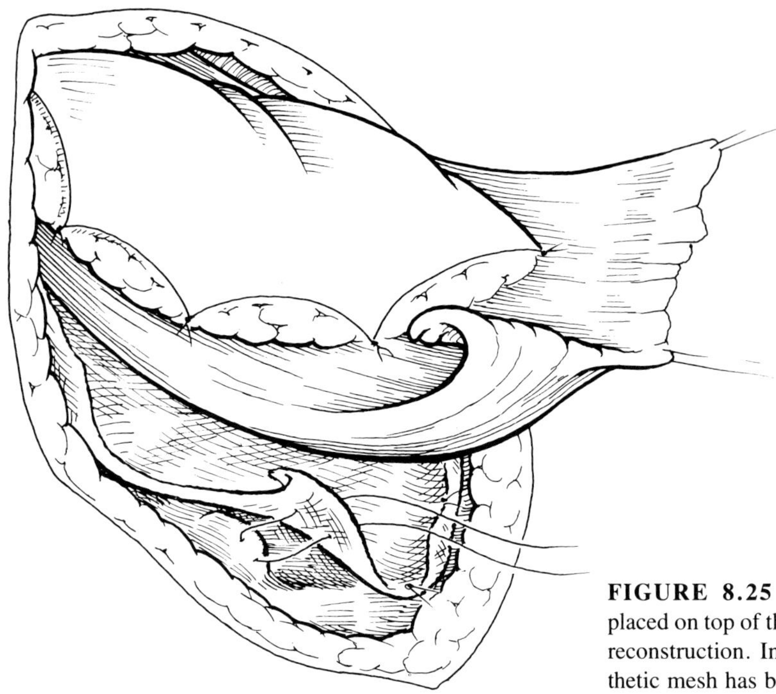

FIGURE 8.25 The flap is placed on top of the skeletal layer reconstruction. In this case, synthetic mesh has been used.

additional range, but there must be no tension on or torsion of the vascular pedicle. After any final adjustments and reconstruction of the skeletal layer (Figure 8.25), the muscle is sutured to the fascial layer of the defect with interrupted sutures (Figure 8.26). It is not necessary to suture the muscle within the subcutaneous tunnel. After hemostasis is accomplished at the donor site, a soft suction drain is placed under the posterior skin flaps and brought out through a stab incision in the axilla or inferior to the original

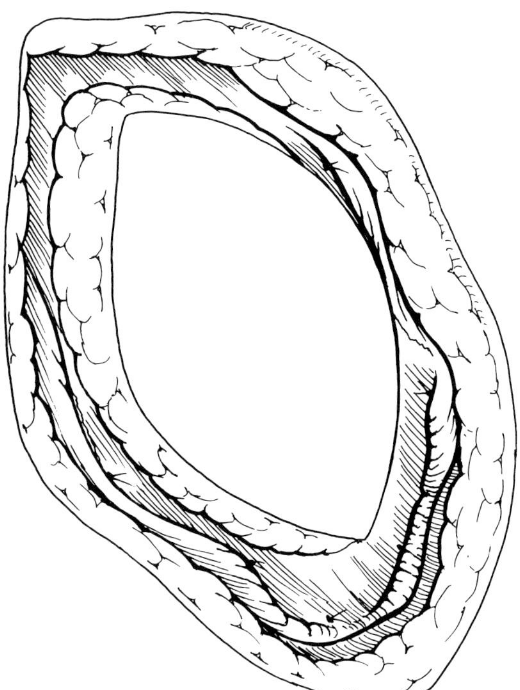

FIGURE 8.26 The muscle is sutured to the fascial layer of the defect.

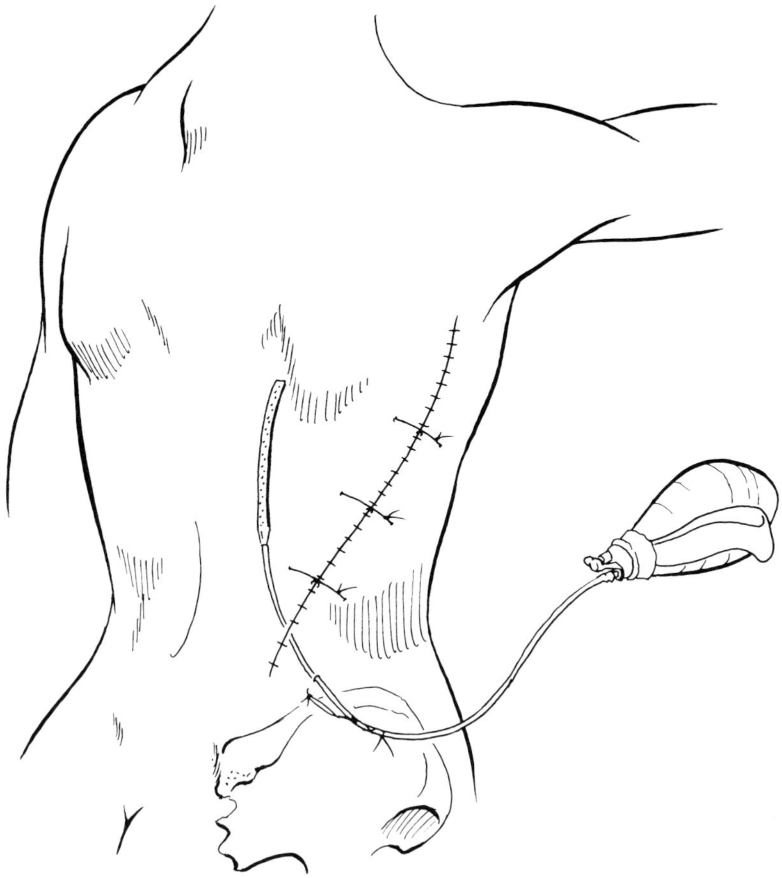

FIGURE 8.27 A soft suction drain is placed under the posterior skin flaps.

incision (Figure 8.27). The drain will remain in place for several days until the serous drainage decreases. When the drain is removed, however, the seroma will again accumulate. This will gradually recede over the ensuing weeks and only rarely requires aspiration.

The donor site is closed primarily if possible. Depending on the size of the skin island removed, the gap can usually be closed by further mobilizing the skin and subcutaneous fat at the level of the deep fascia and ribs laterally. Segments wider than 10–12 cm may require skin grafting. Far-near-near-far retention sutures with number one monofilament are helpful in attaining a safe closure.

Returning to the operative defect, the surgeon removes the dermis-fascial tacking sutures from around the skin island and sutures or staples the skin to the margins of the defect (Figure 8.28). If extra skin is needed for coverage of the muscle, or in the opened tunnel as discussed above, a split-thickness skin graft can be applied to the muscle. If this is to be done, any residual fat is excised from the surface of the muscle in preparation for the graft, and an intermediate-thickness graft is harvested from the buttock/thigh area. The graft is meshed 1.5 to 1 and applied unexpanded so that it will easily conform to the contours of the muscle and allow drainage, yet will heal as a sheet of skin for greater durability. The graft is meticulously sutured to the muscle with fine chromic sutures both around the periphery and at multiple points over the grafted area to ensure good, uniform contact with the recipient bed. It is loosely compressed with saline-soaked coarse sponges for 3–4 days to keep any uncovered interstitial areas moist until they are epithelialized with skin from the graft. The sponges are gently removed at that time, and the graft is lubricated with an antibacterial ointment for several weeks. This will minimize encrustation around the graft and scaling due to the temporary absence of sebaceous activity in the grafted skin.

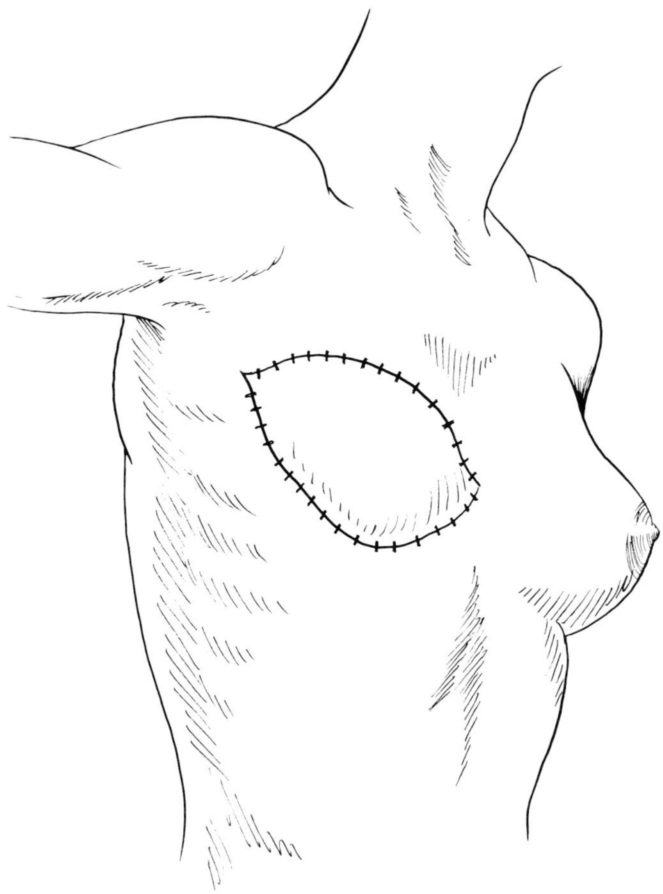

FIGURE 8.28 The skin is closed and no dressing is applied anteriorly. Posteriorly an absorbent dressing is loosely applied.

Mobilization of the Muscle-Only Flap

In certain cases, it is desirable to use the muscle alone rather than the composite flap of skin and muscle. The muscle is approached through an incision close to and parallel with its anterior margin (Figure 8.10). The skin flaps are dissected away from the superficial aspect of the muscle, as described in the previous section, exposing the entire surface of the muscle. The mobilization and transfer of the latissimus is then identical to the previous description except that the skin island is not included. If skin coverage is required after the muscle is transposed to the defect, a meshed skin graft is applied as described in the last section (Figure 8.29).

Consequences of Removal of the Latissimus

Strong extension and internal rotation of the arm, as well as forceful coughing, and depression of the shoulder, may be impaired in the absence of the latissimus. This seems to be temporary, however. These deficits may manifest themselves as weakness in opening twist-off lids and in ironing clothes. One patient described weakness in doing sit-ups with the fingers locked behind his head. However, this seemed to be related to touching the knees with the elbows, which includes adduction of the humerus. In one of our studies, patients having the entire latissimus removed as a free flap underwent

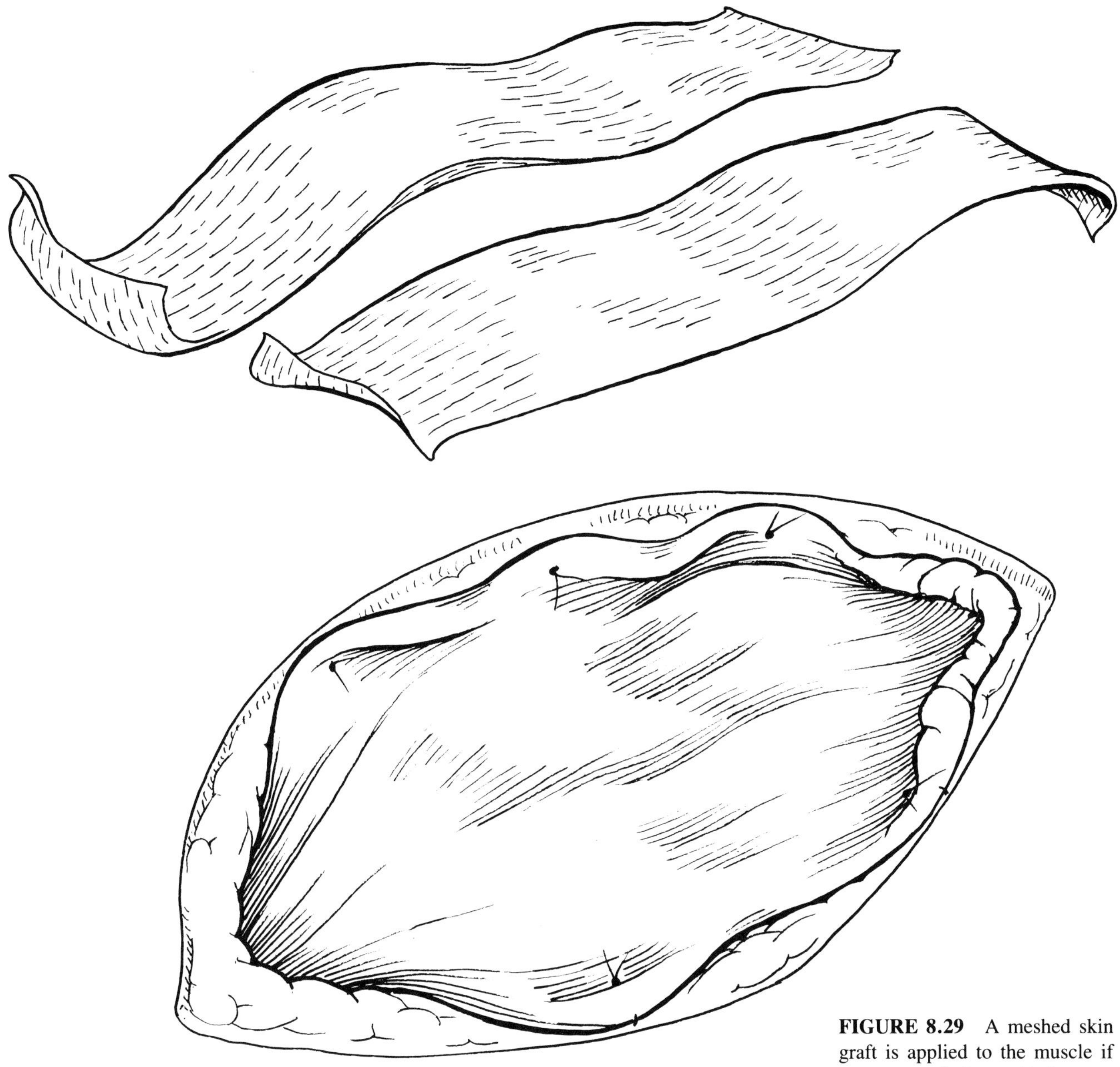

FIGURE 8.29 A meshed skin graft is applied to the muscle if necessary. It is applied unexpanded and secured at multiple points with individual chromic sutures. It is kept moist for three days (saline-soaked gauze dressing) then lubricated with an antibacterial ointment.

computerized muscle strength testing before and after surgery. They were found to regain full strength by the 6th to 8th postoperative week. There has likewise been no observable disability with crutch-walking in young, healthy patients when the latissimus has been removed. However, this has been tested only in adult patients who had no upper extremity problems prior to removal of the latissimus.

ILLUSTRATIVE CASE

A 67-year-old male presented with a partially excised aggressive liposarcoma of the scapular region (Figure 8.30). The lesion was widely excised including the infraspinous portion of the scapula and attached muscles (Figure 8.31). The entire latissimus with its

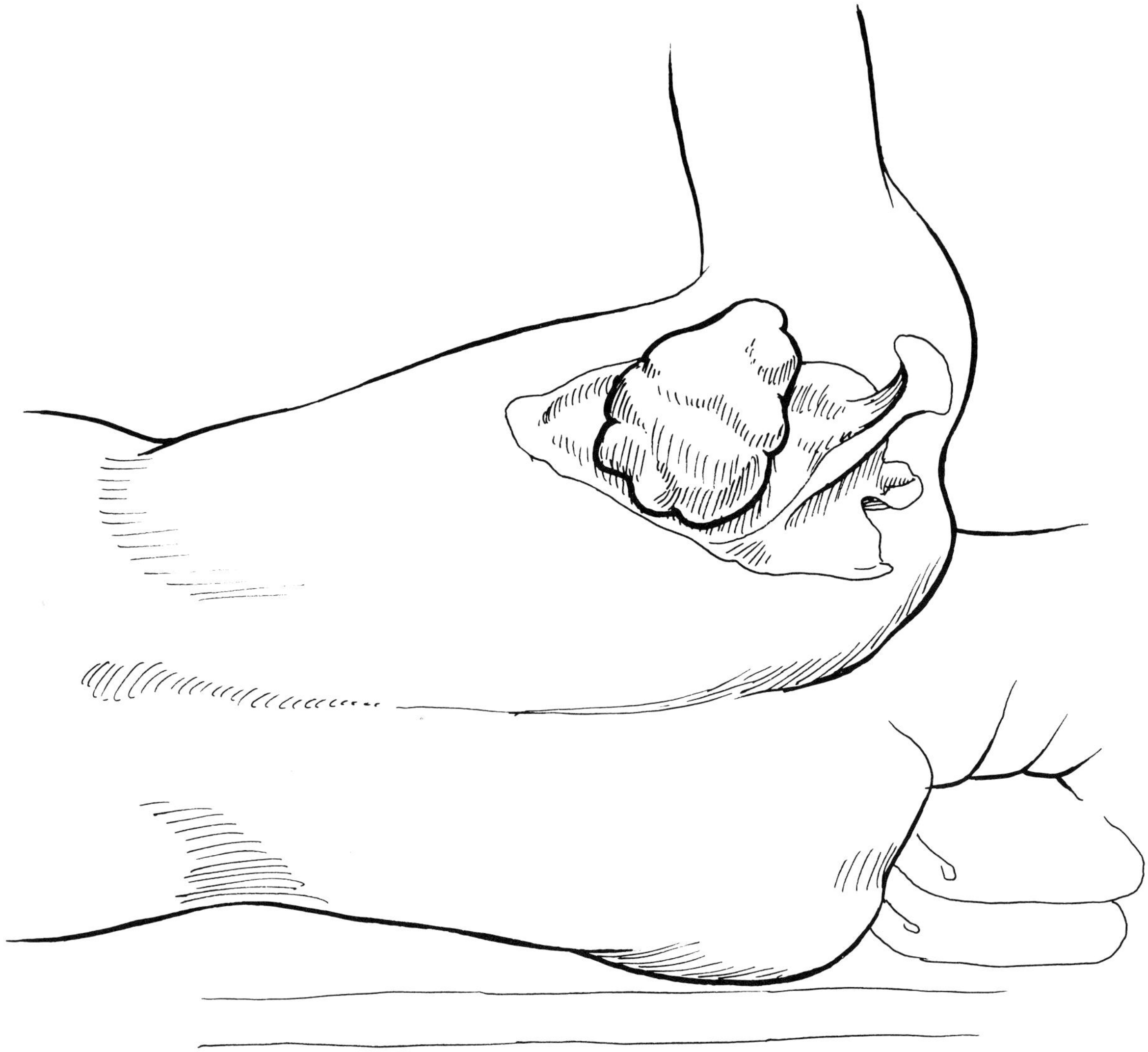

FIGURE 8.30 This patient presented with a partially excised aggressive liposarcoma of the left scapular region.

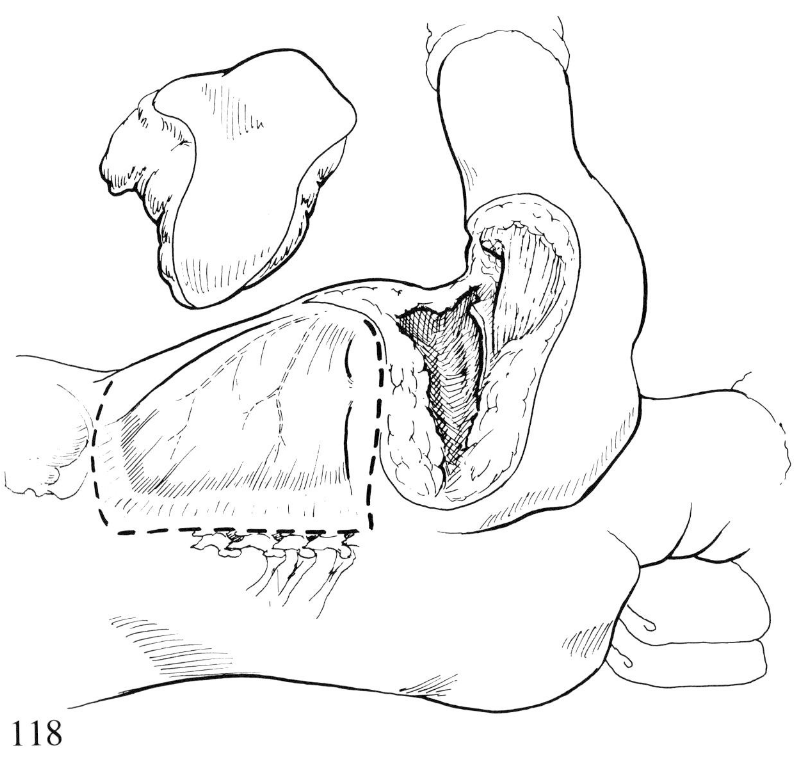

FIGURE 8.31 The lesion is widely excised, including the bony and muscular elements.

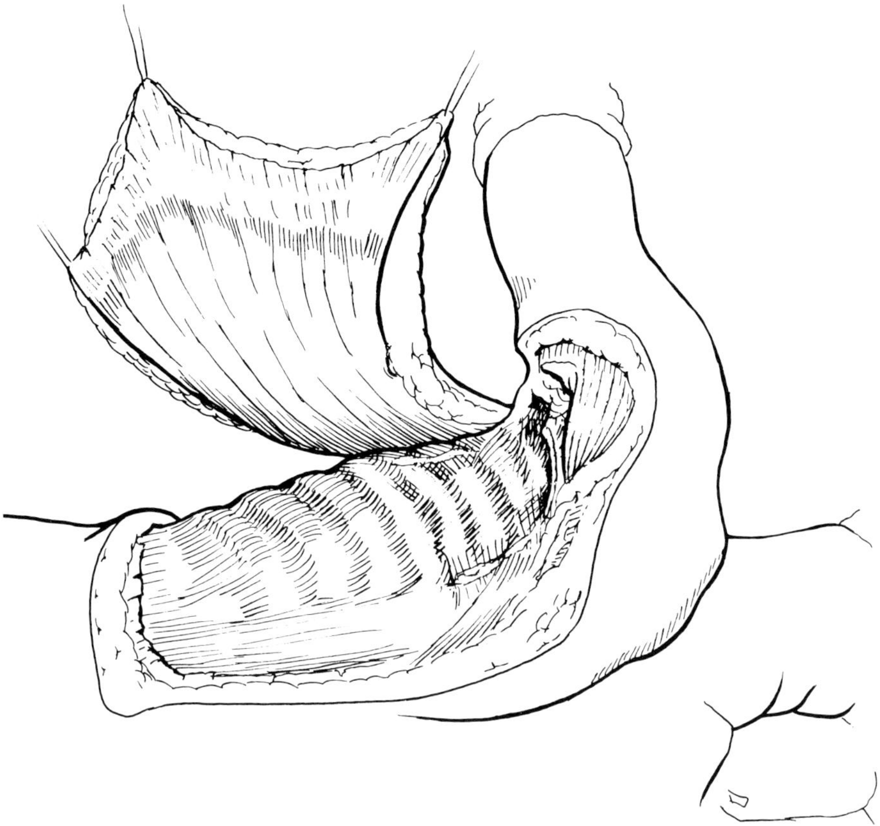

FIGURE 8.32 The entire latissimus and overlying skin are mobilized.

overlying skin was chosen to cover the defect. The combined flap was mobilized as described in the text (Figure 8.32) and transposed to the operative site (Figure 8.33). This large flap allowed the tension to be dissipated over the entire closure. The donor area defect was easily closed primarily and skin-grafting was not needed (Figure 8.34).

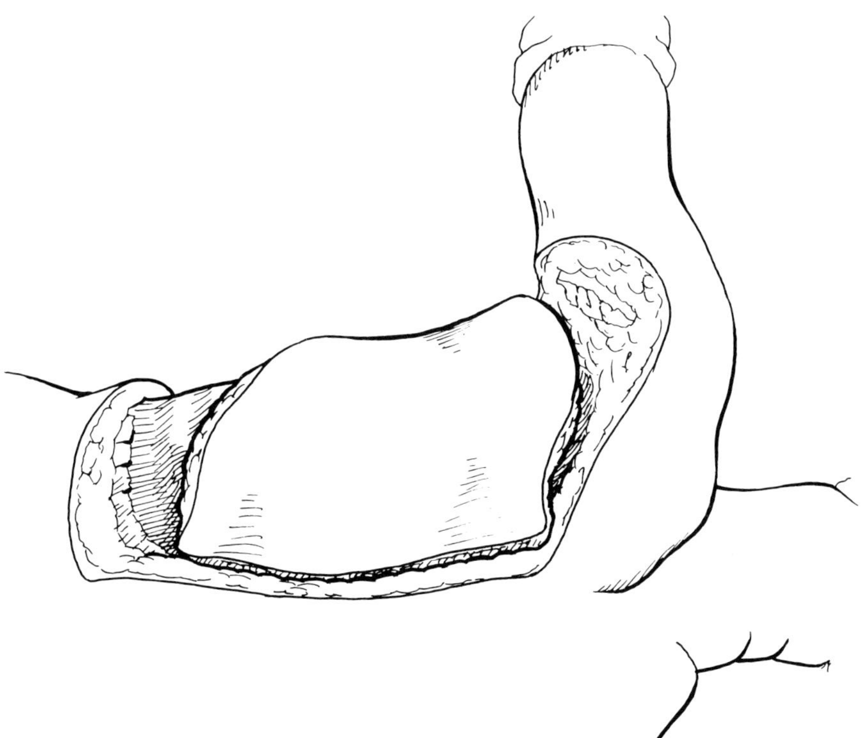

FIGURE 8.33 The flap is transposed to the site of the operative defect.

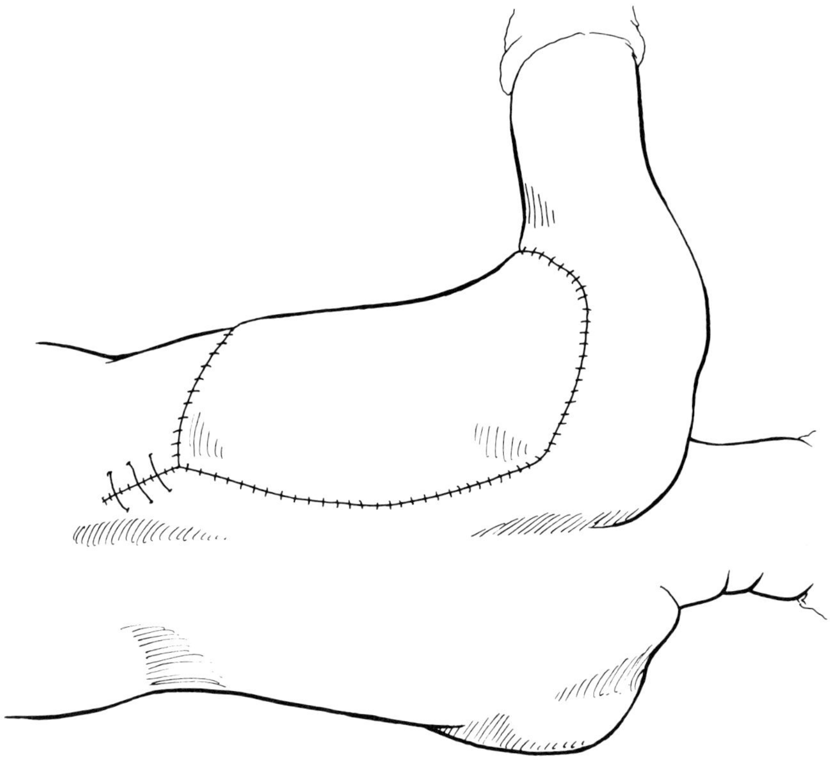

FIGURE 8.34 The donor defect is closed primarily. If tension exists, a skin graft is applied at the donor area.

This provided the area with thick and durable coverage which readily withstood the high-dose postoperative radiotherapy. If skin grafting were required, this less durable tissue would be applied over the iliolumbar donor region, well away from the area that may later be irradiated.

9

The Pectoralis Major Muscle and Musculocutaneous Flaps

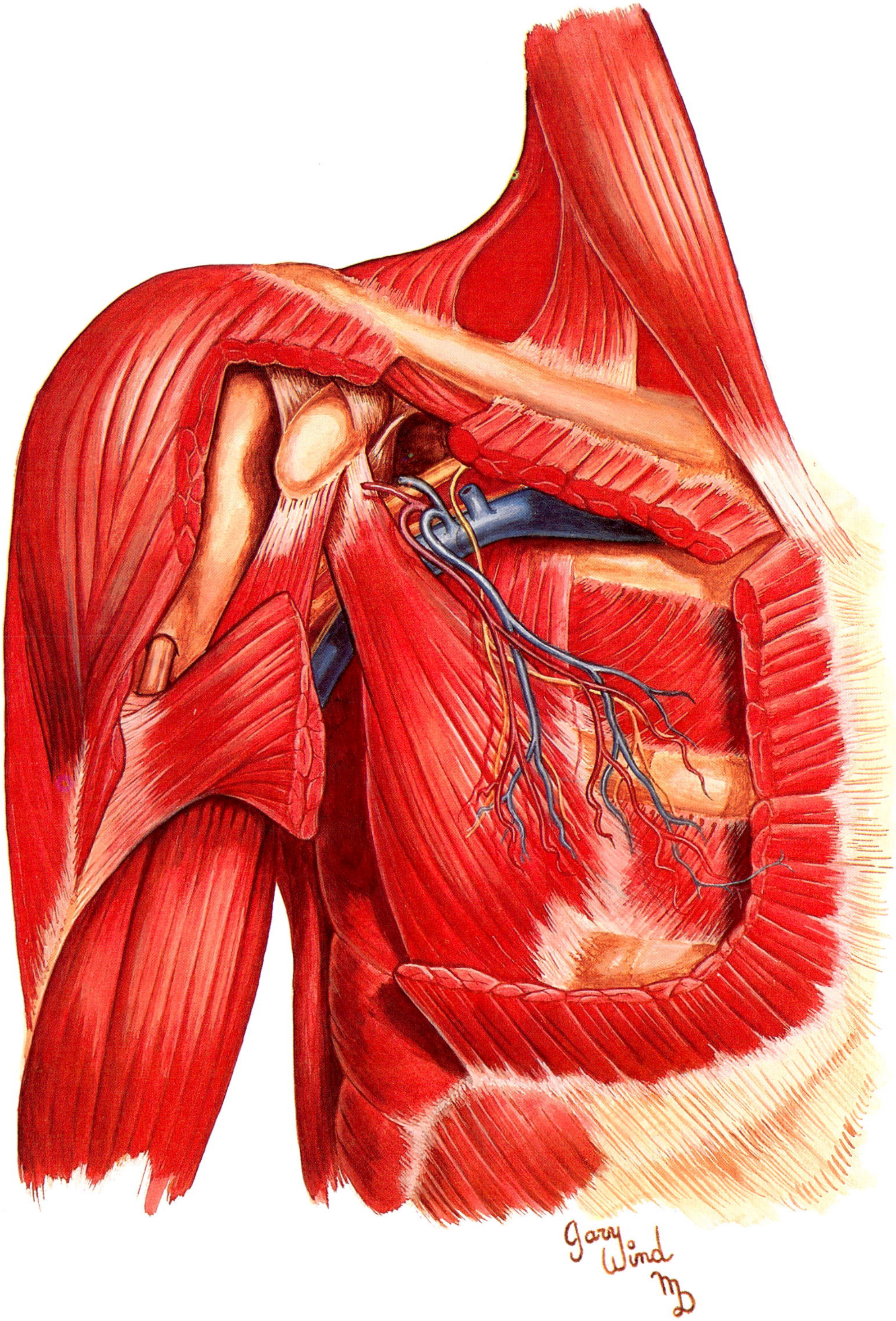

The bulk of the pectoralis major muscle and a portion of the deltoid have been removed to reveal the underlying dominant neurovascular pedicle originating just medial to the coracoid process of the scapula.

PLATE 9.1 The dominant neurovascular pedicle to the pectoralis major muscle is depicted. The bulk of the pectoralis major, its fascia, and the clavipectoral fascia are removed to expose the origin of the thoracoacromial artery inferomedial to the coracoid process, just above the border of the pectoralis minor. The cephalic vein runs between the pectoralis major and the deltoid before arching down to join the axillary vein. The pectoral branch of the thoracoacromial artery and its accompanying vein form an axis beneath the muscle which travels toward the xiphoid. The lateral pectoral nerve arises from the lateral cord of the brachial plexus and joins the vessels within the posterior layer of pectoral fascia. The ancillary neurovascular supply from lateral thoracic artery and medial pectoral nerve are not depicted as they do not contribute to the pectoralis major flap. Penetrating branches of the internal thoracic artery, which are also sacrificed in mobilizing the flap, lie beneath the remaining sternal portion of the muscle.

Anatomy

The pectoralis major muscle originates from the medial half of the clavicle, the sternum, and adjacent costal cartilages and from the external oblique aponeurosis at its junction with the rectus sheath. The muscle fibers converge in a flat bilaminar tendon to insert into the crest of the greater tubercle of the humerus, which forms the lateral lip of the bicipital groove. The more caudal fibers spiral around the inferior edge of the tendon to form the posterior lamina, with the last fibers terminating most cephalad. The tendon passes anterior to the coracobrachialis, short head of the biceps, and tendon of the long head of the biceps and is covered at its insertion by the anterior fibers of the deltoid. The cephalic vein runs in the cleft between the pectoralis major and deltoid muscles.

The deep fascia splits to enclose the pectoralis major and is joined to adjacent fascia and bony prominences. In the posterior layer of fascia, a fat pad contains the neurovascular bundle supplying the muscle. A separate layer called the clavipectoral fascia encloses the underlying pectoralis minor and bridges the gap between the medial border of that muscle and the clavicle.

The dominant blood supply to the pectoralis major is via the pectoral branch of the thoracoacromial artery with contributions from perforating branches of the internal thoracic artery medially and from the lateral thoracic artery. The thoracoacromial artery arises from the axillary artery medial to the proximal border of pectoralis minor and penetrates the clavipectoral fascia approximately 2 cm medial to and 2 cm caudal to the coracoid process of the scapula. It then divides into four branches. The large pectoral branch with its accompanying vein forms the dominant vascular pedicle to the pectoralis major. The vessel follows a somewhat diagonal axis toward the xiphoid, enclosed within the posterior layer of pectoral fascia. Terminal branches of this vessel penetrate the muscle and anterior fascia to supply the overlying skin.

Innervation to the pectoralis major is supplied by the medial and lateral pectoral nerves (named for the cord of the brachial plexus from which they arise, not for their anatomical position). The lateral pectoral nerve, carrying fibers from C5–7, emerges anterior to the axillary artery, penetrates the clavipectoral fascia, and accompanies the major vessel described to supply the cephalad and major portion of the muscle. The medial pectoral nerve with fibers from C8 and T1 passes beneath the axillary artery, supplies the pectoralis minor, and finally penetrates or skirts the lower border of that muscle to terminate in the lower fibers of the pectoralis major.

The two dominant functions of the pectoralis major are adduction and medial rotation of the arm. The muscle pulls the arm anteriorly and medially across the chest and, because of its attachment lateral to the intertubercular groove, medially rotates the arm. Because of the fan-shaped disposition of the fibers, the upper and lower portions of the muscle act along different vectors and effect special actions according to the position of the arm. Surprisingly, despite its great bulk, absence of the pectoralis major is almost totally compensated for by the deltoid, coracobrachialis, latissimus dorsi, and rotator cuff muscles.

General Principles

The pectoralis flap is most useful for anterior defects, specifically those of the upper three-fourths of the sternum. It has been most widely used as a musculocutaneous flap after ablative operations of the head and neck, where it satisfies the reconstructive requirements to provide lining of the oropharynx or external skin coverage.

It is reliable and can provide a thick, well-vascularized closure to both superficial and cavitary defects. It is thus well suited to protect vital mediastinal structures in the absence of the sternum. It can be used as a muscular flap, with or without skin grafting, or it can be used as a combined musculocutaneous flap with the muscle functioning as a carrier for the skin. Either alternative can contribute to a durable closure.

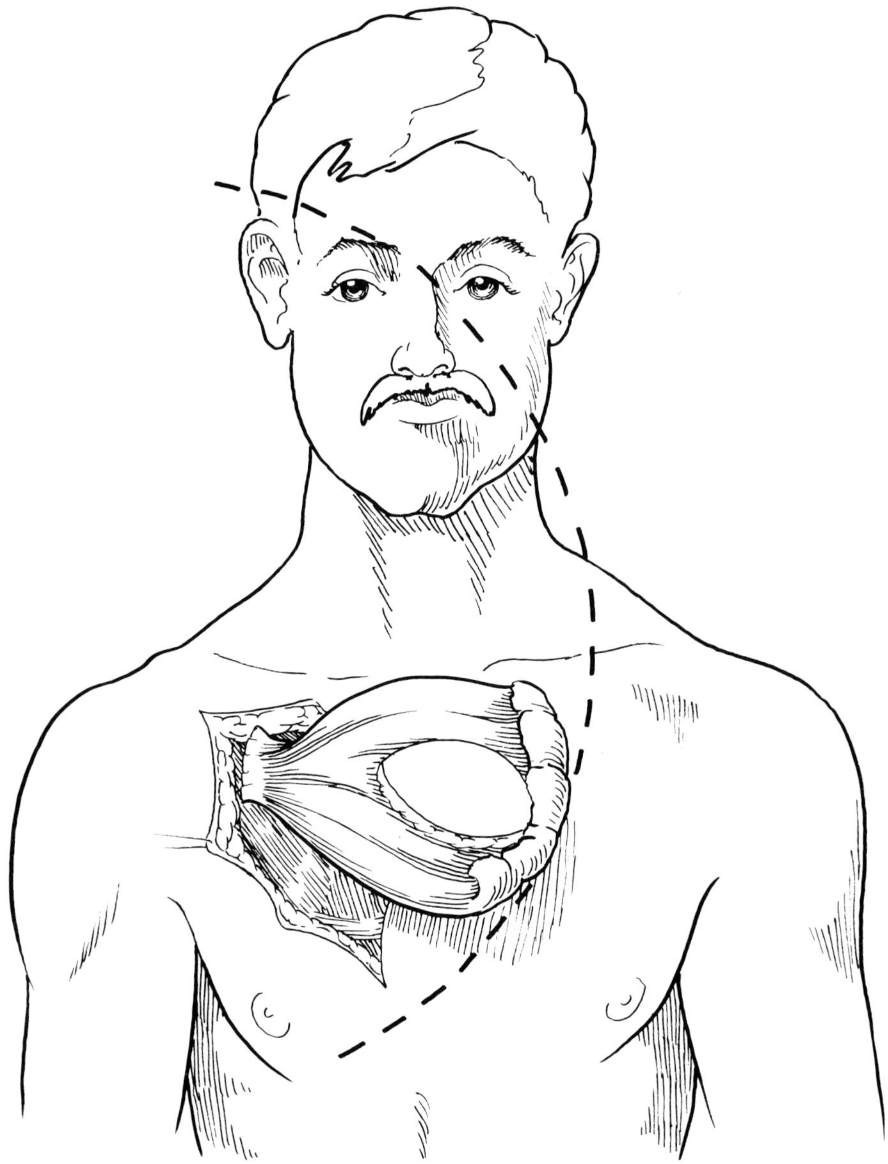

FIGURE 9.1 The range of the pectoralis muscle flap is indicated by the dotted line. In chest wall reconstruction, it is most useful for upper sternal defects.

Due to the location of the vascular pedicle, its arc of rotation is primarily upward and away from the xiphoid region (Figure 9.1). This is the basis for its wide use over the upper chest wall and in head and neck reconstructions. As the flap is brought toward the xiphoid region, however, the pedicle is subjected to increasing tension. Such tension violates the principle of tension-free closure and also places the thoracoacromial vessels in jeopardy.

The flap can be safely mobilized to reach the ipsilateral regions of the lower orbit, the external ear, and mastoid areas, intraorally down to the cervical esophagus, the manubrium and upper body of the sternum, the medial third of the opposite clavicle, and, with proper exposure, the trachea at the level of the sternal angle. As expected, if the procedure related to the defect includes ablation of the thoracoacromial artery (e.g., clavicular resection for tumor), an alternative flap must be chosen.

Bilateral pectoralis flaps may be required for sternal and skin defects in which only the xiphoid remains. In this instance, the upper abdominal tissues can be mobilized to close the skin over the xiphoid while the pectoralis flaps are used for the remaining upper defect. Preparation should be made for the recruitment of other flaps to assist in closure if any tension is anticipated. The principle, again, is to shift this tension well away from the

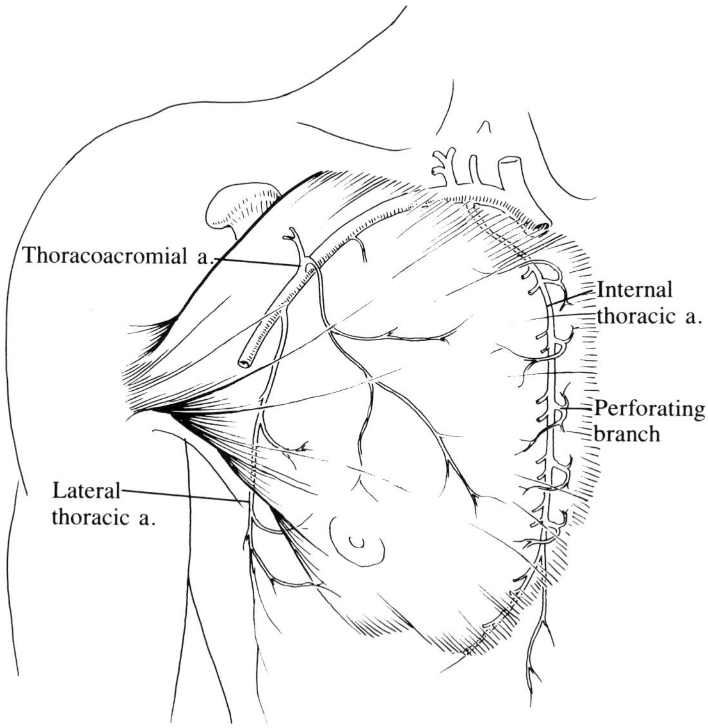

FIGURE 9.2 The thoracoacromial artery, lateral thoracic artery, and perforating branches of the internal thoracic artery supply blood to the pectoralis major muscle and overlying skin.

full-thickness gap in the chest wall and move it to the area from which the flap was harvested. In this way, if a skin dehiscence should occur, it is in an area protected by intact parietes.

The skin overlying the pectoralis major muscle is well supplied by three arterial sources (Figure 9.2). The most important with regard to chest wall reconstruction is that from the perforating arteries of the thoracoacromial system. These vessels, which are transmitted to the dermis through the underlying muscle, exit the pectoralis fascia in a random fashion several centimeters apart before arborizing up into the skin. If a skin segment is to be successfully carried with the muscle, it must be large enough (5–7 cm) in diameter to include at least one of these arterial feeders. If it does not, the skin segment undergoes necrosis in spite of a viable muscle. Second, the perforating anterior intercostal branches of the internal thoracic artery and vein also provide nutrition to the skin of the upper anterior chest wall. This vascular system supports the deltopectoral skin flap, which has been used extensively for head and neck reconstruction (Figure 9.3). Finally, there are contributions to this region from the lateral thoracic artery.

The vascular territory of the skin supplied by the thoracoacromial system overlies the entire pectoralis major muscle and extends several centimeters caudal to its inferolateral border (Figure 9.4). This territory also includes segments of underlying ribs that can be transposed with the muscle. The most reliable area of skin that can be carried with the muscle is the skin overlying the muscle itself, with a 1- to 2-cm margin outside the muscular border. If the harvested skin segment measures much in excess of 8 cm in width, the donor site may require skin grafting for safe closure. Such grafts, applied to the fascia overlying the ribs, heal readily.

An alternative application of this muscle flap is its use without the thoracoacromial vascular pedicle. This choice, based medially on the perforating intercostal branches of the internal thoracic artery, has been used for some sternal defects. In raising this flap, the pectoralis muscle is mobilized in all sectors except those about its sternal attachments. It is then folded toward the sternal defect to fill the gap (Figure 9.5). Usually, both pectoralis muscles are used with this method. To date, we have not found use for such an alternative since the internal thoracic artery has usually been unavailable or of

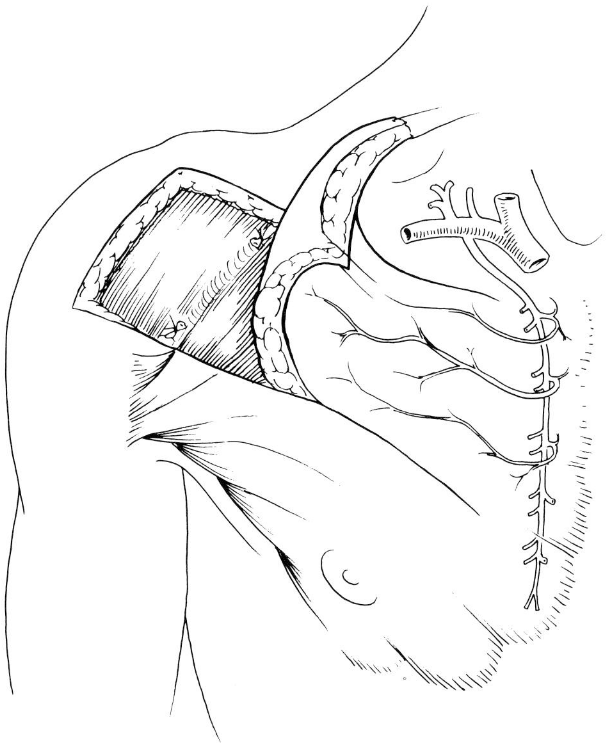

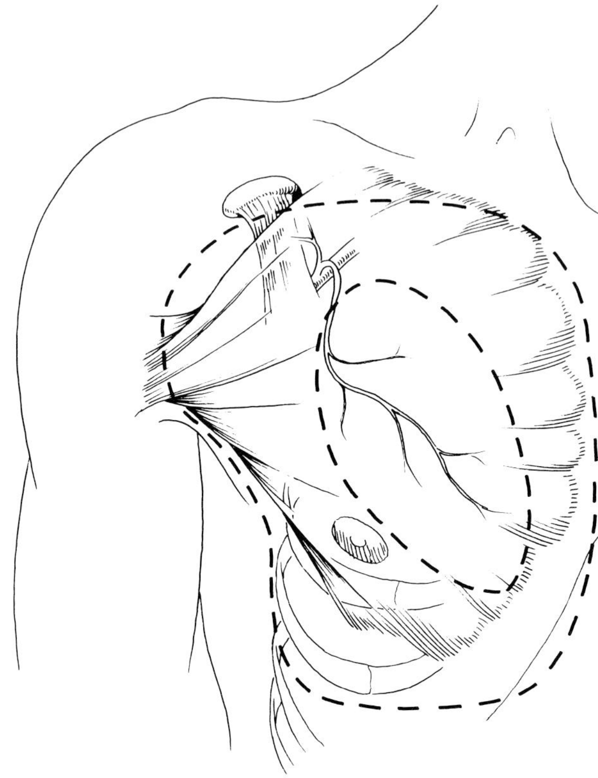

questionable condition after the primary chest wall procedure has been completed. When such muscle coverage is needed, it is our preference to widely mobilize both pectoralis major muscles on the thoracoacromial trunks, transect the humeral insertions and clavicular attachments, and to slide both flaps medially for coverage of the defect. In this way, the same coverage is provided, utilizing the most reliable pedicle.

FIGURE 9.3 The blood supply to the deltopectoral skin flap comes from internal thoracic perforators, particularly the large second intercostal branch.

FIGURE 9.4 The vascular territory, safely based on the thoracoacromial vascular pedicle, is included within the outer dotted line. The inner dotted line shows a safe area to plan the skin paddle.

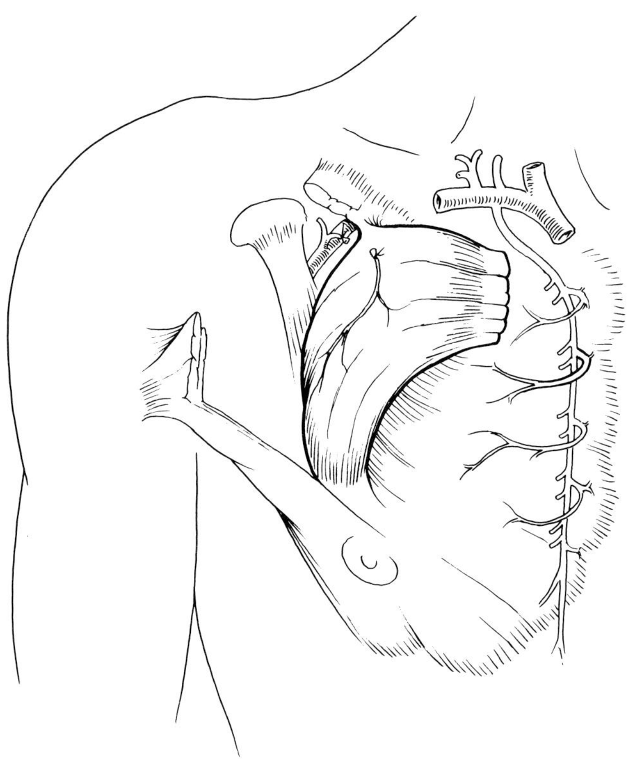

FIGURE 9.5 A reverse pectoralis major muscle flap can be based on internal thoracic perforating vessels. This option is not as versatile as basing the flap on its main blood supply, the thoracoacromial artery.

Another goal of chest wall reconstruction is to supply fresh, richly vascularized tissue to fibrotic or radiation-damaged regions so that primary healing can occur. The pectoralis major flap readily fulfills this requirement in dealing with damaged sternal or parasternal areas. If mantle radiation has been administered over the thoracoacromial vasculature, the pectoralis major flap can still be safely used in the majority of patients.

In elderly patients, the muscle may be quite thin. In young men, the muscle is bulky. These local factors may be advantageous or may present technical difficulties according to the requirements of the reconstruction.

Preoperative Planning

As with the other flaps, the decision to use the pectoralis major is based on the tissue requirements and size of the defect relative to the range of the pectoralis flap. The patient is asked to place the palms of the hands against each other in front of the chest and to push (Figure 9.6). This causes the pectoralis muscle to contract so that it is palpable from

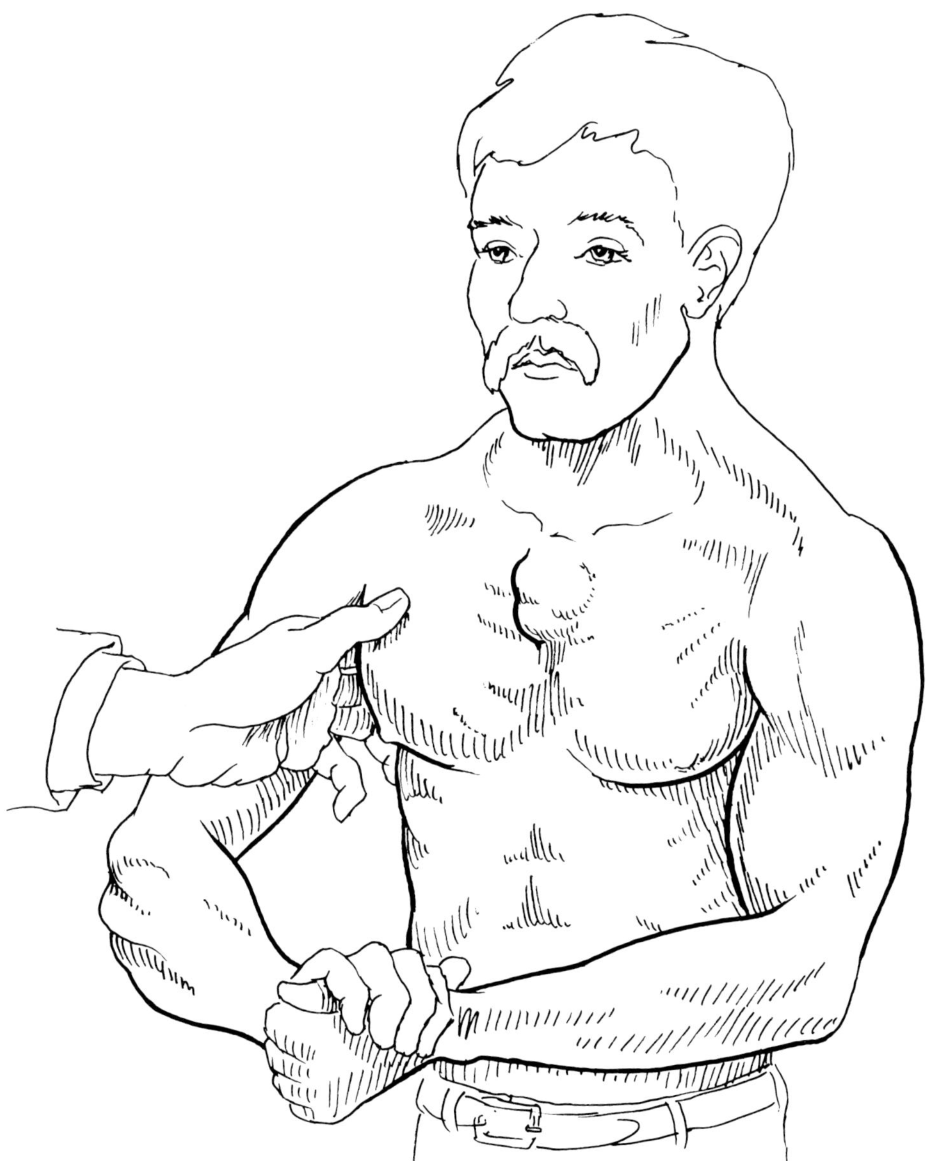

FIGURE 9.6 The integrity of the pectoralis major is tested by having the patient forcefully contract the muscle. It can then be palpated and assessed for use in the reconstruction.

origin to insertion. In feeling the muscle with the fingers and thumb, a quick assessment of its size and thickness are made while mentally picturing the anticipated depth of the defect that it is expected to fill.

An area of particular interest is at the xiphisternal junction, since these muscle fibers represent the distal-most point of the muscle flap. The borders of the muscle are marked with a marking pen, as well as the sternal notch, clavicles, and coracoid process of the scapula. The coracoid is an important landmark and is palpable as a round, firm prominence projecting forward beneath the laternal end of the clavicle just medial to the humeral head. The thoracoacromial vessels exit the clavipectoral fascia approximately 2 cm medial to and 2 cm inferior to the coracoid process. This point is also marked. The vessels (and lateral pectoral nerve) run along the deep surface of the pectoralis major muscle and pursue a roughly diagonal course toward the xiphoid. This course can be marked along an imaginary line from the acromion to the xiphoid. However, the vessels often meander laterally before turning in a medial direction. They may be injured, with subsequent loss of the flap, if this is not kept in mind.

A measuring tape is placed at the origin of the thoracoacromial pedicle medial and inferior to the coracoid process. This is the stationary or pivot point of the flap. The other end of the tape is placed on the distal-most muscle fibers just lateral to the xiphisternal junction (Figure 9.7). This distance represents the range, or reach, of the muscular portion of the flap. This end of the tape is moved to the anticipated defect in the chest wall and should cover the area with room to spare. The closure must be free of any tension. If there is any question, the opposite pectoralis is measured in the same way, and any additional flaps are planned as necessary to provide for a loose closure. If skin is missing or is to be removed at the defect, it may be necessary to include a skin segment with the flap to provide serviceable epithelium for the closure.

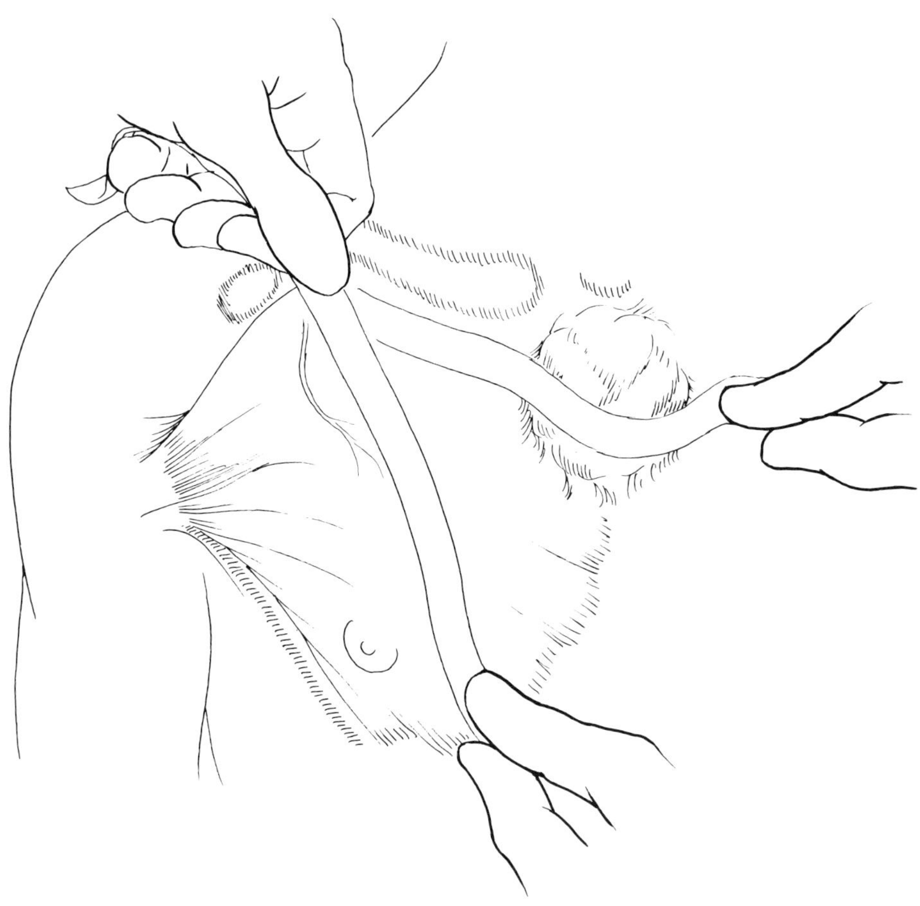

FIGURE 9.7 A measuring tape is used to compare the length of the proposed flap with the distance to the outermost limits of the anticipated defect.

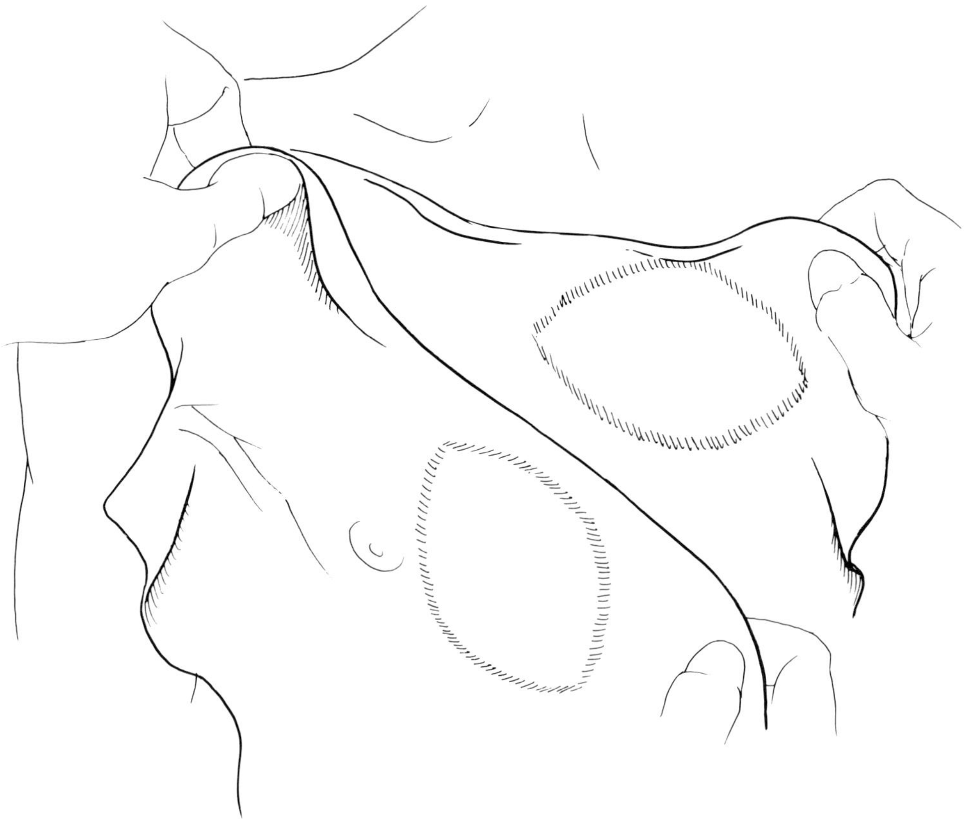

FIGURE 9.8 The outline of the skin island is marked on a towel, and the towel is pivoted on the vascular pedicle to confirm that the island will cover the defect without tension.

A hand towel, which may be cut to resemble the muscle, is placed over the pectoralis major to represent the muscle-skin flap (Figure 9.8). One end, over the pivot point, remains stationary as described. The other end is moved to the defect. The skin island is drawn on the cloth and the distal portion of the cloth flap moved into the anticipated defect. The towel may have to be placed somewhat more cephalad than the tape measure in order to accommodate the skin island over the muscle. This is done several times, with adjustments in the skin island being made so that it will easily fit into the defect. The skin segment is then outlined on the patient's chest. Of course, these markings may require adjustment during the operation after the completion of the surgery related to the defect. The measurements can also be done again at that time.

Preparation for the possible use of other flaps should always be done preoperatively. In this way, the additional flaps can also be assessed, measured, and marked for possible use. (See Chapter 5 for multiple flaps.) This not only avoids errors but makes it possible to prepare and drape the patient in a way that facilitates the use of the additional flaps.

Although this muscle is important in adduction of the humerus, its use in reconstruction has not significantly interfered with the daily activities of our patients. There seems to be adequate compensation for its activity by other muscles.

Mobilization of the Pectoralis Muscle-Skin Flap

When this flap is used, it is usually for anterior defects of the chest wall, anterior intrathoracic reconstructions (such as tracheoesophageal fistula), or to provide lining or coverage for head and neck defects. In dealing with the latter, it can provide lining for the floor of the mouth, palate, hypopharynx, and cervical esophagus. It can also provide coverage for the external ear region, cheek areas, and anterolateral neck. For these reconstructive operations, the patient is usually supine with the trunk and head slightly elevated. For anterior chest wall defects, the patient is also supine with the arms abducted. This stretches the pectoralis muscles and makes the dissection easier. A rolled towel is usually placed between the scapulae.

After urethral catheterization and insertion of the appropriate venous and arterial lines, the head, neck, thorax, upper abdomen, and shoulders are prepared and the drapes stapled to the skin. The anterior thigh is also prepared in case a skin graft is needed. After the defect has been established, an appropriately sized skin island is planned as before and drawn over the pectoralis muscle to reconfirm the preoperative assessment. The skin and subcutaneous tissues around the margin of the skin island are incised down to the pectoralis fascia, and the edges of the skin island are tacked to the pectoralis fascia with temporary sutures (Figure 9.9). These sutures ensure that the skin and muscle move to their new location as a unit, without shearing the vascular perforators supplying the overlying skin.

The dissection then continues away from the undisturbed skin island in all directions, uncovering the remaining superficial aspect of the pectoralis major muscle. The inferolateral border of the muscle is located, and the muscle is split in the direction of its fibers, about an inch away from its free margin (Figure 9.10). Preserving this edge of the muscle may help to retain the contour of the axillary fold postoperatively and avoid an unappealing cosmetic deformity related to total removal of the inferior border of the muscle. This maneuver does not compromise the flap size. The pectoralis major muscle above this edge is then elevated to allow the finger to enter the plane beneath the muscle. Here, the ribs can be easily felt. The fascia under the muscle is easily separated from the ribs with blunt, finger dissection in this areolar plane, sweeping upward to the clavicle and then caudally along the sternum and down to the xiphoid (Figure 9.11). The muscle thins out in this inferior area and can be torn if dissection is forceful.

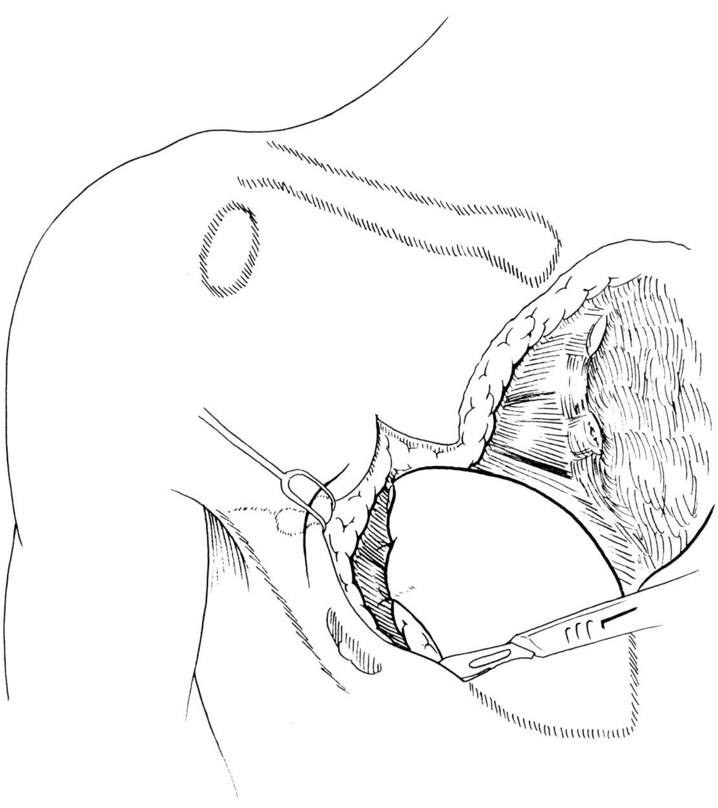

FIGURE 9.9 The sternal lesion has been removed and the skin island over the pectoralis major is incised. The dermis of the skin island is temporarily sutured to the deep fascia to prevent shearing of the perforating vessels to the skin.

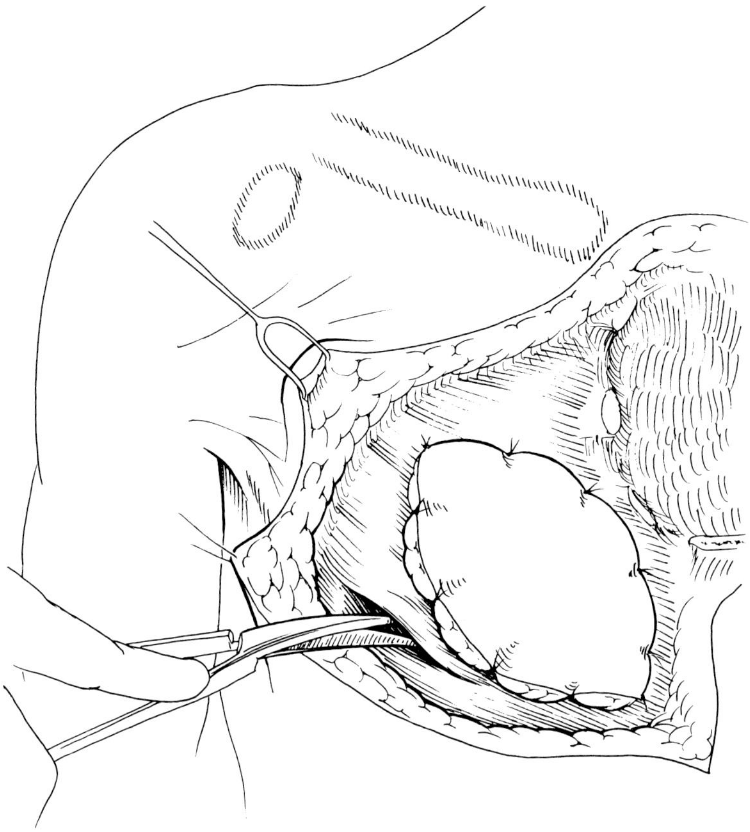

FIGURE 9.10 The lowermost fibers of the pectoralis major are left in situ as mobilization of the muscle begins. The submuscular plane is entered.

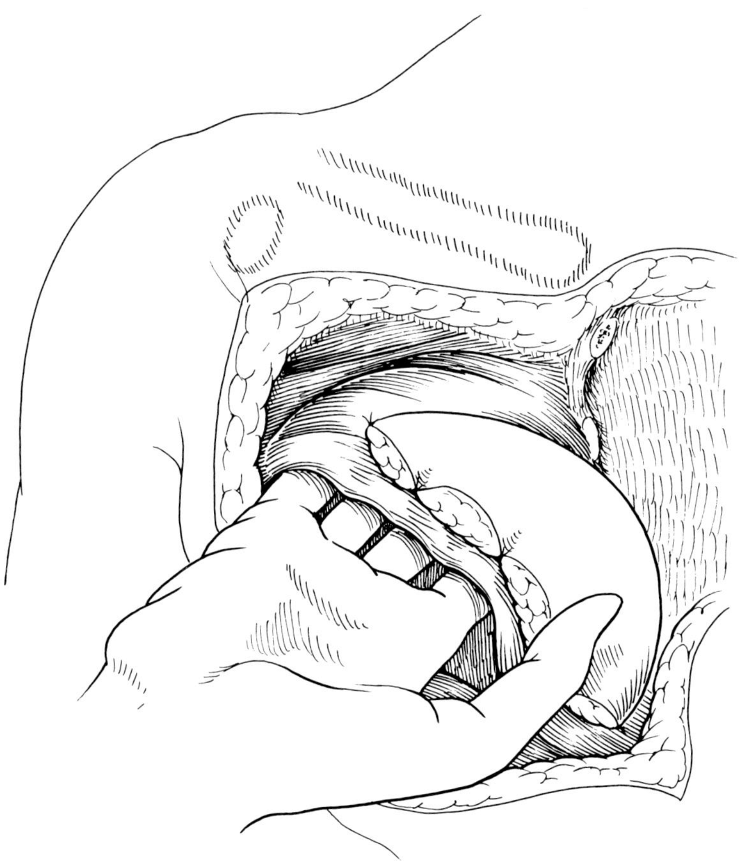

FIGURE 9.11 The areolar submuscular plane is easily dissected with the finger, lifting the muscle off the ribs.

Attention is then turned to sharply dissecting the thick muscular attachments along the body of the sternum (Figure 9.12). This can be done safely and rapidly with scissors or the cutting electrocautery. Here, the large perforating branches of the internal thoracic artery can be seen and ligated before transection. After the muscular origin along the sternum is divided, the muscle can be elevated to search for the thoracoacromial vascular pedicle. The index finger of the surgeon gently palpates the deep aspect of the muscle, between the thumb and forefinger, just medial to the coracoid process of the scapula, and the arterial pulsations can be felt (Figure 9.13). The course of the artery is gently traced as it clings to the deep surface of the muscle, so that its course will be remembered during the remaining dissection. The inferior border of the muscle is preserved as noted, and the dissection is carried toward the humeral insertion of the muscle. The muscle near the insertion is divided at a convenient level, again preserving the most caudal fibers (Figure 9.14). Care must be taken to avoid injury to the brachial plexus and the axillary vessels. During this maneuver, the pedicle is frequently checked so that its position is known at all times.

After division of the muscle near the insertion, the musculocutaneous unit can be turned upward so that the vascular pedicle can be directly visualized (Figure 9.15). Several large silk sutures are placed in the caudal border of the muscle so that it can be retracted upward atraumatically for direct visualization of the pedicle. The clavicular attachments can now be safely divided, working toward the pedicle from both medial and lateral directions. With the pedicle directly visualized, this fascia is slowly divided with the Metzenbaum scissors little by little, cutting only the remaining filmy attachments. The flap is now connected to the body only by its thoracoacromial vessels. It is gently brought to the defect and allowed to fit comfortably therein without tension or torsion of the pedicle (Figure 9.16). If both pectoralis major flaps are used in the reconstruction, the same technique for mobilization is used on the opposite side. The skeletal layer is reconstructed as deemed necessary, and the muscular layer is sutured

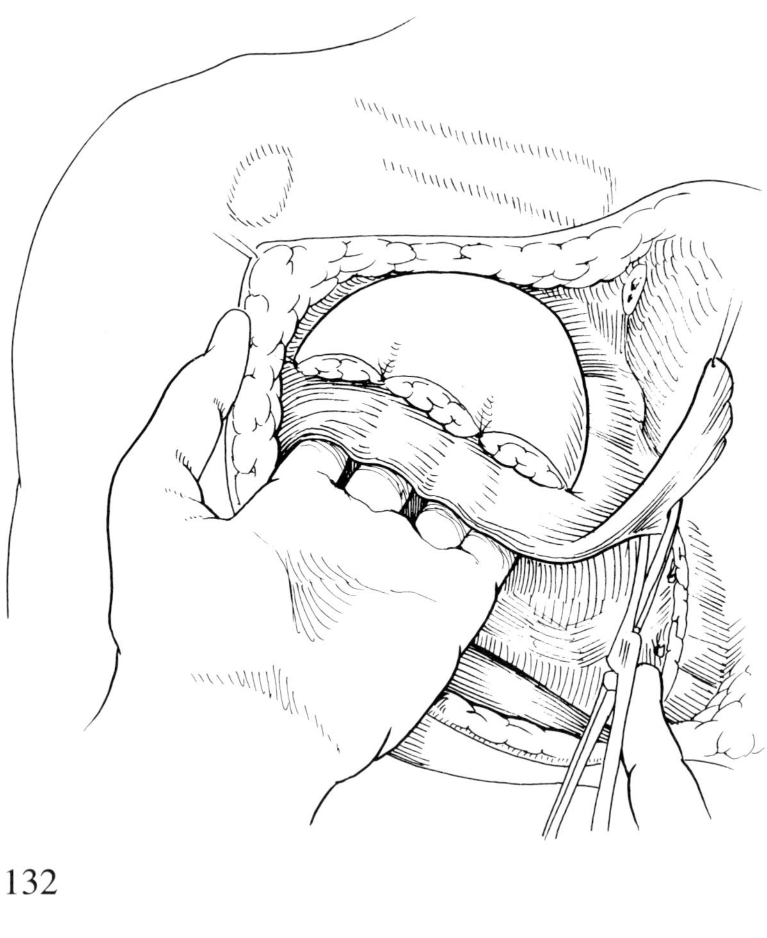

FIGURE 9.12 The medial attachments of the pectoralis muscle are divided, taking care to ligate the perforating branches of the internal thoracic artery.

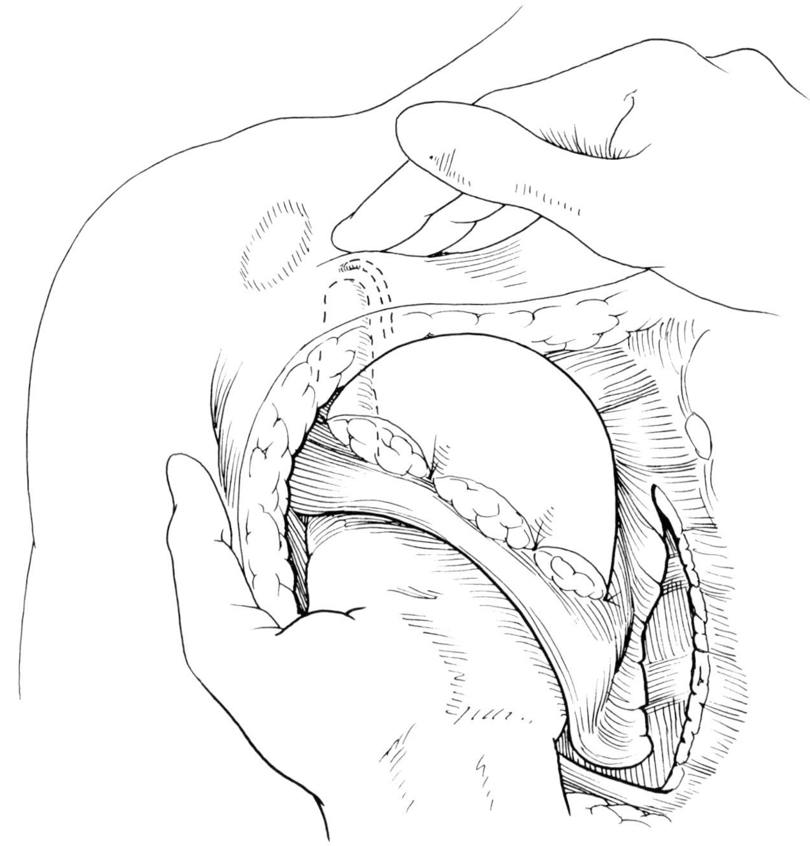

FIGURE 9.13 The surgeon gently palpates to locate the pulsations of the vascular pedicle. Its course is traced so that it will be protected throughout the dissection.

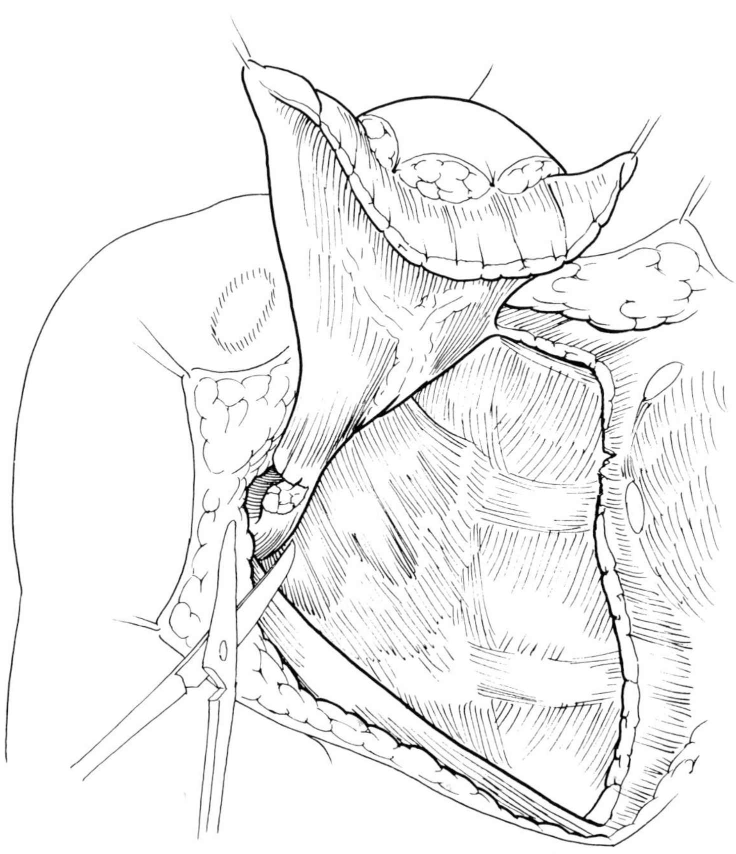

FIGURE 9.14 The medial clavicular attachments are divided along with the insertion of the muscle on the lateral side of the pedicle.

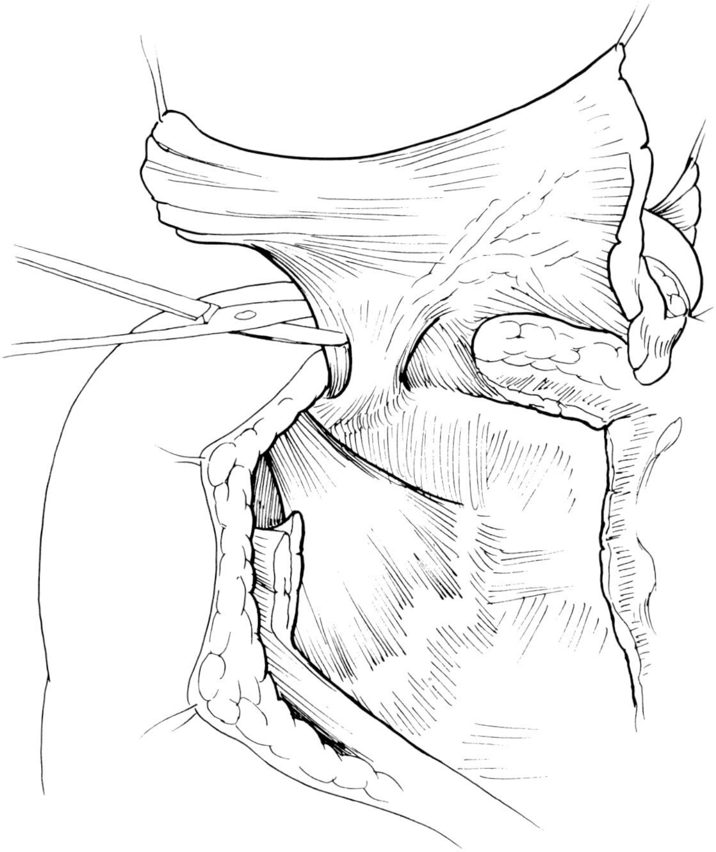

FIGURE 9.15 With the pedicle under direct vision, the remaining clavicular attachments of the muscle are divided.

into position with chromic sutures. The tacking sutures in the skin island are removed, and the skin edges are approximated with staples. The donor defect from which the skin island was harvested can usually be closed primarily with the aid of ample mobilization of the skin and subcutaneous fat at the level of the deep fascia (Figure 9.17). Far-near-near-far sutures of heavy nylon may aid in this closure as retention sutures to take tension off the skin edges.

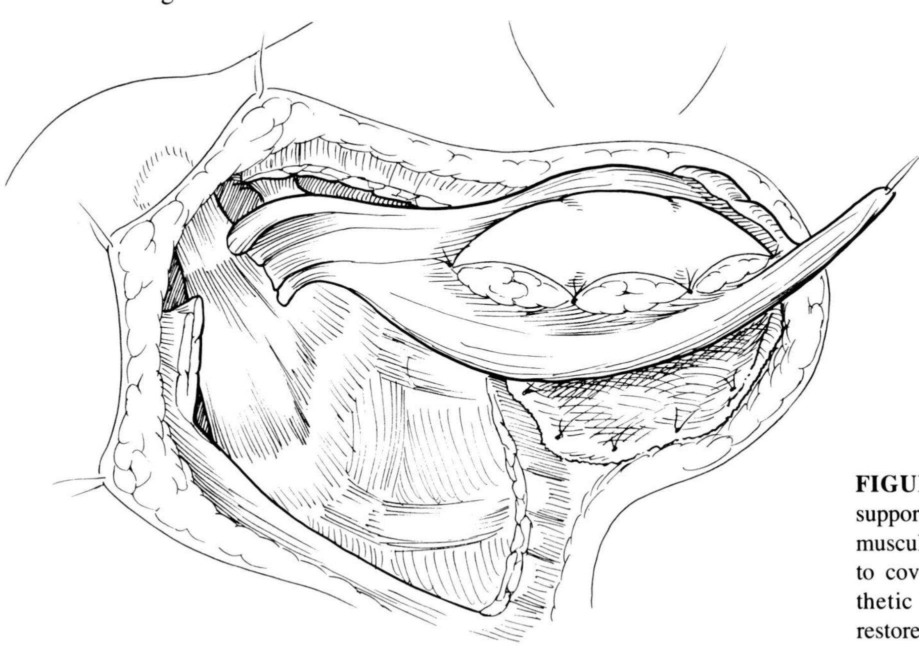

FIGURE 9.16 After skeletal support has been established, the musculocutaneous unit is shifted to cover the defect. Here, synthetic mesh has been used to restore the musculoskeletal layer.

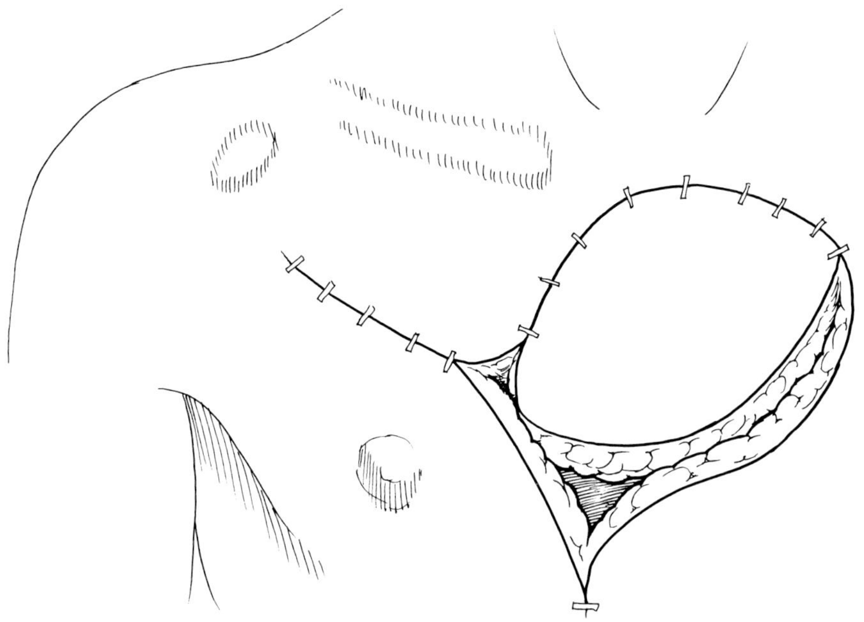

FIGURE 9.17 The tacking sutures in the skin island are removed and the skin is closed. Here, the donor site has been closed by mobilizing adjacent skin flaps.

If excessive tension prevents an easy closure of the central portion of the donor defect, a split-thickness skin graft is used to complete the repair. This sheet graft, of intermediate thickness, is stented for 5 to 6 days with a glycerine-cotton-bolus tie-over dressing. If the defect is a contaminated wound, the graft should be meshed 1.5 to 1.0 to allow drainage and applied unexpanded. It should be sutured to the underlying fascia with fine chromic sutures at many points and kept moist with saline-soaked sponges for 3 to 4 days. In this way, the interstitial area is readily epithelialized from the grafted skin. As with any skin graft, antibiotic coverage against streptococcus is routinely considered.

Mobilization of the Muscle Flap Alone

If skin replacement is desired but a skin island is not practical, serviceable epithelium can be provided over the muscle flap alone with meshed, unexpanded skin grafts (Figure 9.18).

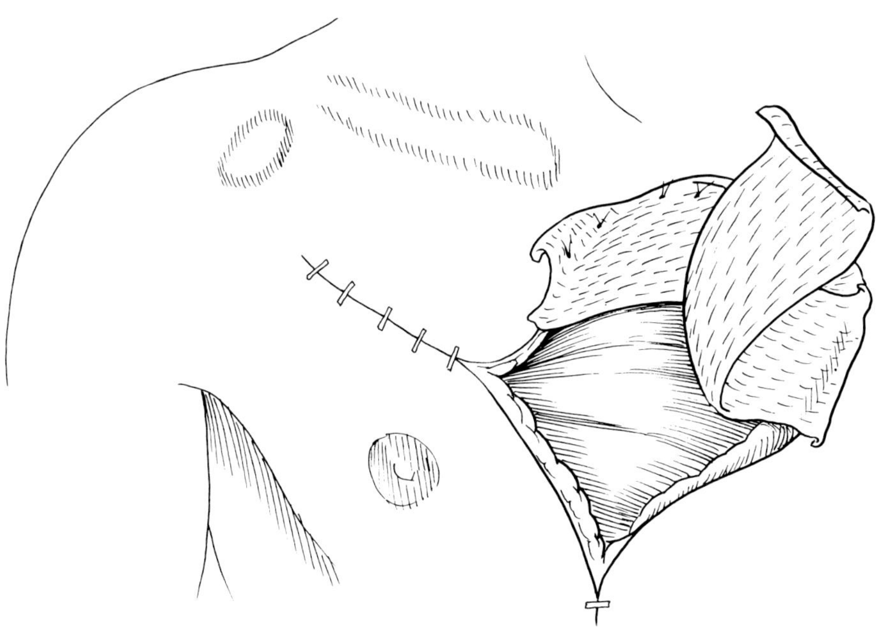

FIGURE 9.18 If muscle alone has been used, any necessary epithelial coverage is completed with meshed, unexpanded split-thickness skin grafts. The meshing allows the grafts to conform to the recipient muscle, and, if unexpanded, heals as a sheet.

When the reconstruction does not require skin replacement (e.g., for sternectomy through a median sternotomy incision or for sternal debridement procedures), the pectoralis major muscles can be mobilized through the midline incision. The dissection is exactly the same as described except that a skin island is not preserved over the muscle.

One or both muscles can be mobilized and easily shifted medially to fill the defect after removal of the sternum. The skin, which has been widely dissected during the mobilization of the pectoralis flaps, usually closes easily over the muscle layer. This procedure is described in the following illustrated case.

ILLUSTRATIVE CASE

This 61-year-old male presented with a slowly enlarging mass in the upper sternal region over a 4-month period (Figures 9.19–9.24). The mass was firm and nontender and did not appear to involve the skin (Figure 9.19). Preoperative evaluation showed a tumor of the manubrium consistent with chondrosarcoma. En bloc resection of the manubrium was accomplished including the sternal angle and upper body, along with the medial third of each clavicle and the medial portions of the attached ribs to ensure free margins (Figure 9.20). The margins were confirmed and the skeletal layer was reconstituted with split rib grafts (Figure 9.21). Both pectoralis major muscles were widely mobilized, the humeral insertions of each were transected (Figure 9.22), and the muscle flaps easily shifted to the midline for loose closure (Figure 9.23). Chest tubes were inserted before the rib graft placement, and the skin was closed without tension (Figure 9.24).

The endotracheal tube was removed on the second day and the patient made an uneventful recovery. Despite aggressive therapy, he expired from metastases 2 years later. There was no evidence of local recurrence during this interval.

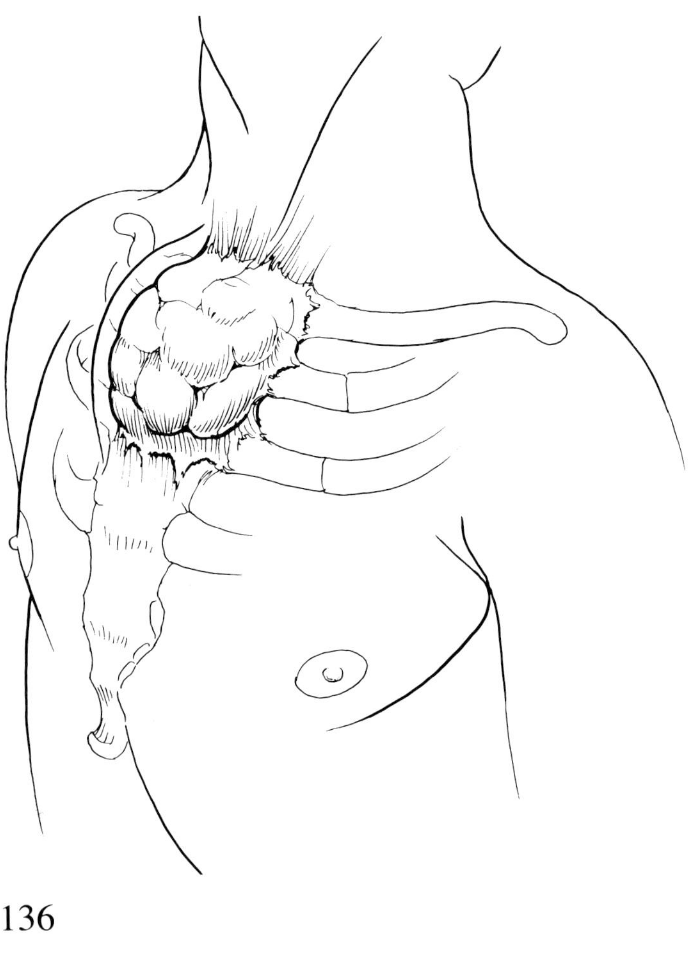

FIGURE 9.19 A 61-year-old male presented with a slowly growing, firm upper sternal mass consistent with chondrosarcoma. The skin was not involved clinically.

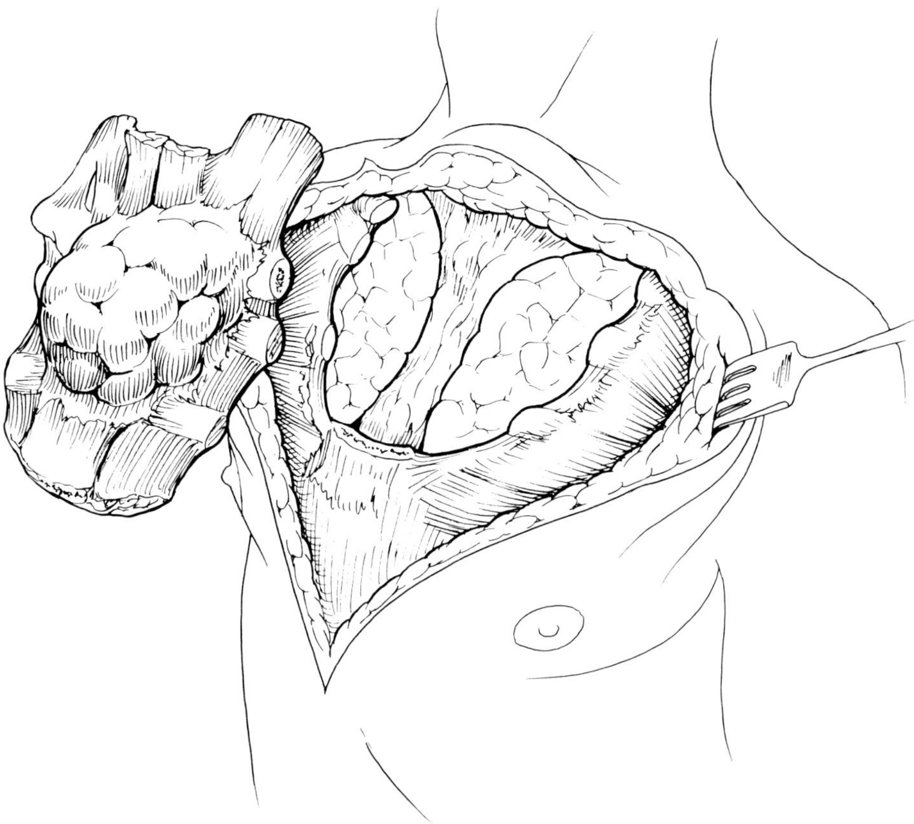

FIGURE 9.20 En bloc resection includes the manubrium and upper body of the sternum, along with portions of the adjacent clavicles and ribs.

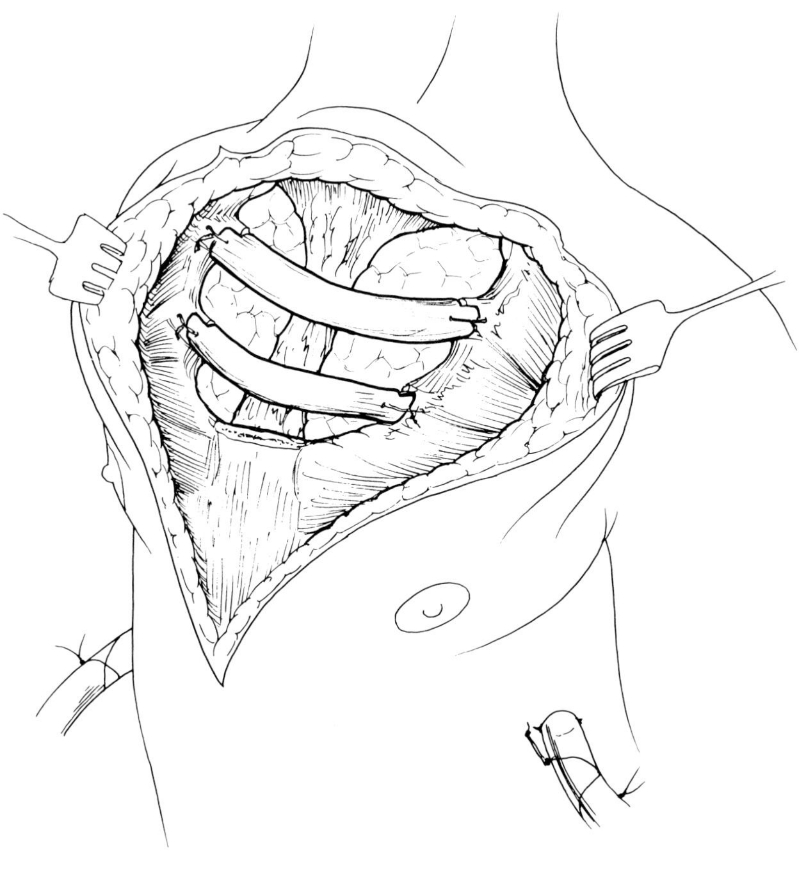

FIGURE 9.21 Chest tubes were inserted and the skeletal layer was reconstructed with rib grafts obtained bilaterally through the primary incision. The ends of the rib segments were modified as described in Chapter 5.

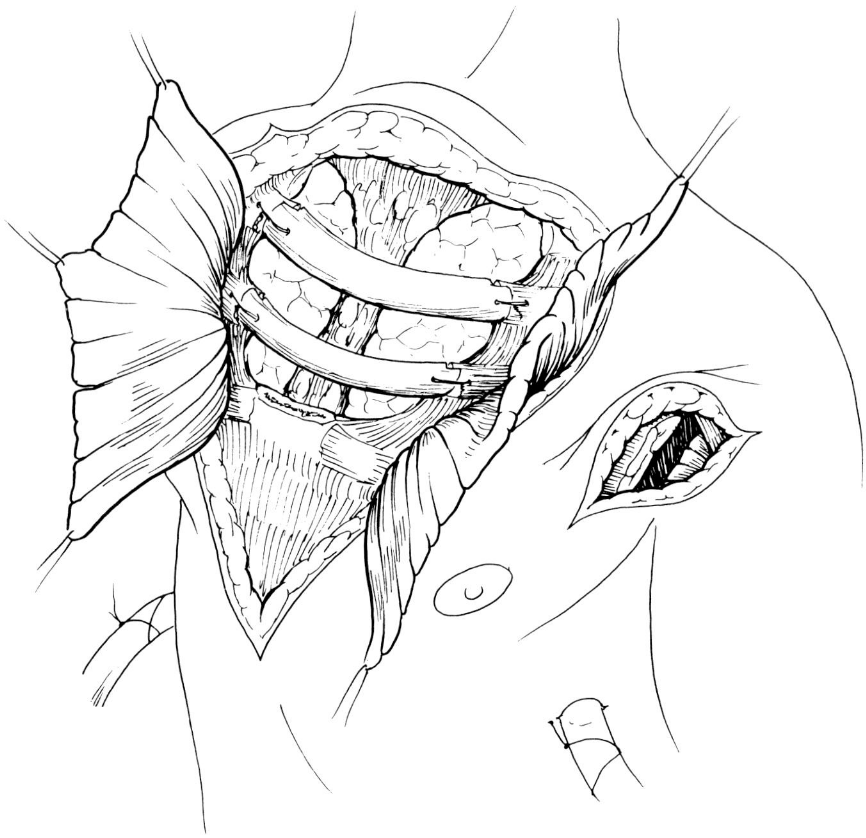

FIGURE 9.22 Both pectoralis major muscles were widely mobilized, the humeral insertions were transected through separate incisions, and the muscle flaps easily shifted to the midline for a loose closure.

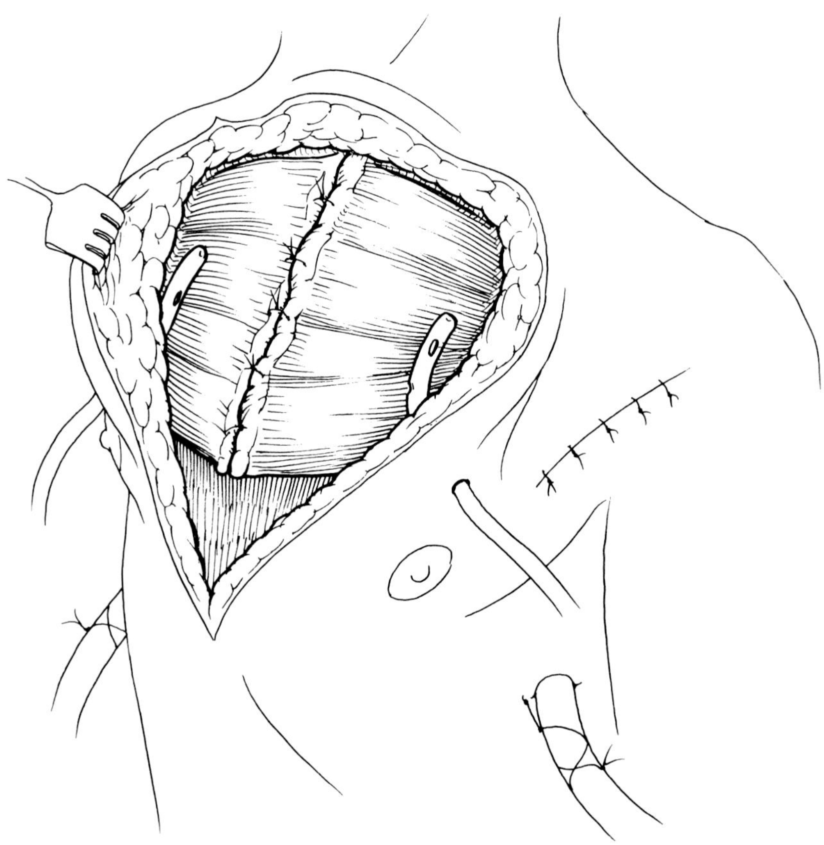

FIGURE 9.23 Closed suction drains were placed in a subcutaneous position.

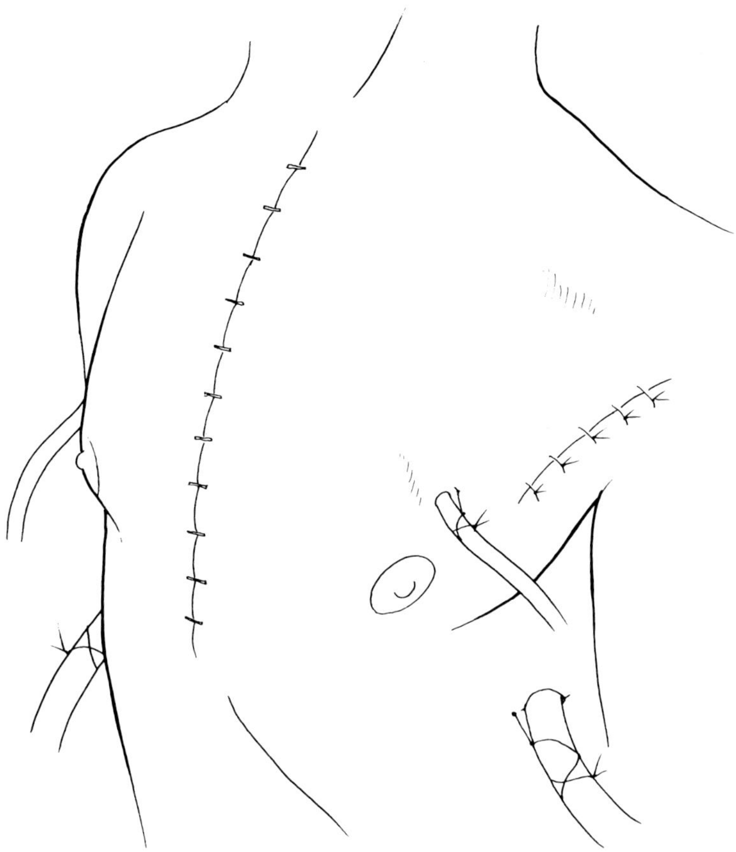

FIGURE 9.24 The skin was closed without tension. Since no skin had been removed, a loose closure was easily accomplished.

10

The Omentum

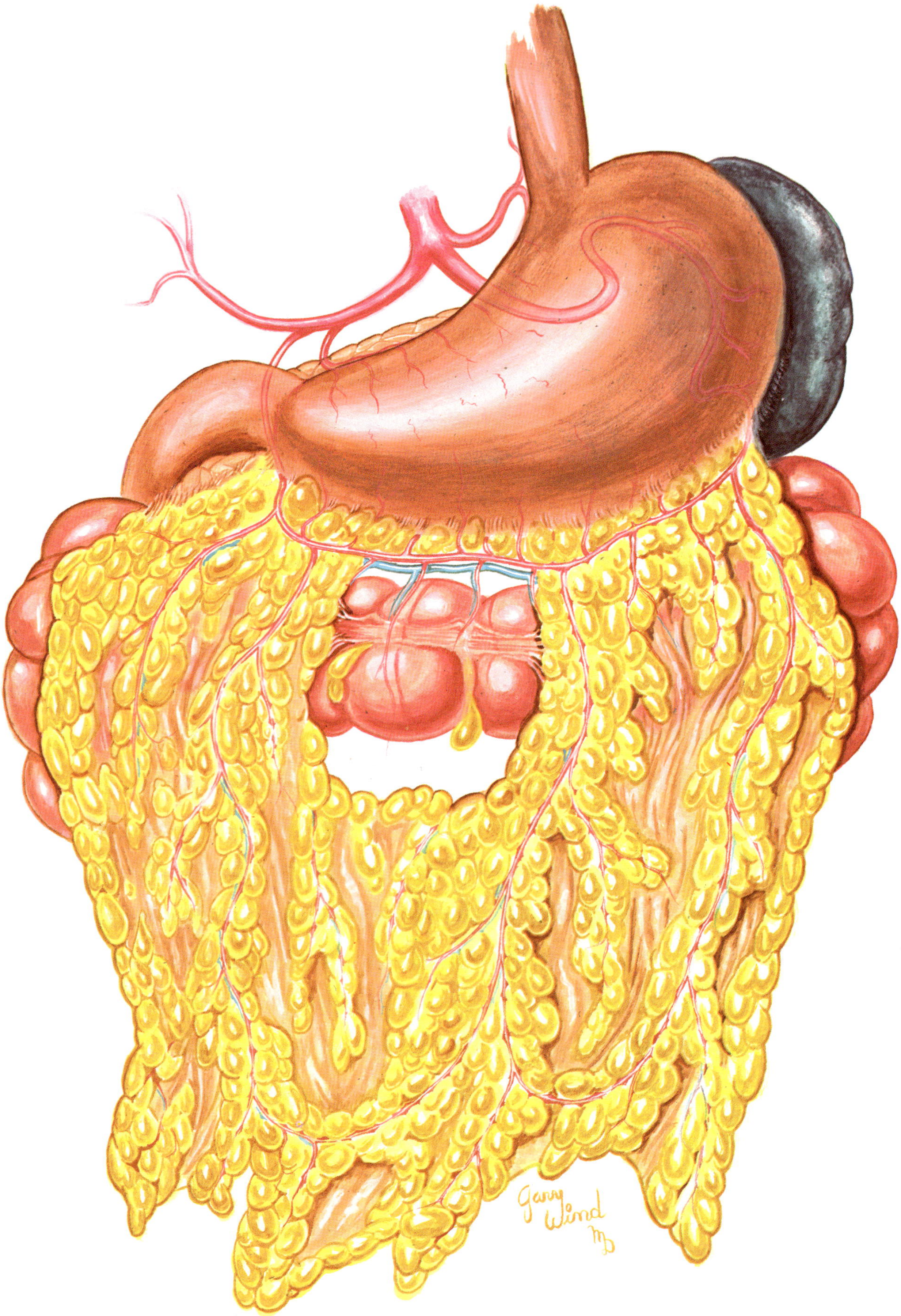

A window has been cut in the upper central portion of the omentum to show the relationship of the underlying transverse colon. The organs are rendered semi-transparent to trace the origin of the gastroepiploic arcade at both its extremities.

Anatomy

The greater omentum is formed embryologically by the relatively rapid growth of the dorsal mesogastrium, which occurs as the greater curvature of the stomach rotates to the left (Figure 10.1A). As the two double layers of the resulting sac continue to grow, they pass over the transverse colon and fuse together distally (Figure 10.1B). The cephalad leaf of the unfused proximal part of the sac becomes the gastrocolic omentum (Figure 10.1C). The caudad leaf fuses with the transverse mesocolon. The degree of fusion is variable, and care must be exercised in mobilizing the gastrocolic portion of the omentum since it, too, may be adherent to the transverse mesocolon (Figure 10.1D). In that case, both the omental and middle colic vessels are subject to injury.

The omental apron lies between the anterior parietal peritoneum and the coils of the small intestine (Plate 10.1). Proximally, the right margin of the greater omentum arises at the first portion of the duodenum. The left margin blends into the gastrosplenic ligament. The omentum may be transparent and diaphanous in the thin patient or weighted with fat in the obese. It is richly vascularized and is a common site for metastatic implants of abdominal malignancy.

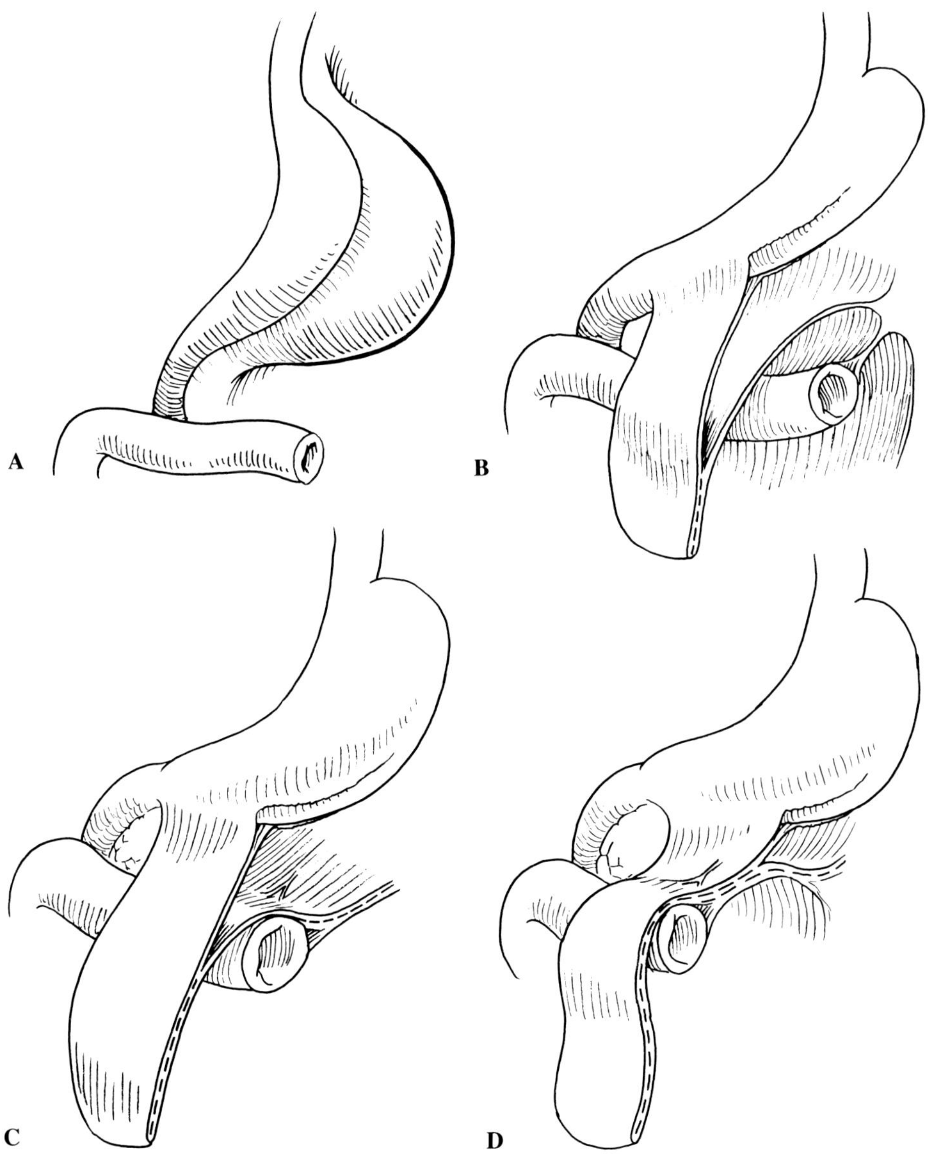

FIGURE 10.1A The greater omentum is formed by the rapid growth of the dorsal mesogastrium as the greater curvature of the stomach rotates to the left. As the stomach grows, the greater curvature becomes situated more caudally.

FIGURE 10.1B As the double layers of the sac continue to grow, they pass over the transverse colon and fuse distally.

FIGURE 10.1C The cephalad leaf (of the unfused proximal part of the sac) becomes the gastrocolic omentum. The caudad leaf fuses with the transverse mesocolon.

FIGURE 10.1D The degree of fusion is variable, and care must be exercised in mobilizing the gastrocolic portion of the omentum since it may be adherent to the transverse mesocolon. In that case, both the omental and *middle colic* vessels are subject to injury.

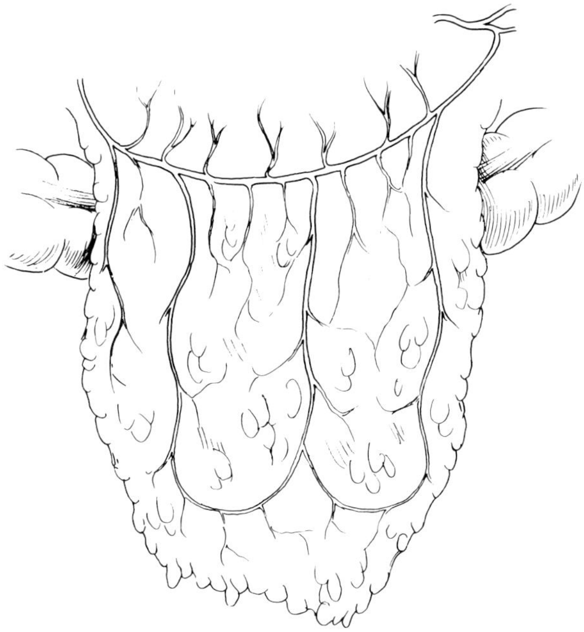

FIGURE 10.2 The blood supply to the greater omentum is based on the arcade formed by the left and right gastroepiploic arteries, which reside between the layers of the gastrocolic omentum. The vessels anastomose along the greater curvature of the stomach.

The blood supply to the greater omentum is based on the arcade formed by the right and left gastroepiploic vessels. The right gastroepiploic artery is the larger of the terminal branches of the gastroduodenal artery and emerges beneath the first portion of the duodenum just distal to the pylorus. Occasionally, it arises from the superior mesenteric artery. The smaller left gastroepiploic arises from a branch of the splenic artery before that vessel penetrates the spleen. The two vessels lie between the layers of the gastrocolic omentum and anastomose along the greater curvature of the stomach. This arch gives rise to ascending and descending branches. The multiple parallel ascending branches split at the greater curvature to supply the anterior and posterior walls of the stomach. The descending branches include dominant vessels that follow a fairly consistent pattern of right, middle, and left trunk (Figure 10.2). In addition, an accessory vessel arises near the origin of the right gastroepiploic. The middle omental vessel bifurcates, usually distally, and the branches join the right and left omental vessels. Rarely, the middle vessel is absent and the right and left vessels join directly (Figure 10.3A). Another rare occurrence is an incomplete gastroepiploic arch with the left vessel arising directly from a splenic branch (Figure 10.3B).

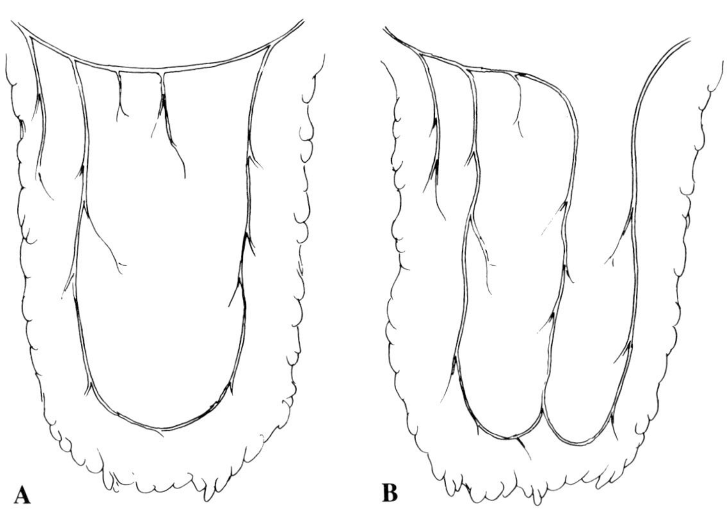

FIGURE 10.3 There may be variations in the blood supply to the omentum. The middle vessel may be absent (Figure 10.3A) or the gastroepiploic arch may be incomplete (Figure 10.3B).

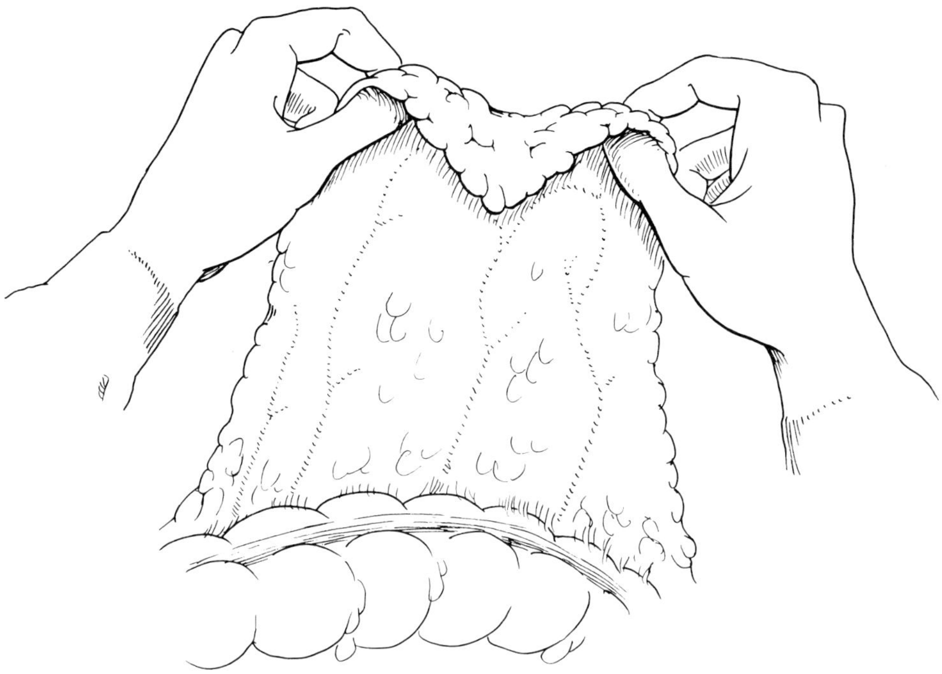

FIGURE 10.4 If the omentum contains too much fat to allow direct visualization of the vessels, they may be seen by holding the tissues up to the light (transillumination).

When the omentum contains too much fat to visualize these vessels directly, they may be seen by holding the omentum up to the light (Figure 10.4). The venous drainage of the omentum follows the pattern of the arterial supply. The left gastroepiploic vein empties into the distal splenic vein or one of its tributaries. The right gastroepiploic usually drains into the superior mesenteric and occasionally into the splenic or portal vein.

Engorged omental veins may signal unsuspected portal hypertension. Portal pressure can be measured directly by cannulating a vein and attaching a manometer.

General Characteristics

The omentum is a pliable, soft membrane, rich in blood vessels, fat, and lymphatics, that can be used for a variety of anterior, lateral, and intrathoracic defects. In the absence of adhesions, it can be rapidly mobilized and, especially in obese patients, can be voluminous. Due to its ample blood supply, it readily supports the healing of skin grafts applied to its surface, and its pliability can be useful in filling cavitary and irregular defects. It is of greatest value in the reconstruction of open and chronic wounds, especially of the sternum, and can reach all areas of the anterior thorax (Figure 10.5). It is usually chosen when muscle flaps are unavailable or when it is needed to augment the use of other flaps in dealing with large defects.

Its disadvantages include its lack of inherent strength and the necessity of opening the abdomen for harvesting the tissue. Ventral hernia, although a legitimate concern, has not been a problem.

Mobilization of the Omentum

A routine bowel preparation is administered according to the preference of the surgeon. For anterior defects, the patient is usually in the supine position on the operating table. After endotracheal anesthesia, a Foley catheter is inserted and the dressing, if any, is removed from the thoracic lesion. In dealing with an open defect, the wound is

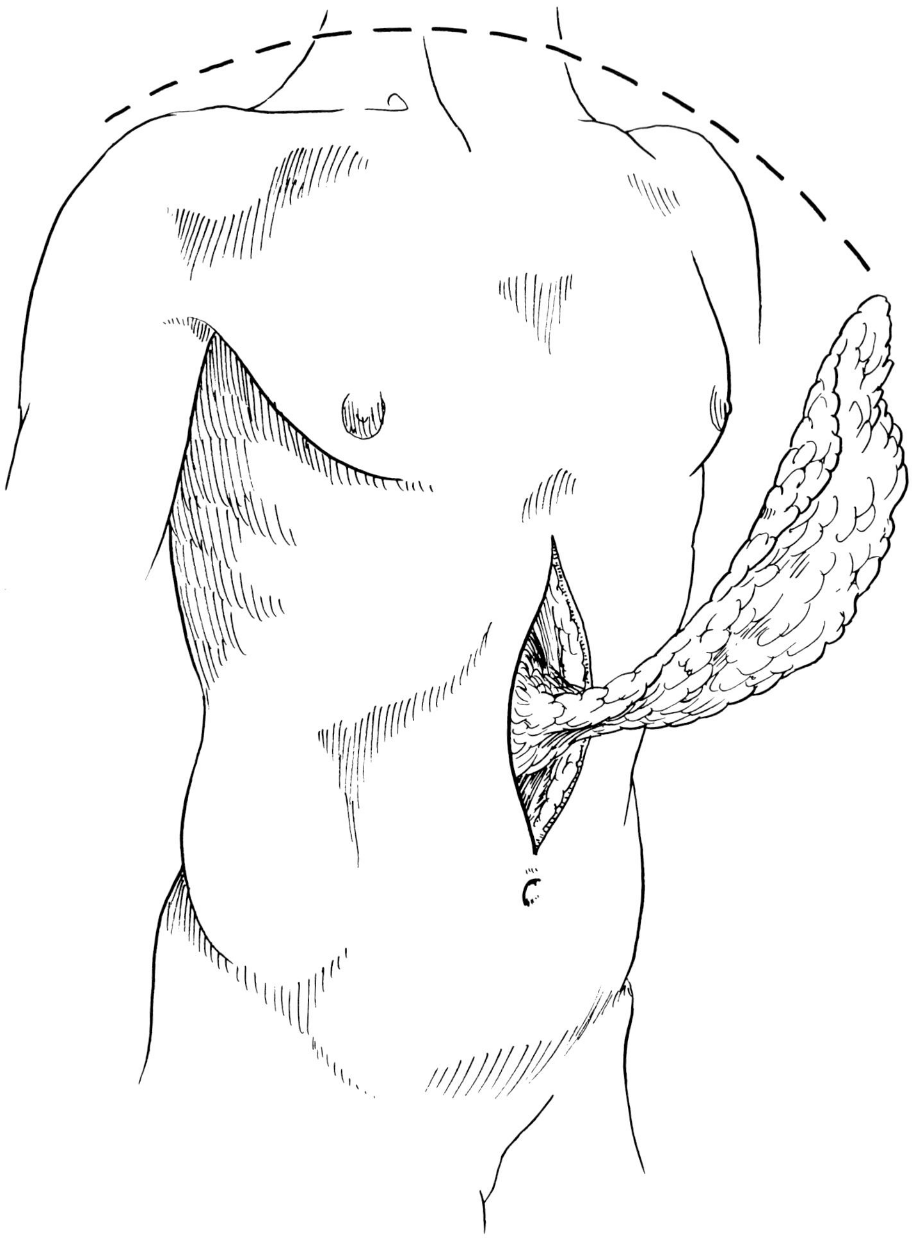

FIGURE 10.5 The range or arc of rotation of the omentum includes virtually all areas of the anterior and lateral thorax. In selected cases, it can also be used for intrathoracic defects.

thoroughly assessed to assure that it is as clean as possible before any closure is considered. If further debridement is necessary, this is accomplished first, and it may be necessary to postpone the reconstruction until conditions are optimum.

The abdomen and thighs are prepared first and the open chest wound last, so that aseptic conditions are as close to ideal as possible. After the chest has been prepared, a dry sterile sponge is placed in the chest wound, and a rubber dam-patch is cut from a sterile surgeon's glove and stapled to the skin around the wound (Figure 10.6). The sponge absorbs any drainage and prevents it from spreading to contaminate other areas. A betadine-steri-drape (adherent) is then placed over the chest, further sealing it from the abdominal area, and the abdomen reprepared. The entire area is then draped, including the thighs as the donor sites for skin grafts.

The abdomen is entered through an upper midline incision that extends to just below the umbilicus. A nasogastric tube is inserted and its position checked from within the abdomen. After a brief exploration, attention is turned to assessing the omentum. The vessels are easily injured and care is taken to handle this tissue gently. It is lifted

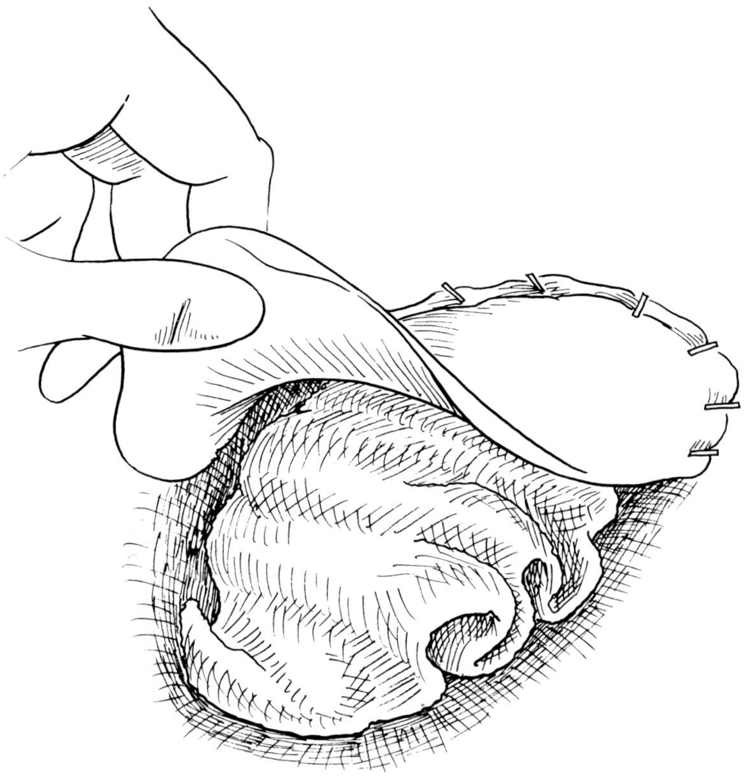

FIGURE 10.6 After thorough cleansing of the open chest wound, a sterile cotton sponge is placed in the defect and a rubber patch is stapled over the defect. The area is then reprepared with antiseptic solution before draping the patient.

from the colon, and any adhesions are isolated and sharply divided while protecting the viscus from which they are liberated (Figure 10.7). After the omentum is freed, its filmy attachment to the transverse colon is isolated and gradually divided (Figure 10.8). Care is taken to avoid injury to the middle colic vessels within the transverse mesocolon. Likewise, the appendices epiploicae are left intact to avoid crossing diverticula of the

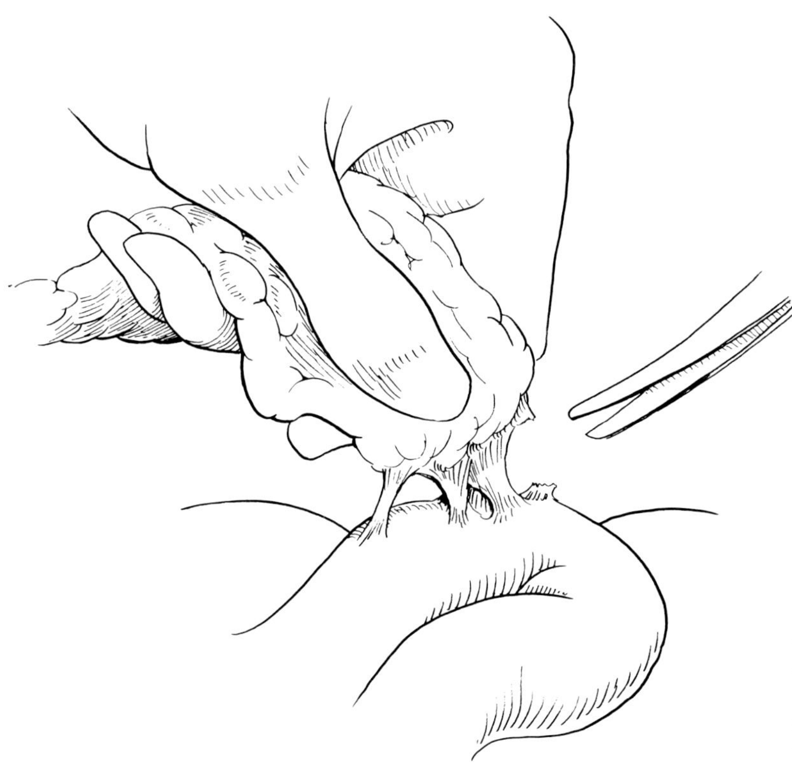

FIGURE 10.7 It may be necessary to divide adhesive bands sharply in order to liberate the omentum from other abdominal structures.

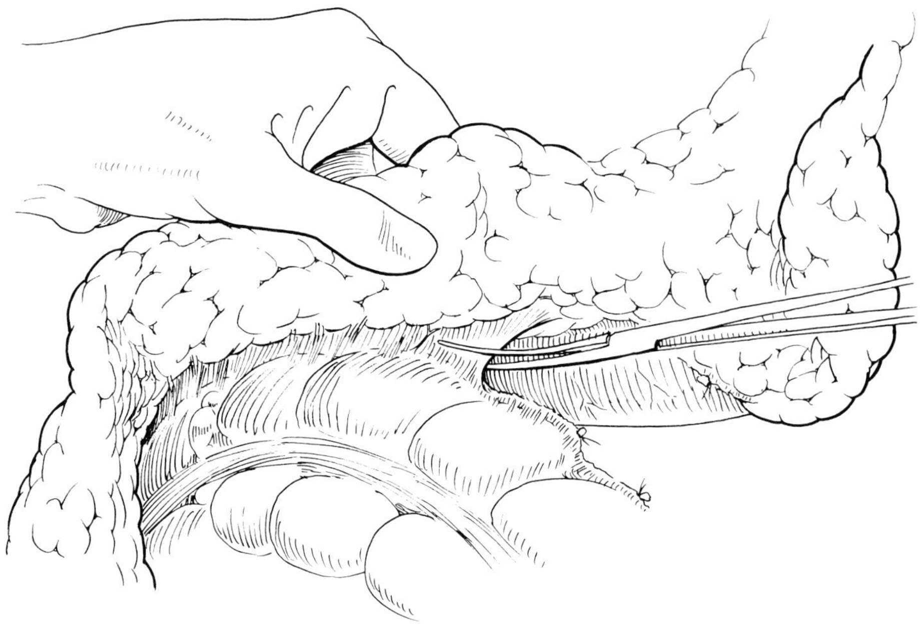

FIGURE 10.8 The filmy bare area that joins the omentum to the transverse colon is located by gently lifting the omentum. It is sharply divided, taking care to avoid injury to the middle colic vessels and any diverticula.

colon. The small blood vessels should be individually clamped with hemostats and immediately ligated with fine silk ties. This will avoid tearing of the blood vessels by the weight of the clamps. If this occurs, a hematoma may develop that can spread rapidly between the leaves of the omentum, making the tissue difficult to use due to loss of pliability.

The short vessels between the gastroepiploic arch and the greater curvature of the stomach are now approached, again segmentally dividing the vessels and ligating them individually (Figure 10.9). An anterior row and a posterior row form a radial pattern around the greater curvature of the stomach, and these are ligated close to the gastric serosa. After this step, the omentum is attached by the left gastroepiploic artery, which arises from a terminal branch of the splenic artery and from the right gastroepiploic

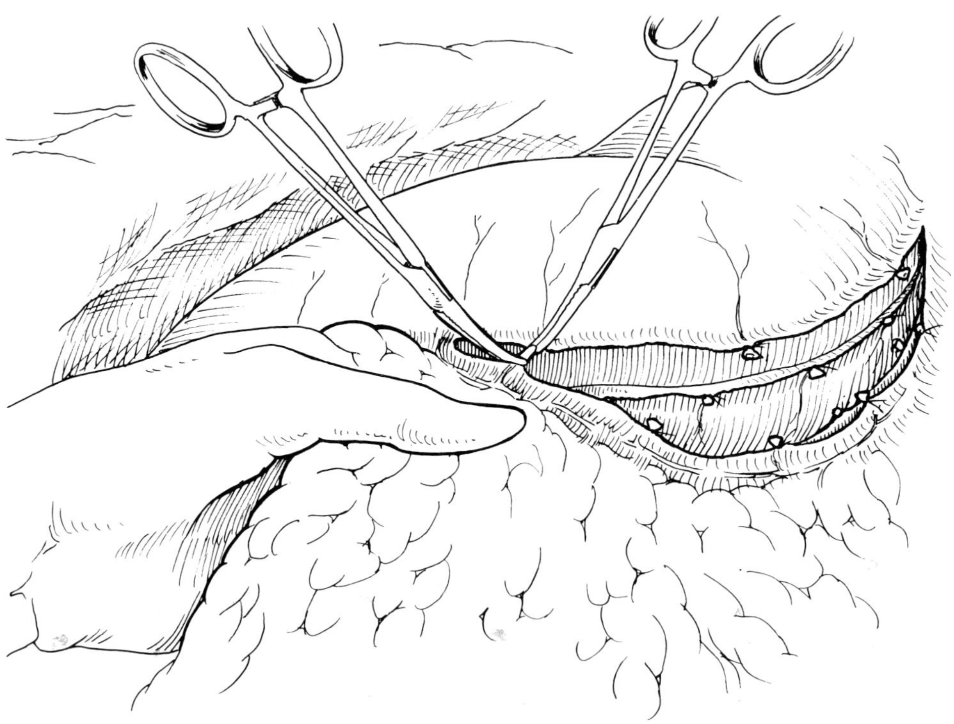

FIGURE 10.9 The short vessels between the gastroepiploic arch and the greater curvature of the stomach are serially clamped, divided, and tied immediately. No clamps are allowed to hang since the vessels may be torn, and the resulting hematoma could make the omentum difficult to use.

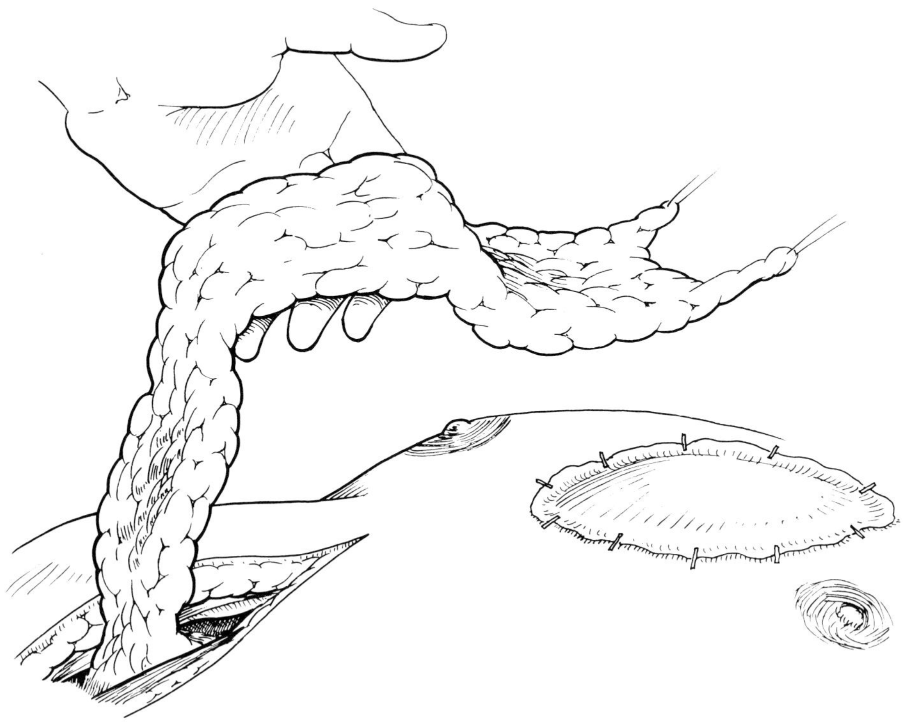

FIGURE 10.10 An assessment is made to ensure that the omentum, still attached to the left and right gastroepiploic arteries, will have sufficient length to reach the defect. It should be redundant enough to easily fill the defect without any tension. If it is too short, it can be lengthened.

artery near the pylorus. Before further dissection, the omentum is lifted from the abdomen and over the chest to ascertain its reach (Figure 10.10). Often, it easily covers the defect without further mobilization. If more length is needed, the left gastroepiploic vessels are divided at a convenient point along the greater curvature, without entering the region of the splenic hilum (Figure 10.11). With this added length, the omentum usually

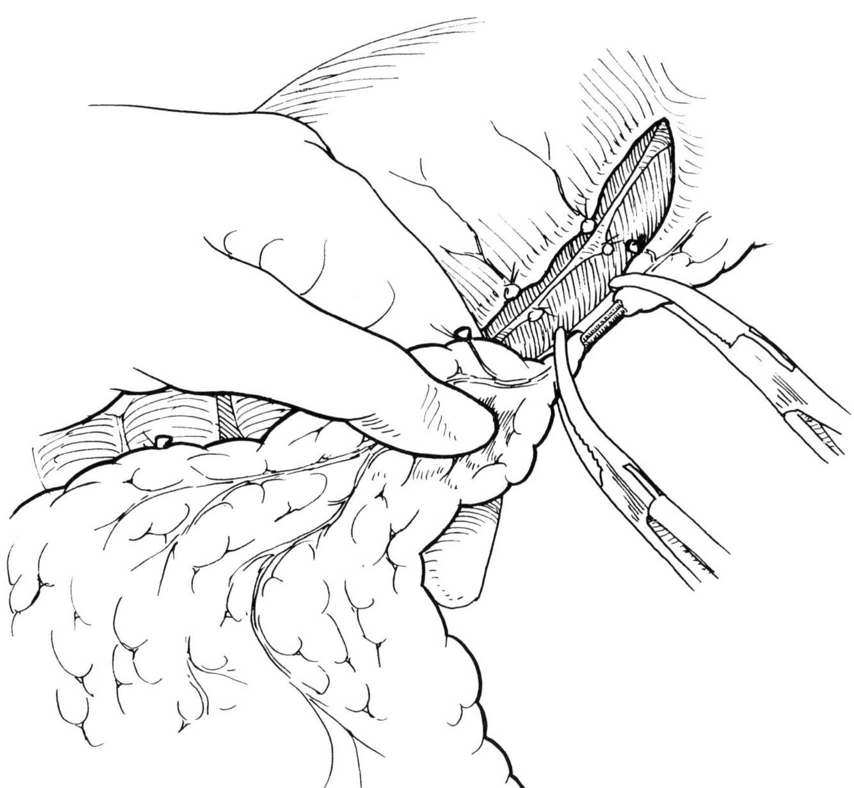

FIGURE 10.11 Lengthening the omentum, the left gastroepiploic artery is divided at a convenient point without disturbing the splenic hilum. This maneuver gives added length with the omental flap based on the right gastroepiploic artery.

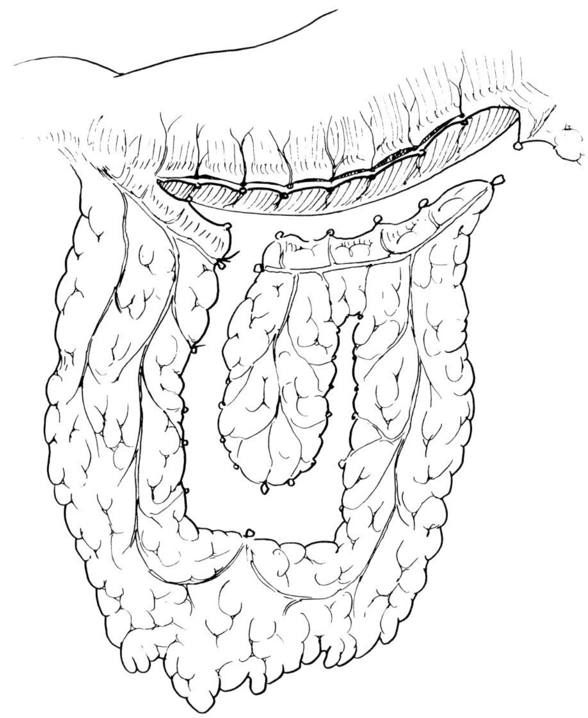

FIGURE 10.12 If more length is needed, the omentum can be unfurled through selected division of its internal vessels; it is still based on the right gastroepiploic artery.

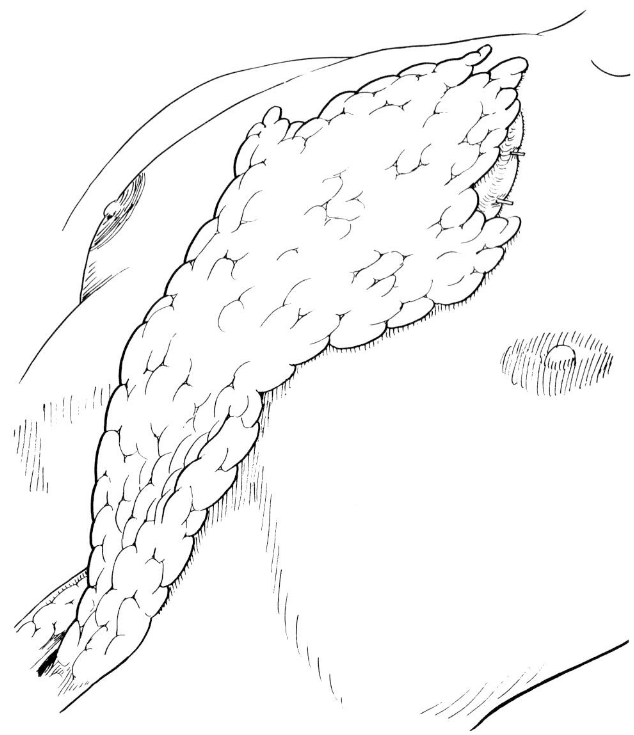

FIGURE 10.13 The omentum should be loose enough to fill the defect with no tension whatsoever.

reaches to the head and neck areas. In the rare case where more length is needed, the vessels can be divided and the omentum unfurled (Figure 10.12).

The omentum should fit loosely into the defect, filling the cavity without tension on the pedicle (Figure 10.13). This maintains free circulation within the pedicle and flap and also prevents gastric outlet obstruction from tethering by the right gastroepiploic vessels (Figure 10.14).

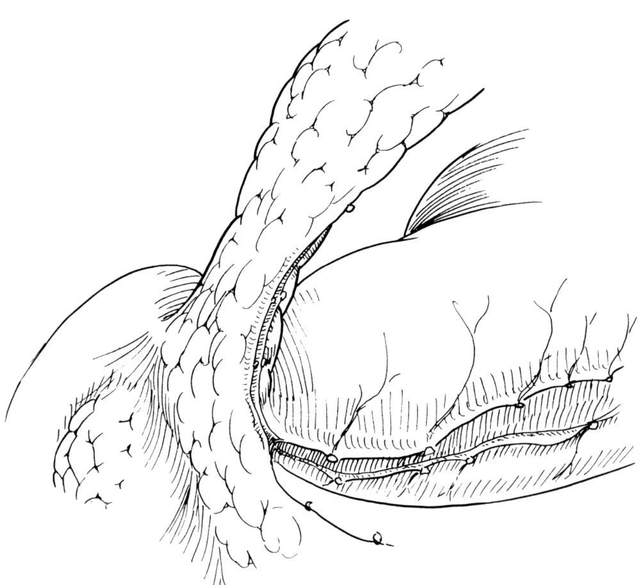

FIGURE 10.14 There must also be no tension on the vascular pedicle. Such tension could result in strangulation of the omental flap or gastric outlet obstruction through tethering of the pyloric area.

In some patients, it is helpful to insert a feeding jejunostomy so that enteral nutrition can be started soon after the operation. This is of great importance in early healing if the patient's caloric intake has been poor and also in certain elderly or debilitated patients. Since nasogastric decompression is a routine part of the early postoperative regimen, the jejunostomy can be of great value in providing nutritional support while gastric decompression is maintained. When a jejunostomy has been decided on, a convenient segment of jejunum is chosen, approximately 18 in. distal to the ligament of Treitz, which allows the tube to exit easily from the left abdominal wall. A routine Witzel-type jejunostomy is performed with a double purse string and a series of Lembert sutures for the serosal seal (Figure 10.15). It is best to use a red rubber catheter (number 18) rather than the trocar and the small catheters that are commercially available since the tube doesn't kink as frequently or obstruct due to inspissation of dietary supplements. A few extra holes are cut in the tube before insertion. The bowel is secured to the anterior parietal peritoneum, and the catheter is secured to the skin. Feeding is begun on the first postoperative day.

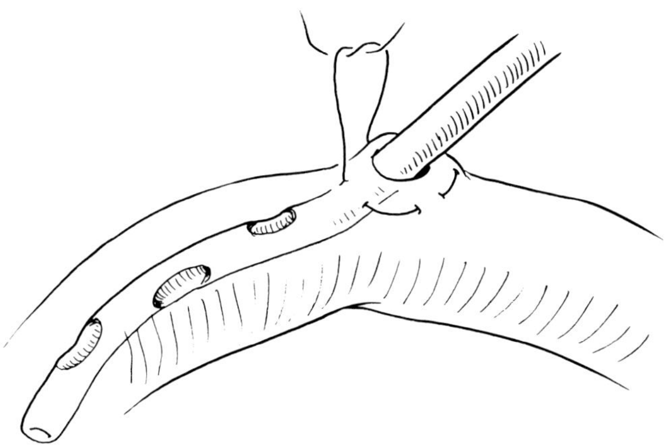

FIGURE 10.15A Jejunostomy can be of great value in providing nutritional support to debilitated patients. The antimesenteric side is entered and a medium rubber catheter (with extra holes cut) is inserted. The purse string is tied.

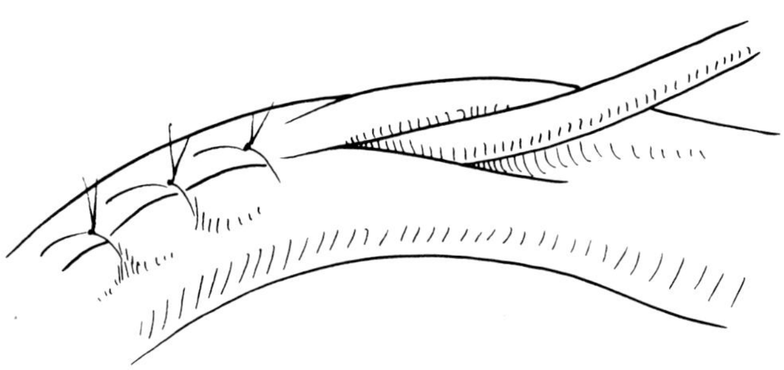

FIGURE 10.15B A serosal tunnel is established (to ensure a good seal) in standard fashion with Lembert sutures.

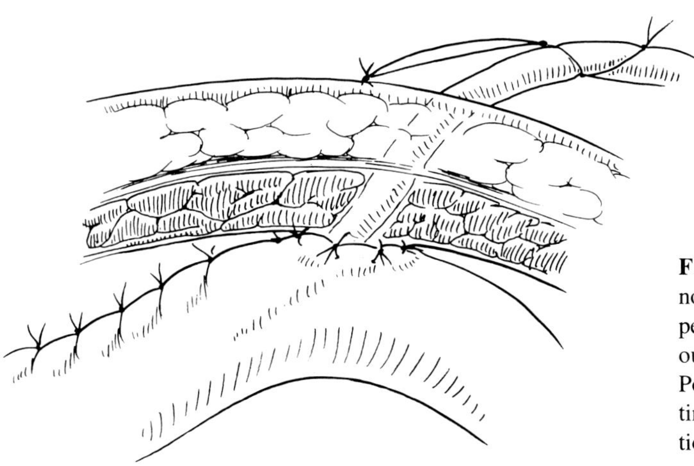

FIGURE 10.15C The jejunostomy is fixed to the parietal peritoneum and the tube brought out through a small incision. Positioning of the bowel is routinely checked to avoid obstruction or volvulus.

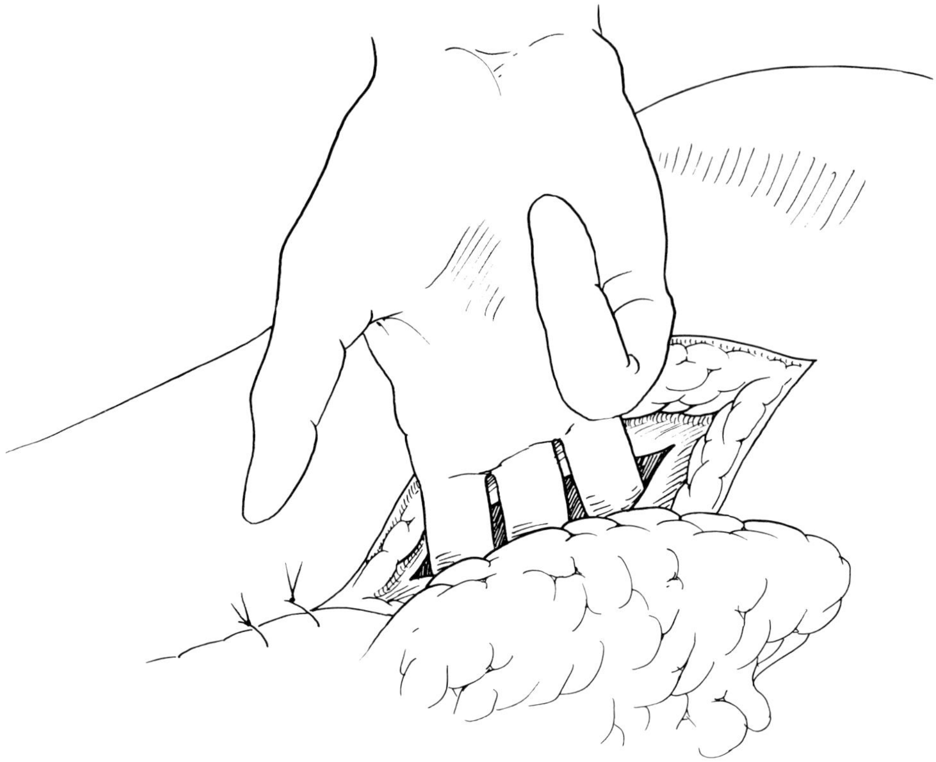

FIGURE 10.16 The abdominal closure leaves a cephalad fascial defect open (3–4 fingerbreadths) to avoid constriction of the omental vessels in their passage to the chest.

The omentum is brought out of the cephalad portion of the wound and laid on the still-draped chest. It is protected from desiccation by moist laparotomy sponges, and the abdomen is closed in layers after assessing the colon, stomach, and jejunum for residual bleeding from the dissection. The fascia of the cephalad portion of the abdominal wound is left open with room to spare (3–4 fingerbreadths) so that there is no constriction of the omental vessels as they cross this layer (Figure 10.16). The skin is closed up to the omentum.

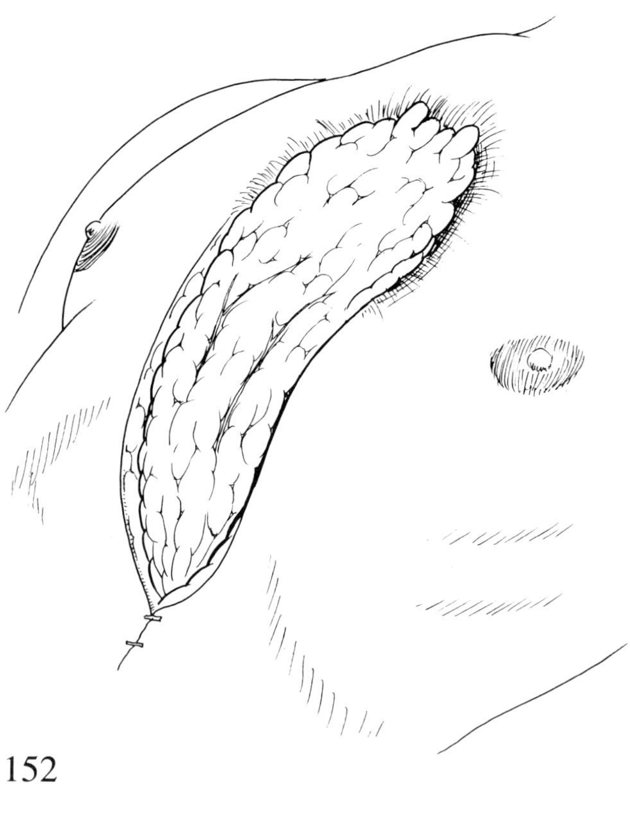

FIGURE 10.17 The intact skin between the abdominal incision and the chest wall defect may be opened and the omental flap positioned in this trough. If this option is selected, a skin graft can be used to cover the exposed omentum.

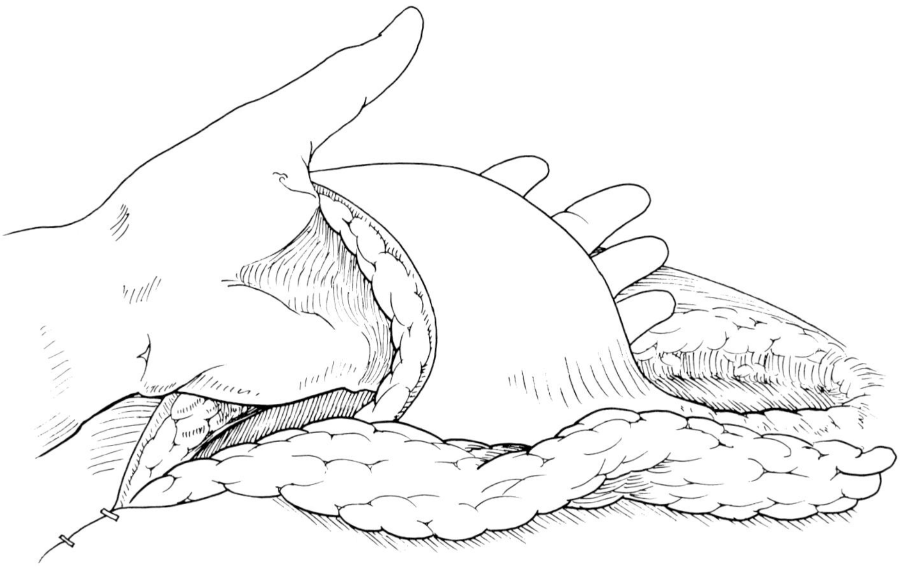

FIGURE 10.18 Another option is the fabrication of a wide (4–5 fingerbreadths) subcutaneous tunnel through which the omentum is drawn in order to reach the chest wall defect. Care is taken to avoid pressure on the vascular pedicle. If there is any question, the tunnel is opened to make a trough for the flap.

The chest is uncovered and any last bit of debridement accomplished as necessary. The intact skin between the abdominal wall and the defect can be incised and the omentum allowed to lie in the opened area with a direct route to the defect (Figure 10.17). If the skin is opened, a skin graft is used to cover the omentum. Alternatively, a large subcutaneous tunnel can be established to allow the omentum to reach the chest wound. If the latter is chosen, there should be room enough to allow the opened hand to go through the tunnel with ease (Figure 10.18). After the tunnel is established, the skin of the abdominal incision is closed.

The chest wall defect may require skeletal support in the form of rib grafts or nylon mesh (Figure 10.19). This is discussed in Chapter 5. After this support is utilized, the omentum is placed in the wound and secured with interrupted chromic sutures to the

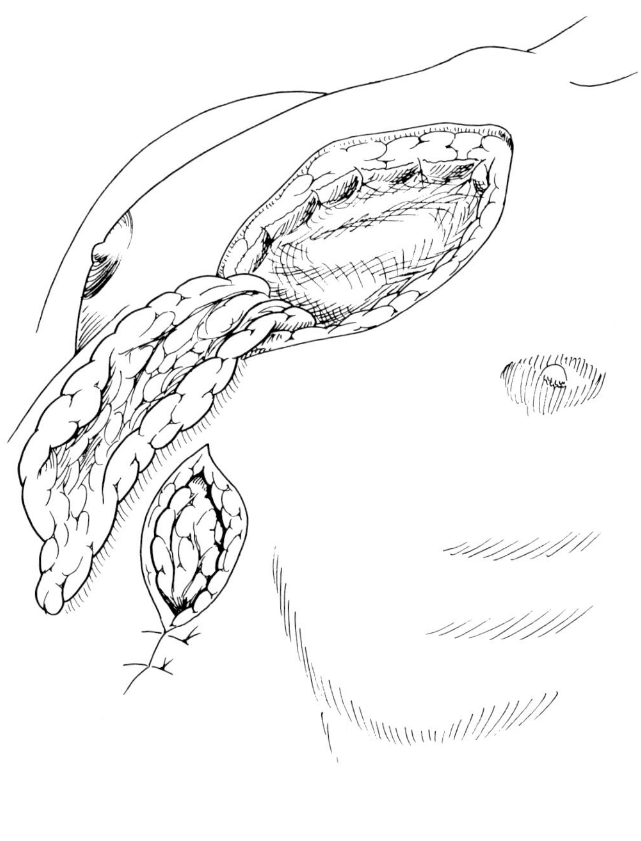

FIGURE 10.19 After reconstruction of the musculoskeletal layer, the omentum is drawn through the tunnel (or placed in the opened trough). Here, the skeletal layer has been reconstructed with a synthetic mesh.

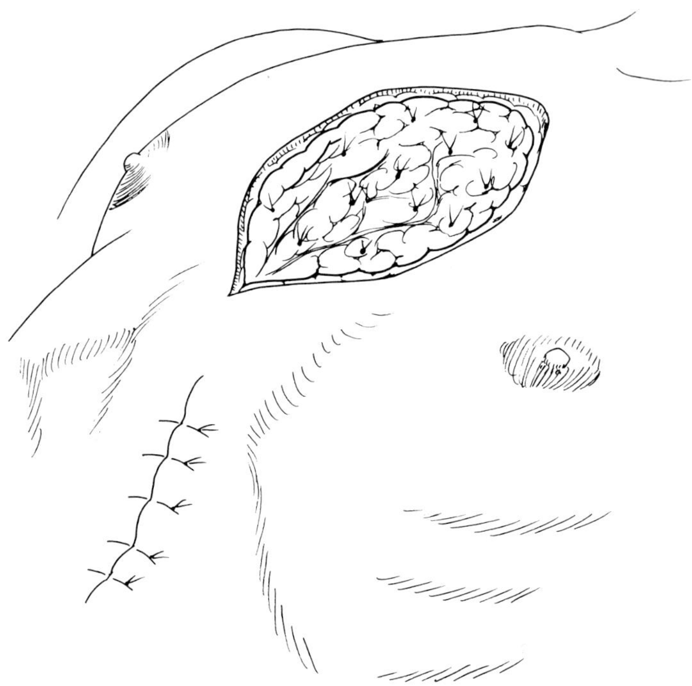

FIGURE 10.20A The omentum is secured to the edges of the defect and to the deeper structures with a few absorbable sutures. Care is taken to avoid injury to the many fine omental vessels. Such injury could cause a hematoma and difficulties with subsequent healing.

deeper structures and skin edges (Figure 10.20A). Care is taken to avoid injury to the omental vessels, which, again, could result in a hematoma and difficulty due to loss of flap pliability or the subsequent healing of the skin graft. A meshed, split-thickness skin graft of intermediate thickness is placed on the omentum. It is meshed 1.5 to 1 and applied unexpanded. The meshing allows collections of serum to drain through the graft without lifting it off its bed. Meshing also allows the graft to fit the irregular contours of the omental flap. Leaving it unexpanded allows it to heal as a sheet of durable skin. A few quilting sutures of interrupted chromic are placed to assure that every part of the graft is secured to the omentum (Figure 10.20B). This assures a better take of the graft.

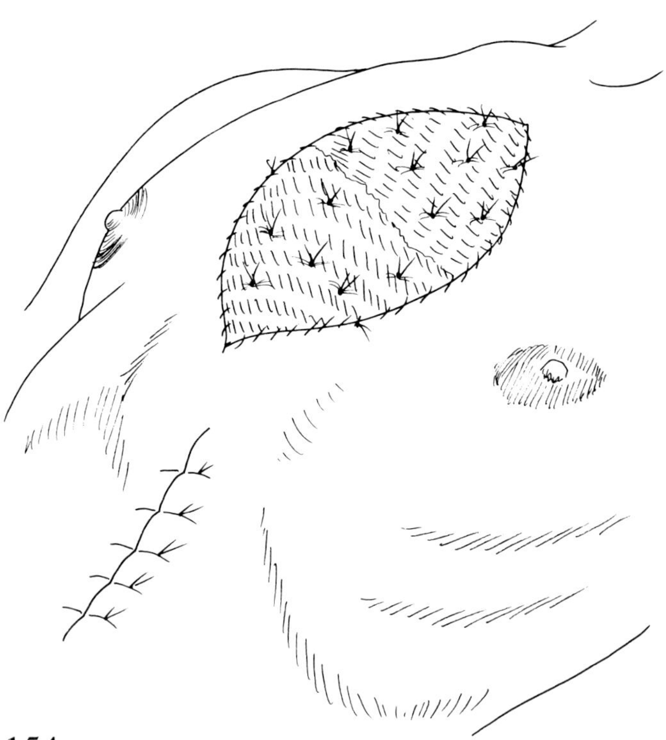

FIGURE 10.20B A meshed split-thickness skin graft is applied to the surface of the omentum flap to provide coverage. The meshing allows it to fit the irregular contours more efficiently as well as provide for drainage of fluid collections (which could lift the graft from its bed). A few quilting sutures are added to ensure good contact between the graft and the omentum.

A fine mesh gauze is placed on the skin graft and covered with saline-moistened cloth sponges. These sponges are kept moist with saline on the ward for 3 to 4 days. This prevents the interstitial areas between the meshed graft from desiccating until epithelialization occurs from the adjacent areas of the skin graft. This growth of new skin usually is accomplished within 4 days, and the dressing can be gently removed. After this, antibacterial ointment is applied directly to the graft to prevent encrustation and scaling. This is done until the graft regains sebaceous activity.

ILLUSTRATIVE CASE

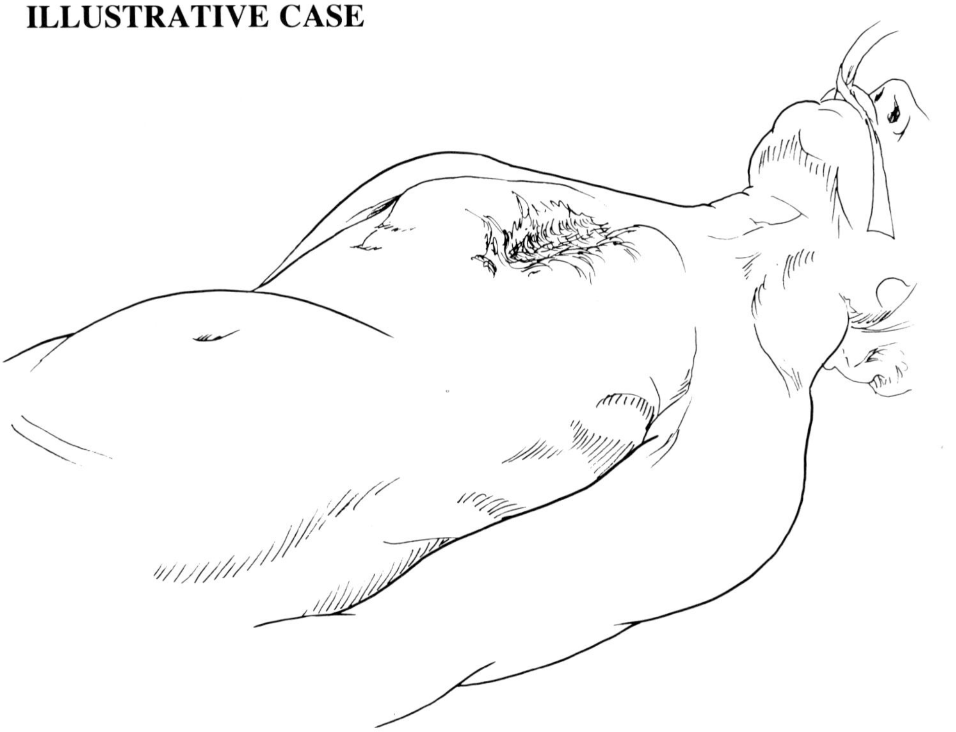

FIGURE 10.21 A 54-year-old female developed central sternal breakdown 20 years after a bilateral radical mastectomy and high-dose radiotherapy. Biopsy of the ulcerated area shows no recurrent cancer.

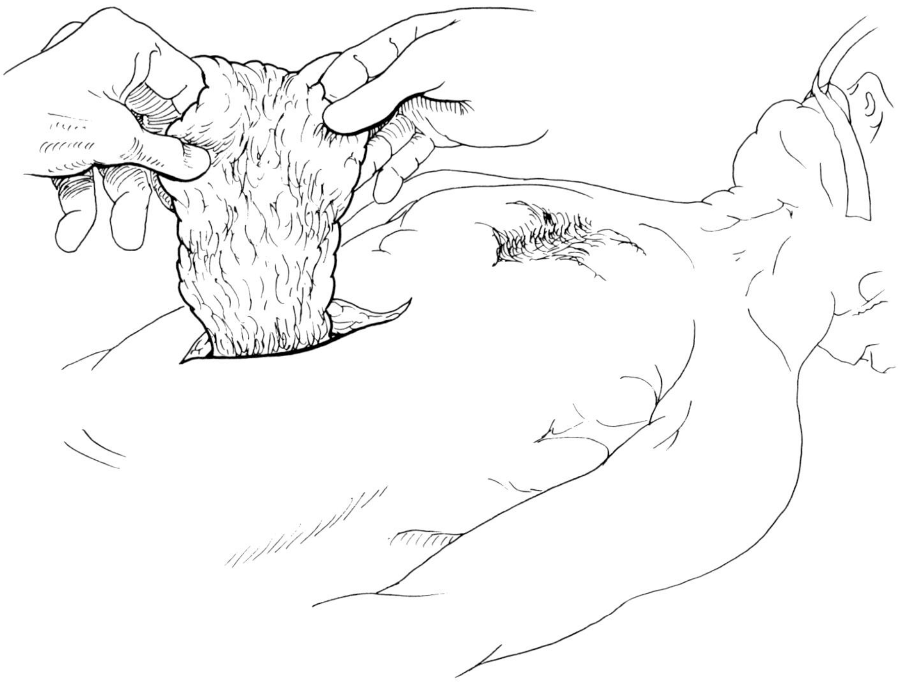

FIGURE 10.22 Because the patient has only one functional latissimus, a weakened shoulder girdle, and arm lymphedema, the omentum is the first choice to fill the postresection defect. Abdominal exploration reveals a voluminous omentum suitable for the purpose.

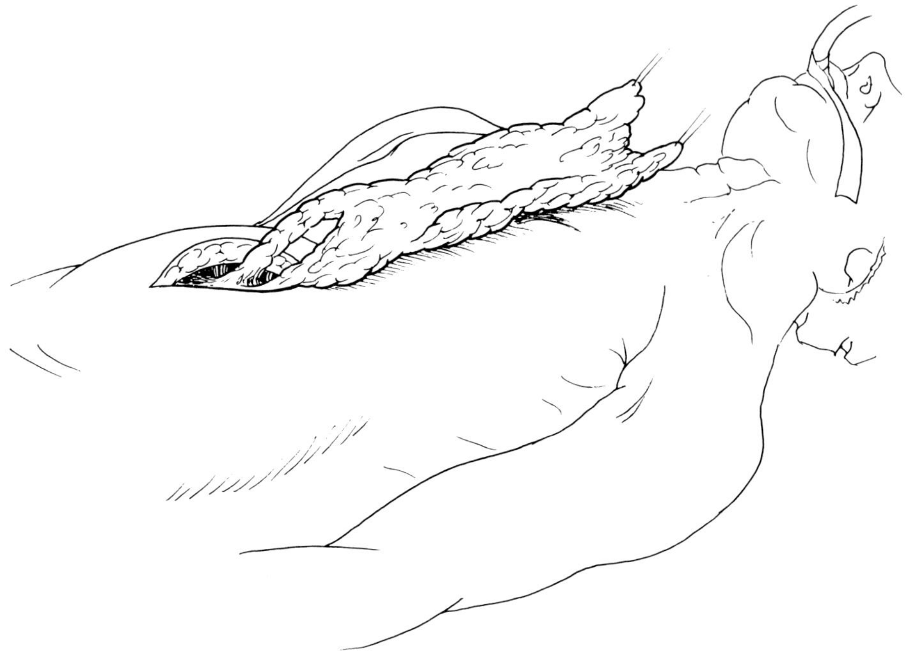

FIGURE 10.23 The omentum easily reaches beyond the defect without lengthening.

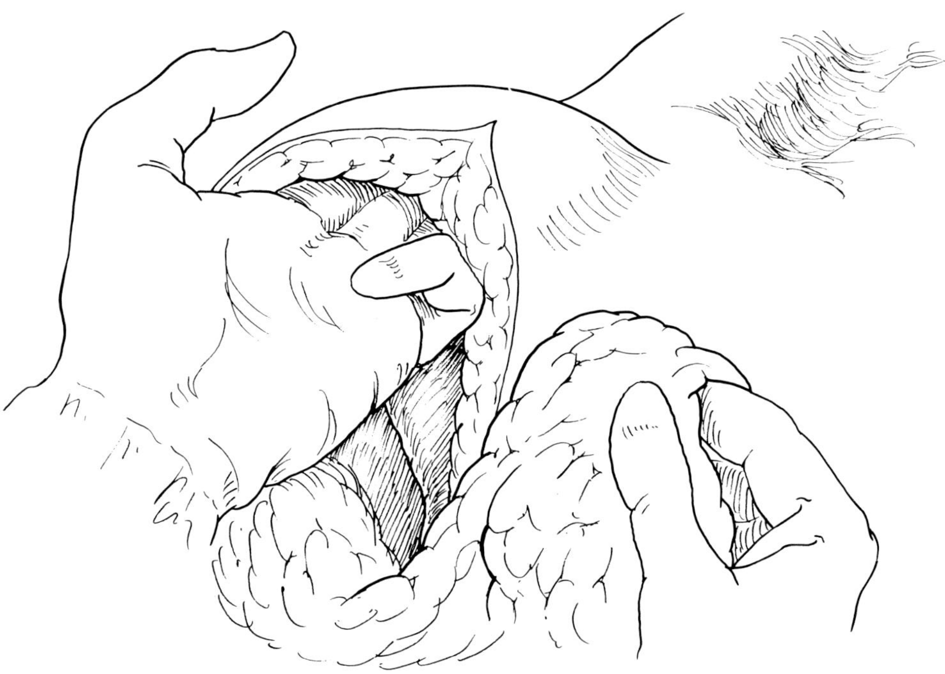

FIGURE 10.24 The lower portion of the subcutaneous tunnel is dissected and the abdomen closed. Attention is then turned to the sternum.

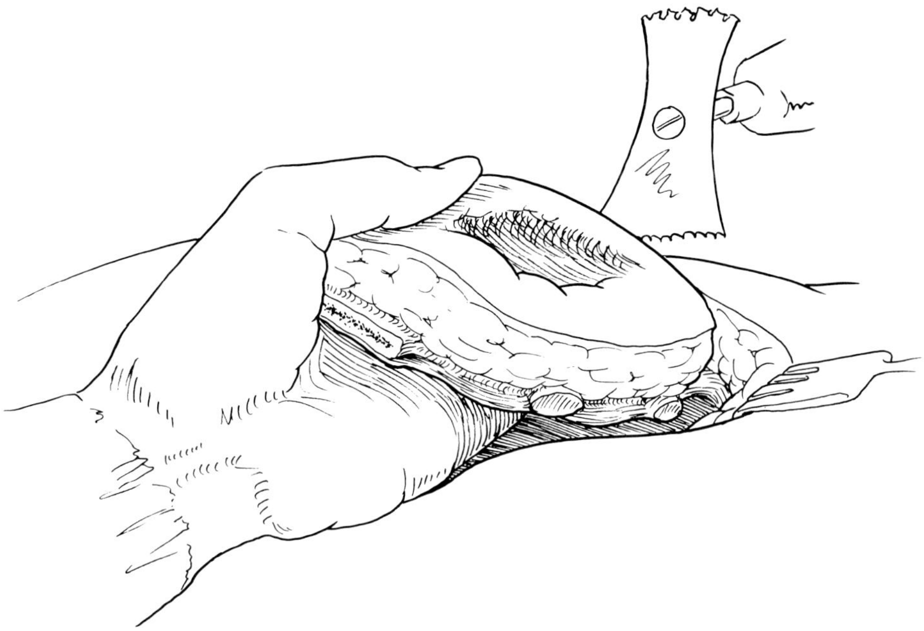

FIGURE 10.25 The necrotic sternum and surrounding tissues are resected beyond the area of tenderness and back to normal tissue.

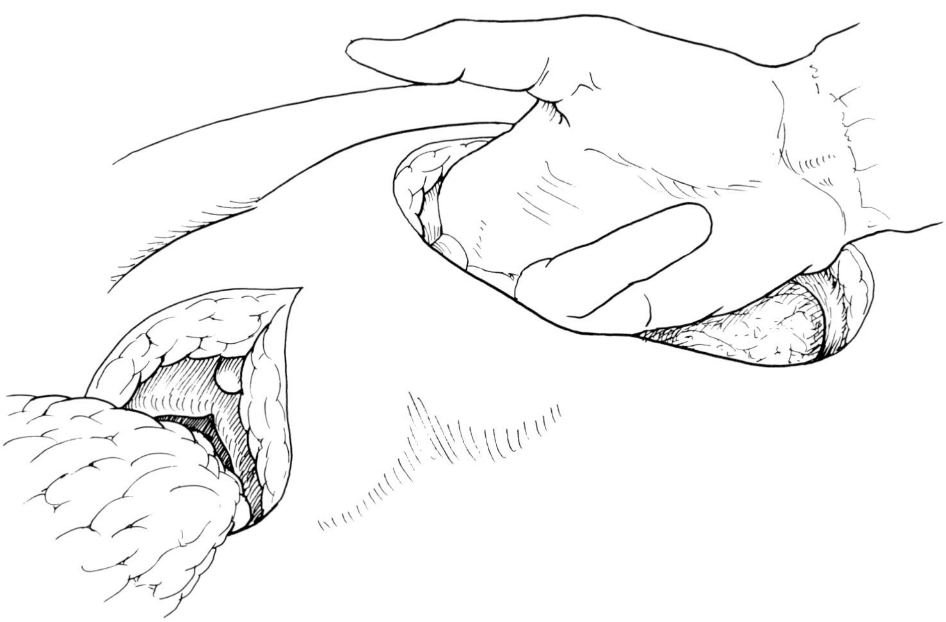

FIGURE 10.26 The cephalad portion of the tunnel is now dissected to allow easy passage of the surgeon's hand.

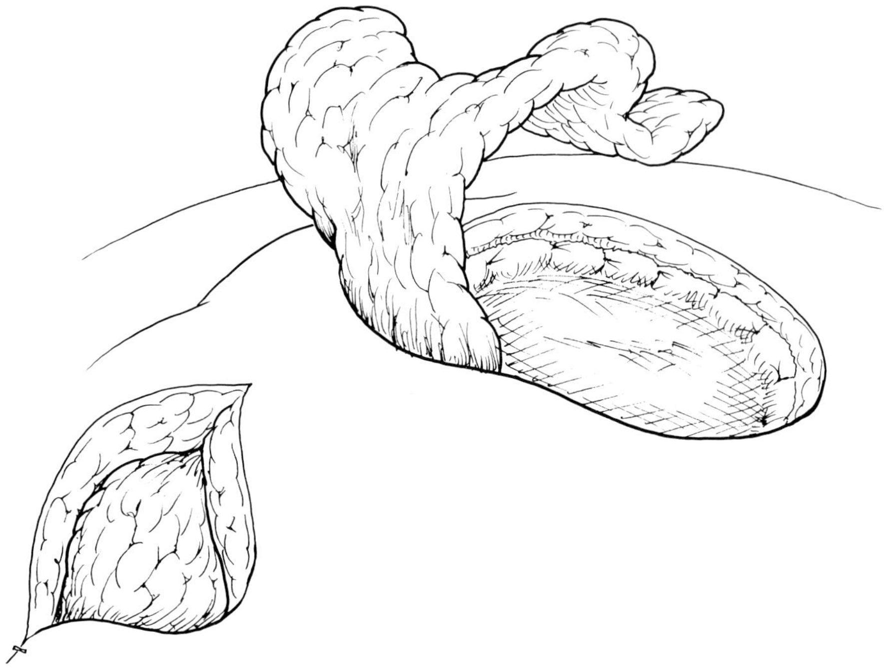

FIGURE 10.27 The musculoskeletal layer is reconstructed with polypropylene mesh to protect the heart and great vessels, and the omentum is passed through the tunnel.

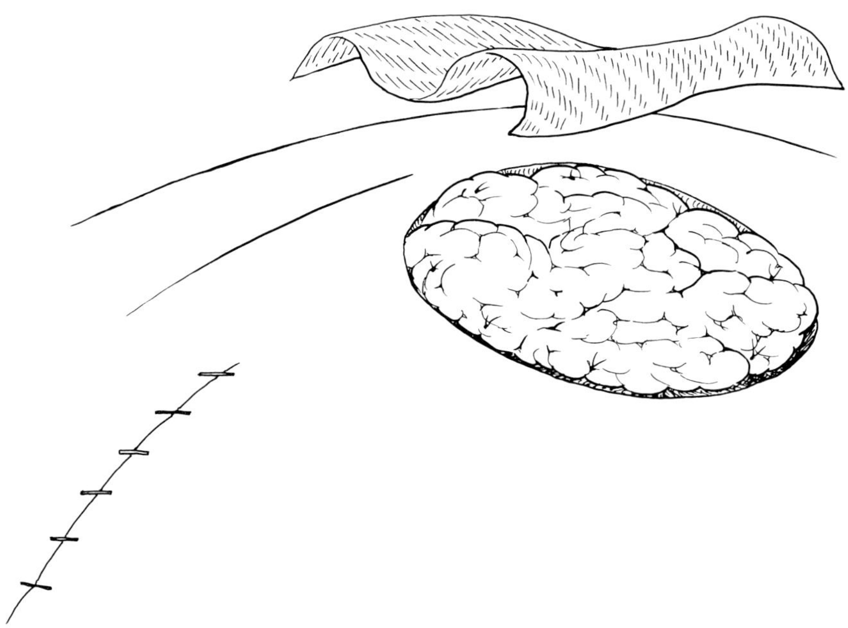

FIGURE 10.28 The omentum is loosely sutured to the margins of the defect and covered with a meshed, unexpanded split-thickness skin graft. The abdominal incision is closed. The patient continues to do well 5 years after the operation. The flap is well healed and soft. The polypropylene mesh, although applied tightly, is now somewhat lax.

11

The Rectus Abdominis Muscle and Musculocutaneous Flaps

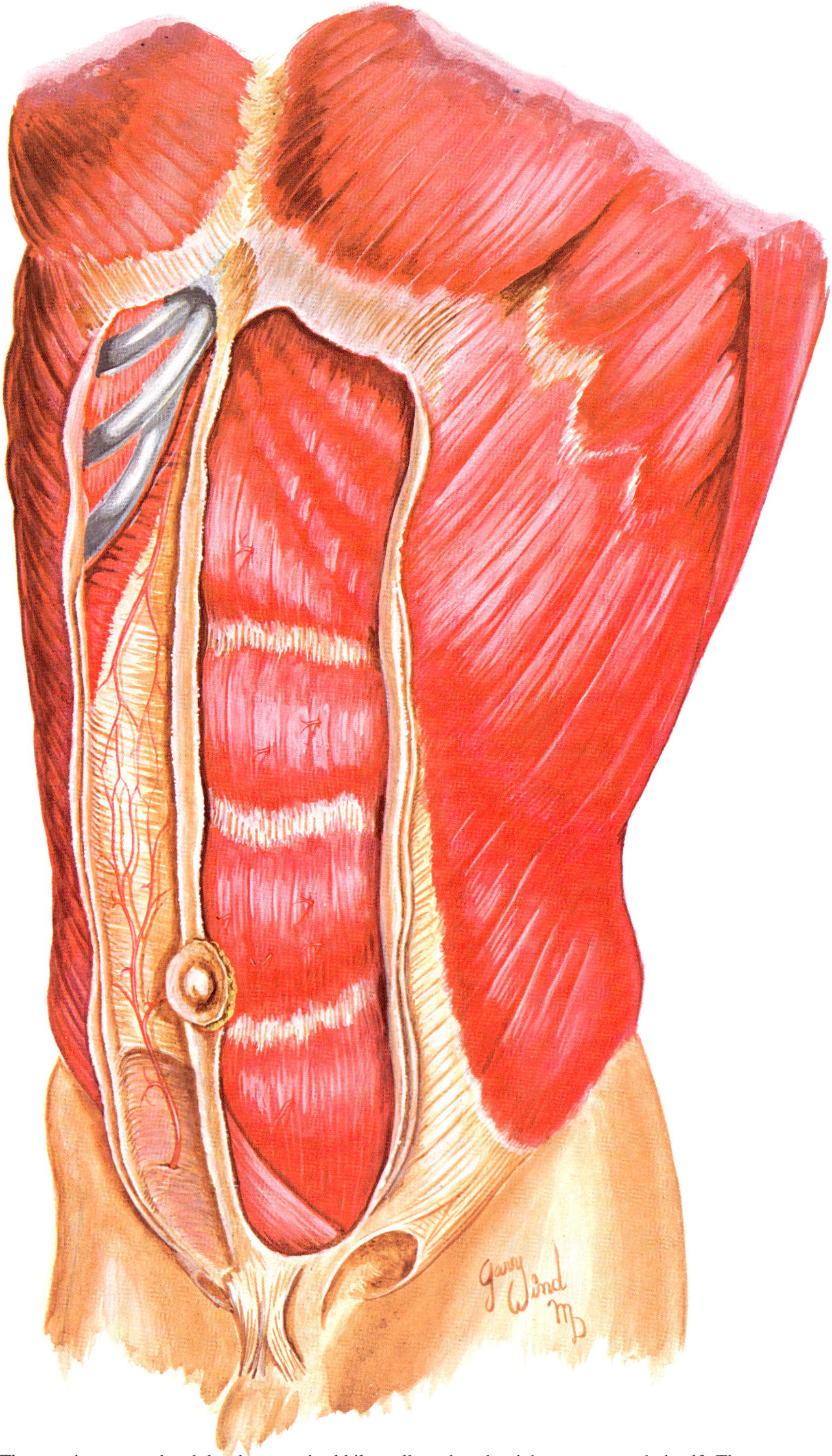

The anterior rectus sheath has been excised bilaterally as has the right rectus muscle itself. The intramuscular plexus of communicating vessels originating from superior and inferior epigastrics can be seen on the figure's right. The anterior perforating branches of these vessels can be seen on the opposite side emerging from the muscle. These vessels, more heavily concentrated around the umbilicus, penetrate the anterior rectus sheath to supply the overlying abdominal skin.

Anatomy

The rectus abdominis is a flat bandlike muscle originating from the crest of the pubis by a short broad tendon whose medial portion interdigitates with its contralateral counterpart (Plate 11.1). The variable, triangular pyramidalis muscle arises just anterior to the rectus origin and inserts into the linea alba between the pubis and umbilicus. At its cephalad end, the rectus becomes flatter and broader before inserting into the fifth, sixth, and seventh costal cartilages. There are usually three irregular fibrous bands crossing the muscle at the xiphoid, the umbilicus, and midway between the two. These segmental bands are variable and often incomplete, rarely passing through the full thickness of the muscle to its deep surface. The bands do form attachments to the anterior rectus sheath, especially at the margins of the muscle, and frequently contain small blood vessels.

The rectus sheath consists of fused layers of aponeurosis from the external oblique, internal oblique, and transversus abdominis muscles. The posterior sheath incorporates the transversus aponeurosis and posterior lamella of the split internal oblique aponeurosis. At the arcuate line situated between the umbilicus and pubis, the aponeurosis of both of these muscles contributes only to the anterior sheath, leaving just the transversalis fascia between the muscle and the peritoneum. The external oblique aponeurosis fuses with the anterior sheath in a diagonal line closer to the midline at the pubis than at the xiphoid.

The rectus muscle and overlying abdominal skin are supplied by a lattice of vascular channels originating in the superior epigastric vessels above and the inferior epigastric vessels below. The superior epigastric artery is the smaller of the two feeding vessels and is the continuation of the internal thoracic after that vessel gives off the musculophrenic artery at the level of the sixth intercostal space. The superior epigastric artery and its accompanying veins penetrate the costoxiphoid attachment of the diaphragm to reach the posterior surface of the rectus muscle, where it frequently divides and penetrates into the muscle.

The larger inferior epigastric vessels arise from the external iliac artery and vein and run between the transversalis fascia and peritoneum past the medial margin of the deep inguinal ring. They penetrate the transversalis fascia and enter the rectus sheath between the pubis and umbilicus. The vessels divide and penetrate the muscle to give off muscular branches, an umbilical branch, lateral segmental branches, and musculocutaneous perforators. Multiple fine (<.5 mm) terminal branches of the two systems anastomose within the muscle midway between the umbilicus and xiphoid. The largest cutaneous branches penetrate directly from the main vascular axis through the anterior rectus sheath to the overlying skin. Smaller branches penetrate through the linea alba and the lateral edge of the rectus sheath. Several lateral segmental branches, arising mostly from the inferior epigastric, anastomose with terminal branches of the lower six intercostal arteries. The majority of the cutaneous branches also arise from the inferior epigastric, and the greatest concentration of these perforators is found around the umbilicus.

Innervation to the rectus and overlying skin is supplied by sensory and motor fibers contained in the ventral rami of T7–T12. These nerves emerge behind the costal cartilages to reach the plane between the internal oblique and transversus muscles, where adjacent nerves freely communicate. The nerves then pierce the lateral margin of the rectus sheath, penetrate the muscle posteriorly, and innervate it before sending terminal sensory cutaneous branches through a series of small hiatuses in the anterior rectus sheath. As a rule, T10 terminates around the umbilicus, T12 reaches the pubis.

The rectus abdominis muscle flexes the vertebral column, bringing the sternum toward the pubis. Absence of the rectus may impair this action and may permit the pelvis to tilt anteriorly, exaggerating lumbar lordosis. A more serious consequence is the potential for ventral herniation, especially if a large portion of the anterior rectus sheath has been removed below the level of the arcuate line. Both of these risks are potentially greater when both rectus muscles are used as flaps.

General Characteristics

The rectus abdominis flap is useful in two ways: (1) as a muscle flap alone and (2) as a musculocutaneous (combined muscle-skin) flap. As a muscle flap, the rectus provides a long strip of vascular tissue that can be used to fill cavitary defects and to increase the capacity for healing in compromised wounds, especially in and around the lower sternum.

As a muscle-skin (musculocutaneous) flap, it affords thick coverage and a variety of options in tailoring the skin segment to meet specific needs. For example, due to the extensive vascular territory (see Chapter 3 for the concept of vascular territories) supplied by the epigastric vessels, a large area of skin on the anterior abdominal wall becomes available for potential use in chest wall reconstruction with the rectus as a carrier for the cutaneous segment (Figure 11.1). Certain areas of this territory are more useful (and reliable) than others. The areas directly over the muscle and those near the umbilicus are safer than other regions due to the higher concentration of vessels to the overlying skin in these locations (Figure 11.2). If thick skin coverage is required, the first choice is the vertical rectus abdominis musculocutaneous flap. Since the skin segment is directly over the muscle, it has the best blood supply and is therefore more reliable. The next choice would be the transverse musculocutaneous flap. If skin coverage is not required, the rectus muscle alone should be considered.

When used as a transverse muscle-skin flap, it is somewhat different from other musculocutaneous flaps in that relatively little bulk is provided by the muscle itself. The greater volume of such a flap, which depends on the underlying strip of muscle for viability, is composed of skin and subcutaneous fat. Such a ratio is different from that of other musculocutaneous flaps, which usually contain more muscle than skin and fat. Having more skin and fat, however, is not necessarily an advantage since the adipose tissue, due to its poorer blood supply, is not as resistant to infection and is generally less hearty than muscle tissue. In dealing with cavitary defects or with tissues compromised

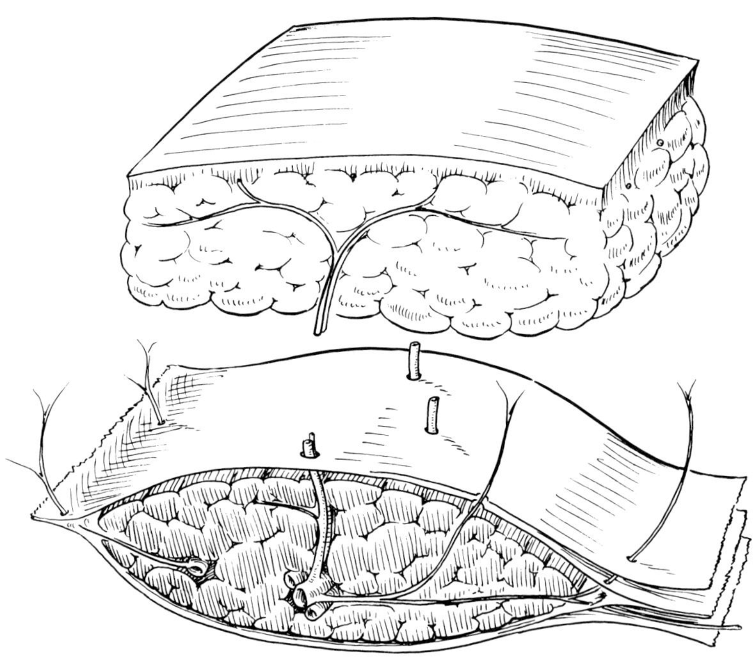

FIGURE 11.1 Vascular territories or specific areas of skin derive their circulation from the underlying muscle. These arterioles perforate the fascia and arborize in the subdermal plexus that nourishes the skin.

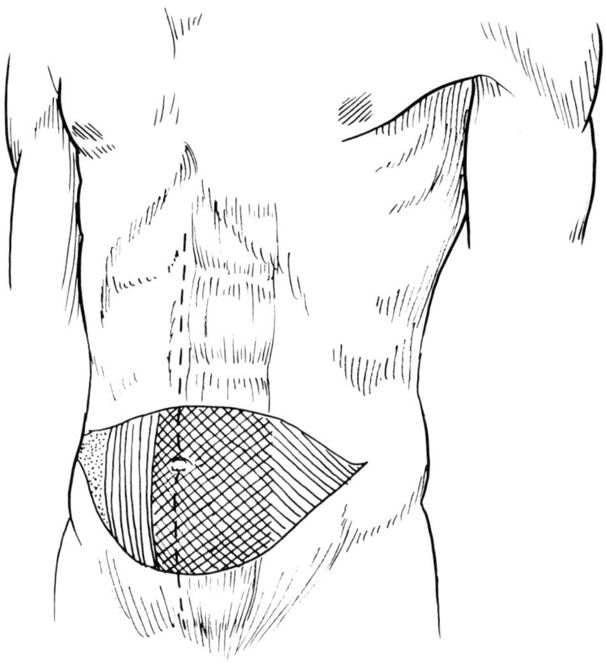

FIGURE 11.2 The most reliable area of the transverse rectus abdominis musculocutaneous flap overlies the muscle itself. Here, this area, overlying the patient's left rectus abdominis muscle, is crosshatched. It contains the greatest concentration of arterioles to the skin. Other areas are not as reliable but can still retain viability. The diagonal and vertical lined regions are in this category. The speckled area is unreliable and should not be used in the reconstruction. For a right-sided flap, the areas are a mirror of the preceding description. A previous midline incision limits the skin territory in that the skin area on the other side of the scar should not be used.

by unfavorable influences (e.g., radiation or infection), muscle tissue or the omentum should be used rather than skin and fat. Despite these disadvantages, this combined flap can provide coverage and healing even under adverse conditions.

The range or reach of the flap, along with the large parcel of tissue it can provide, is its greatest asset. The composite musculocutaneous (transverse abdominal) flap is used most effectively in patients who have a thick (though tight) layer of abdominal fat, especially in the region of the umbilicus and hypogastrium. In these patients, more material is available to fill the defect in the chest wall. However, it should not be loose fat that hangs as an apron. Such laxity or obesity is, in fact, a contraindication to the use of the muscle-skin flap since the blood supply to the fat and skin are much attenuated in these patients. Advanced age is also a relative contraindication for the same reason. A better alternative in these patients would be to use the muscle alone or a vertical rectus flap.

Before selecting this flap, one must be certain that the vascular pedicle is intact. For sternal defects, the internal thoracic artery on which the flap is based must be uninjured. Previous radiation to the artery doesn't necessarily rule it out since the flap can survive despite this insult. However, sternal resections or sternal retention sutures can interrupt its course and render the flap unusable. Likewise, previous cholecystectomy incisions, or any incisions that have divided the rectus muscle, result in necrosis of the flap distal to the point of previous division of the pedicle. If the internal mammary artery has been used to revascularize the heart, this contraindicates its use. If there is any question, arteriography should be obtained. The skin segment which is on the opposite side of the midline is likewise unusable if there has been a previous midline incision.

One of the disadvantages of using the rectus abdominis flap with a transverse island of skin is the length of time required for the meticulous dissection. It is not uncommon for the mobilization and closure of the donor site to take 3 or 4 hours. This must be considered and weighed against the patient's ability to withstand such a procedure safely.

The muscle-only flap or the flap with a vertical skin segment can be harvested more rapidly, and the length of the overall operation is usually much shorter. Also, this vertical flap and the muscle-alone flap are more reliable from a vascular standpoint than the transverse flap.

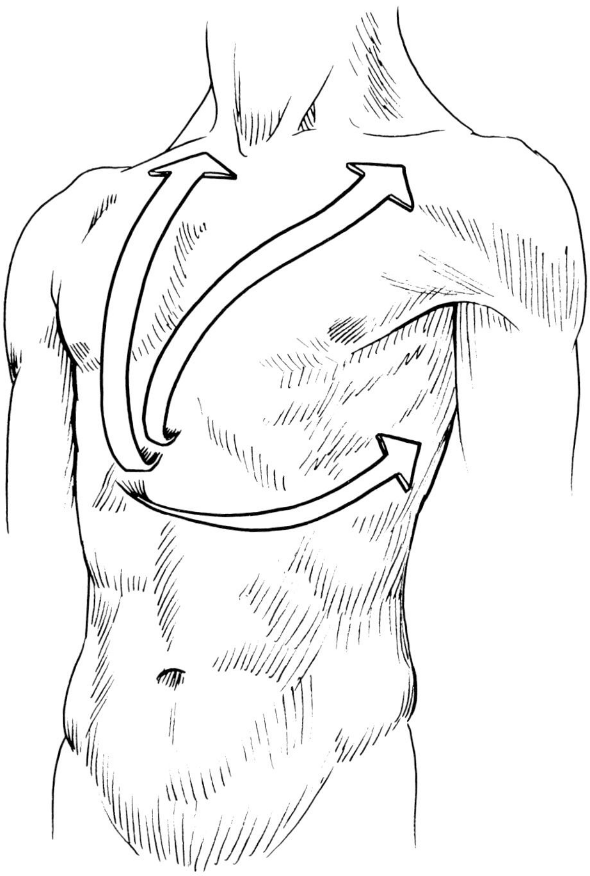

FIGURE 11.3 The arc of rotation or reach of the rectus abdominis muscle and musculocutaneous flap—when based on its superior pedicle, the internal thoracic artery and its continuation, the superior epigastric artery—is most useful for the reconstruction of anterior and anterolateral chest wall defects.

Relative contraindications include patients who are smokers, due to the vasoconstrictive effects of nicotine; obesity, due to the less reliable vascularity associated with a thick panniculus; advanced age; inadequate bulk of tissue over the lower abdominal wall; and previous abdominal incisions that may devascularize the flap.

The flap has two arcs of rotation. One arc is based on the deep inferior epigastric artery and can be used for coverage of lower abdominal, flank, and lower extremity defects as far distally as the upper knee area. The other arc is based on the superior epigastric and internal thoracic arteries. It can be swung upward for lateral, midline, or upper anterior chest wall defects as far as the shoulder and clavicular areas. This latter arc is used for reconstruction of the chest wall (Figure 11.3). It is also possible to use both rectus flaps simultaneously.

Preoperative Planning

The transverse rectus is described first since it is the most difficult to mobilize and since the main principles are applicable to the other two alternatives. It is convenient for the surgeon to sit in front of the patient, who is standing. The anticipated chest wall defect is measured. If an ulcerative radionecrotic defect is present, palpating for tenderness over the bony and cartilaginous segments of the ribs can give an indication of the extent of the upcoming resection. Such tenderness correlates relatively well with the area of necrotic and damaged tissue that should be removed. This perimeter of proposed excision is marked on the skin with a marking pen and its diameter measured (Figure 11.4). The flap of choice is the contralateral rectus rather than the ipsilateral since there is less chance of kinking or constriction of the vascular pedicle.

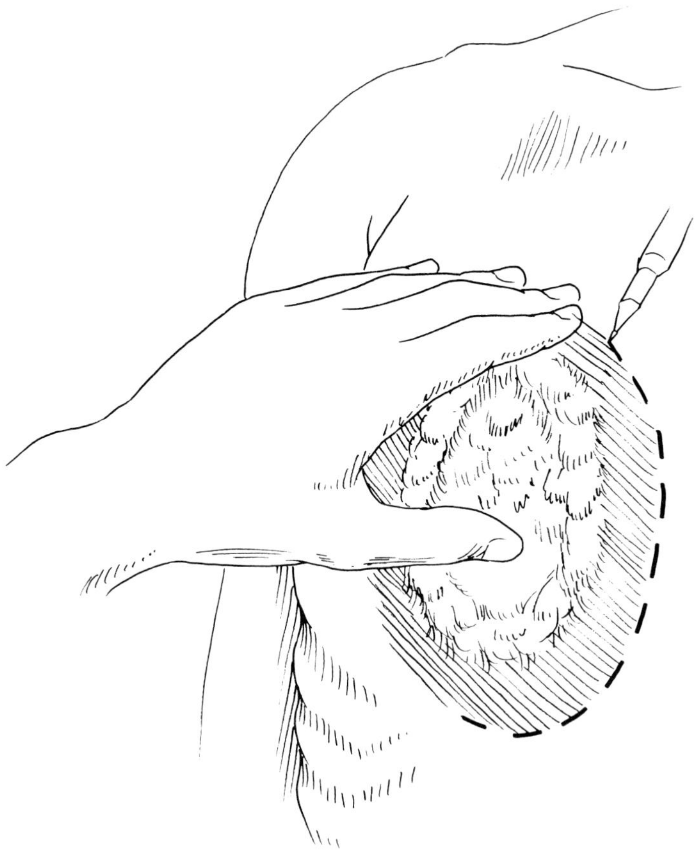

FIGURE 11.4 In planning the extent of the chest wall excision, the margins of the proposed defect are correlated with physical and radiographic findings and marked.

The Transverse Rectus Flap

The anterior superior iliac crests are palpated, and a curved line is drawn between two marks that are situated 5 cm above the crests. The midpoint of the curve is 5–8 cm cephalad to the umbilicus (Figure 11.5). The lower abdominal skin and fat are grasped and stretched to gain a mental picture of the amount of filler that will be available (Figure 11.6). One is reminded that the fat must be ample and the skin area somewhat mobile but not to the point where it hangs loosely. If it is this loose, the blood supply to the fat and skin is unreliable. One end of the tape measure is placed 6–7 cm lateral to the midline, at the level of the xiphoid process, and over the cephalad portion of the selected rectus muscle. This is the pivot point for the flap and represents the fixed part of the vascular pedicle on which the flap will turn to reach the chest wall defect. The other end of the tape is swung from the lower abdomen (about two-thirds of the distance from the umbilicus to the pubis and 2–5 cm above the pubic hair line) up over the proposed chest wall defect (Figure 11.7). This gives a general idea as to the reach of the flap, and the surgeon can get an idea as to how the tissue will fit into the defect.

Another arc is drawn on the patient to complement the first line and to complete a large ellipse. The midpoint of this latter line is 2–5 cm above the pubic hairline and the lateral extensions of the arc sweep upward to meet the ends of the previously marked line, just cephalad to the anterior iliac spines (Figure 11.8). The rectus muscle is drawn in and the defect is again measured. A mental picture of how the flap will swing up to the defect and which portion of the flap will cover the defect is made. This portion of the flap is also measured to assess the width required to repair the defect adequately. The loose abdominal skin and fat is again grasped to get an idea of how the abdominal layers will close after this large segment is removed. It should be fairly loose, even though the extensive mobilization of the abdominal tissue certainly aids in this closure of the donor site.

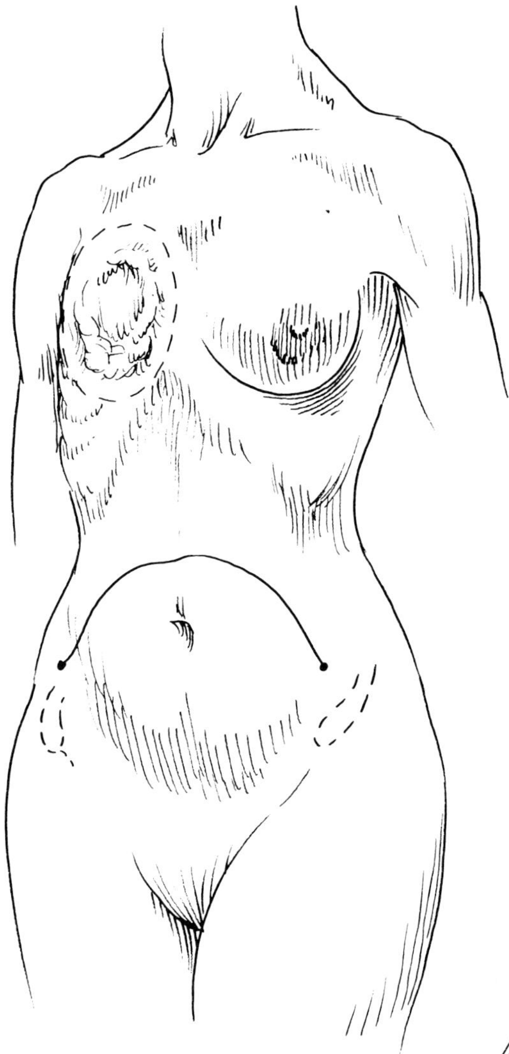

FIGURE 11.5 The upper border of the transverse rectus abdominis musculocutaneous flap is marked. With a standard flap, this corresponds to a line that begins 5 cm cephalad to each anterior superior iliac crest and arcs 5–8 cm cephalad to the umbilicus.

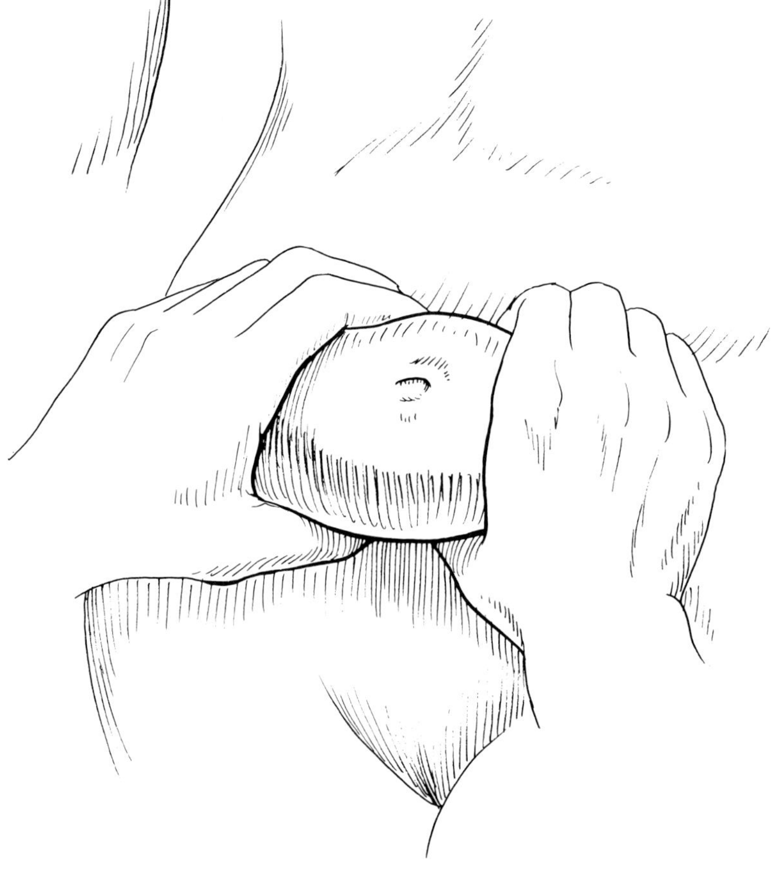

FIGURE 11.6 The lower abdominal skin and fat are grasped to assess the amount of filler available for the chest wall defect. The fatty layer should be thick and somewhat adherent to the fascia. A thin layer of fat and skin that hangs in an apron renders the skin portion unreliable from a vascular standpoint due to the poor condition of the musculocutaneous perforating vessels.

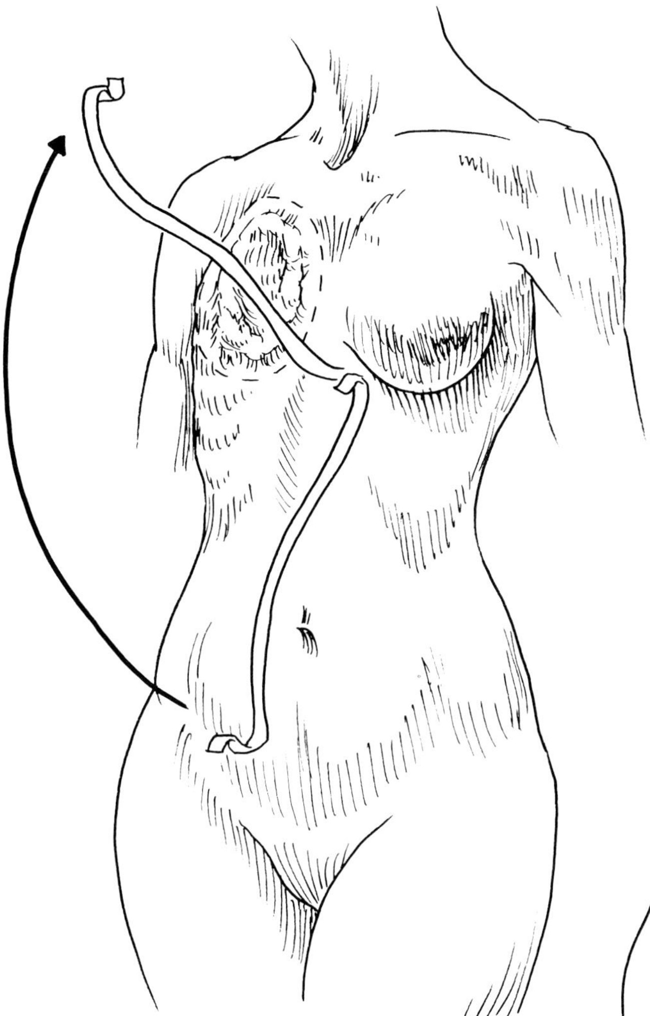

FIGURE 11.7 In checking the arc of rotation or reach of the flap, one end of the tape measure is placed 6–7 cm lateral to the midline and at the level of the xiphoid. This is the approximate location of the vascular pedicle on which the flap will turn in order to reach the chest wall defect (i.e., the pivot point). The other end is placed over the lower reaches of the flap and swung up over the proposed defect. It should overshoot the defect with room to spare.

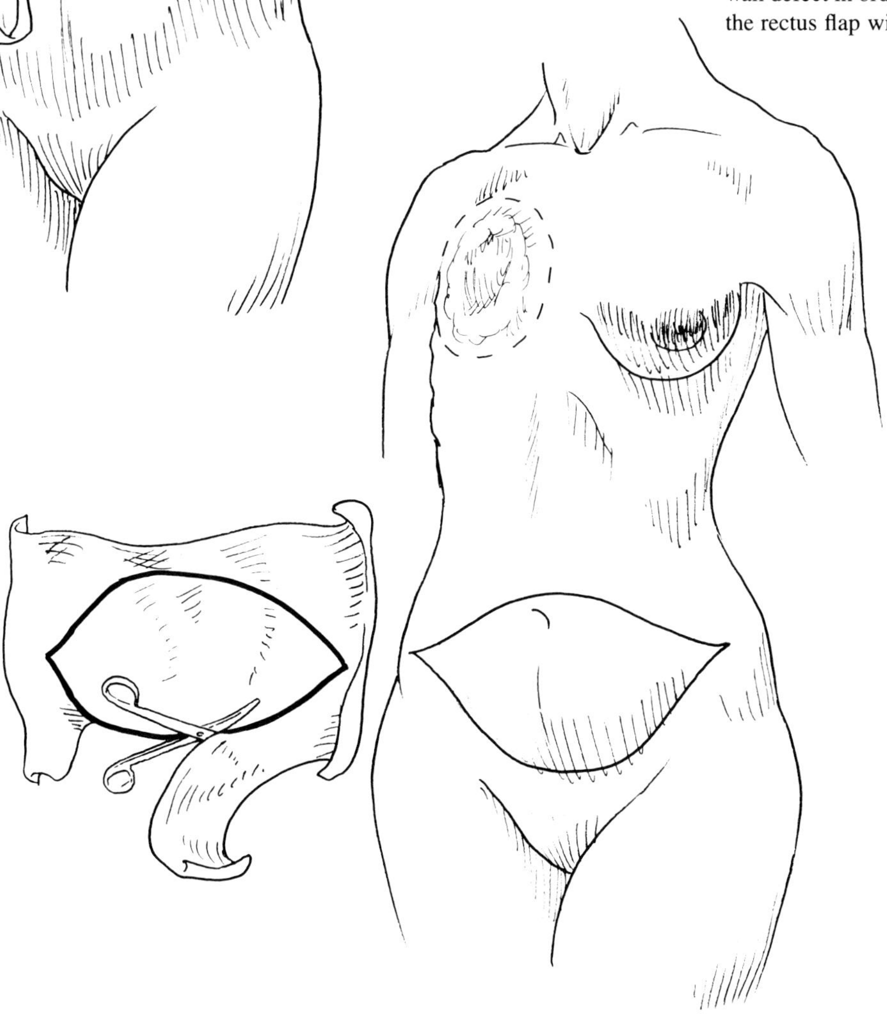

FIGURE 11.8 The lower arc of the flap is drawn in 2–5 cm above the pubic hairline. The flap is elliptical in shape to facilitate closure of the abdominal donor skin defect without lateral redundancy. A cloth flap may be cut and rotated up over the proposed chest wall defect in order to assess how the rectus flap will fit.

It may help to cut a piece of cloth into the shape of the proposed flap and to rotate this cloth flap up into the area of the defect (Figure 11.8). This allows accurate planning as to the size and shape of the final flap. If there is any doubt, plans are made for alternate or additional flaps. The reason for the elliptical shape is for ease in closure of the donor site. This large flap may offer more tissue than needed at the recipient defect, but it can be economically trimmed during the operation so that such waste is minimized. The part of the flap across the midline and away from the pedicle is unreliable. Plans should be made to discard it before setting the flap into the chest wall defect.

Mobilization of the Transverse Flap

The patient is supine on the operating table but is positioned to allow bending at the waist and being brought into a sitting position during the operation. After endotracheal anesthesia and the appropriate lines are in place, and after an initial cleansing of the chest area, the thoracic defect is plugged with absorbent, cotton sponges, and a portion of rubber glove is stapled over the defect to prevent contamination of other areas. The thorax, abdomen, upper arms, and thighs are then reprepared and the field is draped (Figure 11.9).

The upper limb of the previously marked ellipse is entered and the incision carried down to the deep fascia. The incision is beveled away from the planned skin flap to preserve perforating vessels to the skin (Figure 11.10). The skin and fat away from the flap and over the upper abdomen and lower anterior chest wall are elevated from the fascia, cauterizing the perforating vessels before they are divided (Figure 11.11). This prevents subfascial and rectus muscular hematomas that, if large enough, could compromise the flap. After this wide mobilization, the patient is moved to a 45° sitting position, and the mobilized skin and fat are brought down over the undisturbed lower abdomen as in a vest-over-pants maneuver. Skin hooks or sutures are used. At the same time, the

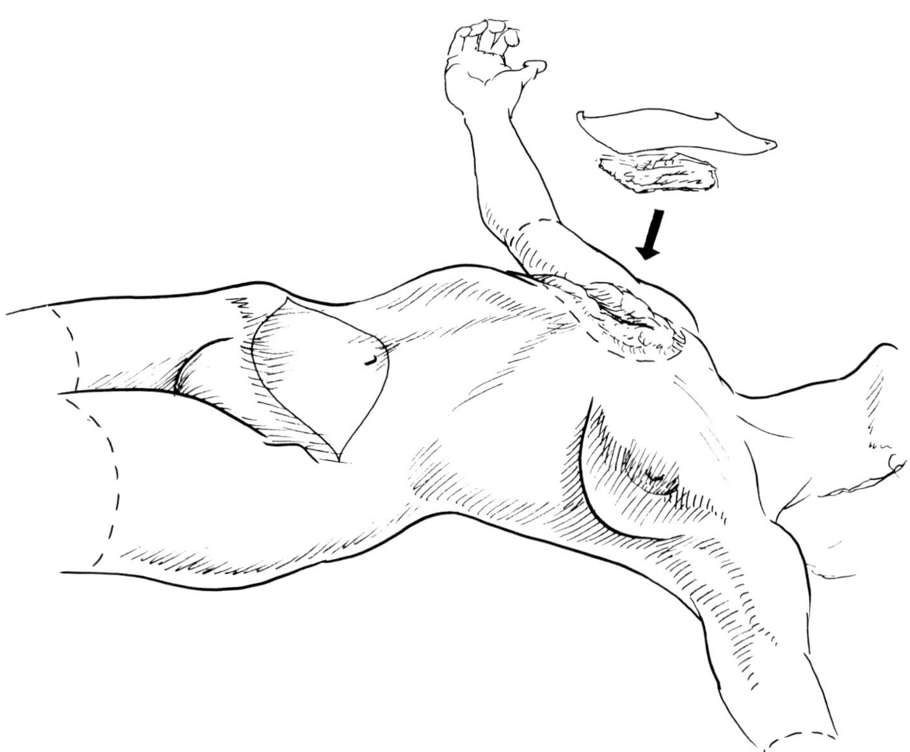

FIGURE 11.9 The patient is supine on the operating table. Appropriate monitoring lines, endotracheal tube, and Foley catheter have been inserted. The area is widely prepared (dotted lines), and a cotton sponge and rubber dam are used to isolate the contaminated chest wall lesion.

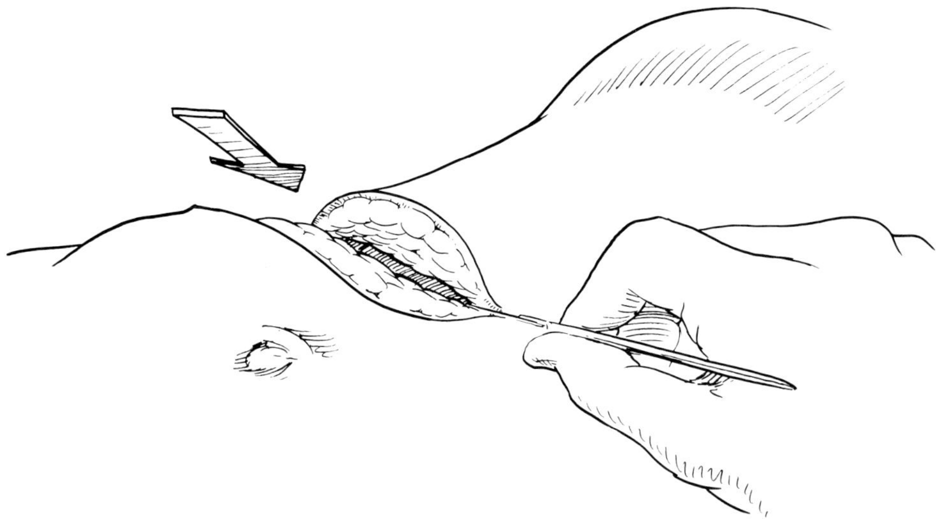

FIGURE 11.10 The upper arc of the incision is entered, beveling the fat away from the umbilicus to preserve any perforating vessels to the skin portion of the flap. The incision is deepened to the anterior abdominal (deep) fascia.

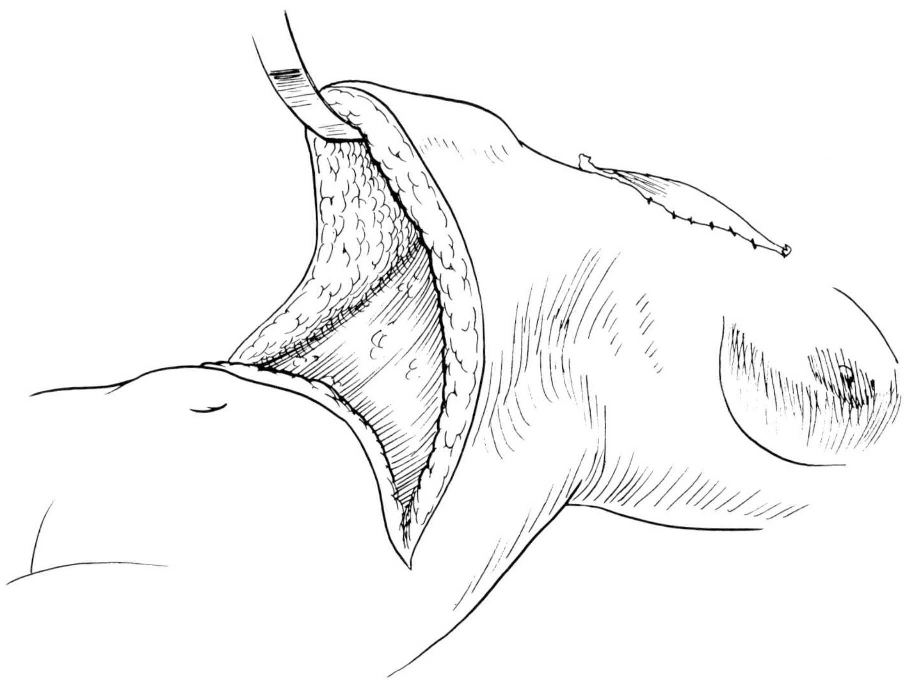

FIGURE 11.11 The skin and fat (away from the flap) are elevated off the deep fascia, cauterizing the abdominal perforating vessels before they are transected. The dissection is carried out over the ipsilateral rectus muscle as well as over the contralateral abdomen and lower chest wall. This wide mobilization facilitates the abdominal skin closure after removal of the rectus flap.

undisturbed lower abdominal tissues are swept upward by external (hand) pressure (Figure 11.12). This allows the surgeon to assess how large a flap of tissue can be removed and still allow safe closure of the donor site. The lower reach of the mobilized tissue is conservatively marked on the undisturbed abdominal skin with a marking pen (Figure 11.12). The new line represents the lower edge of the proposed flap. If preoperative measurements were accurate, the line should coincide with the preoperative marks. The patient is returned to the supine position.

The newly marked, lower margin of the flap is incised down to the deep fascia, again beveling the incision away from the skin flap to preserve the perforating vessels (Figure 11.13). Starting on the contralateral side (away from the rectus muscle that will eventually be the carrier for the skin flap), the skin and subcutaneous fat are separated from the deep fascia (Figure 11.14). The dissection is carried across the linea alba (midline decussation) approximately 1 cm onto the fascia overlying the rectus muscle. Any large perforators along this arbitrary 1-cm line are preserved.

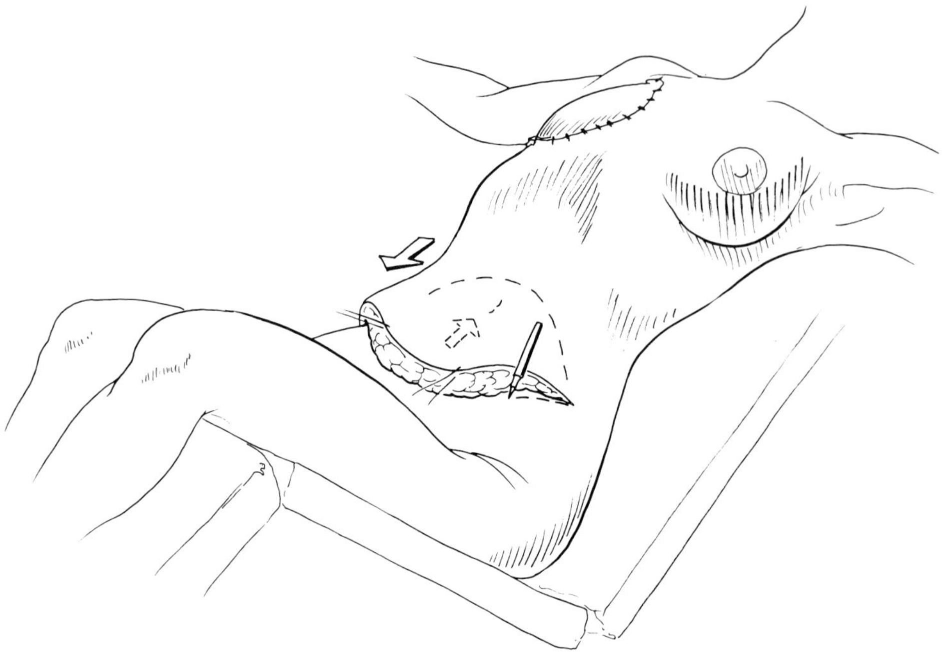

FIGURE 11.12 After the upper abdominal tissues are mobilized up over the costal areas, the patient is bent at the hips and the mobilized tissues are pulled downward toward the pubis (solid arrow). At the same time, the lower abdominal skin is pushed upward (dotted arrow). This gives an idea of how large a flap can be removed and still allow primary closure. The skin is marked along the lower reaches of the mobilized tissues. This line marks the lower boundary of the flap.

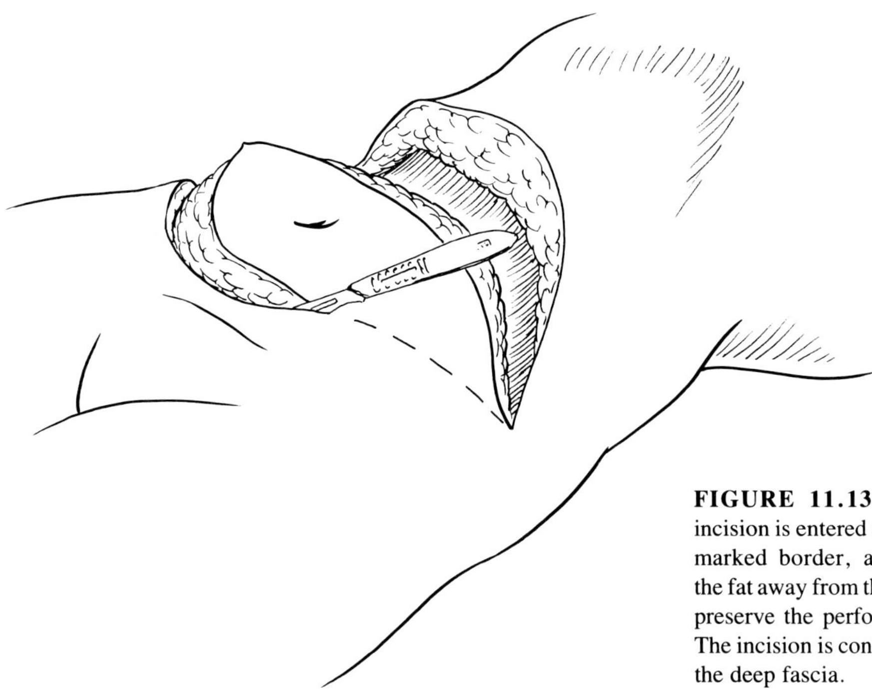

FIGURE 11.13 The lower incision is entered over the newly marked border, again beveling the fat away from the umbilicus to preserve the perforating vessels. The incision is continued down to the deep fascia.

The ipsilateral skin and fat are likewise separated from the deep fascia, starting laterally and moving toward the midline. This is continued onto the rectus fascia up to approximately 1 cm medial to the lateral border of the rectus muscle. Again, any large perforators to the fat are preserved along this margin (Figure 11.14).

The fascia over the rectus in the suprapubic region is incised in a V shape, and the apex of the V is sutured to the dermis of the rectus flap (Figure 11.15). Other areas along the skin are likewise sutured to the fascia over the muscle. This ensures that the fat is not

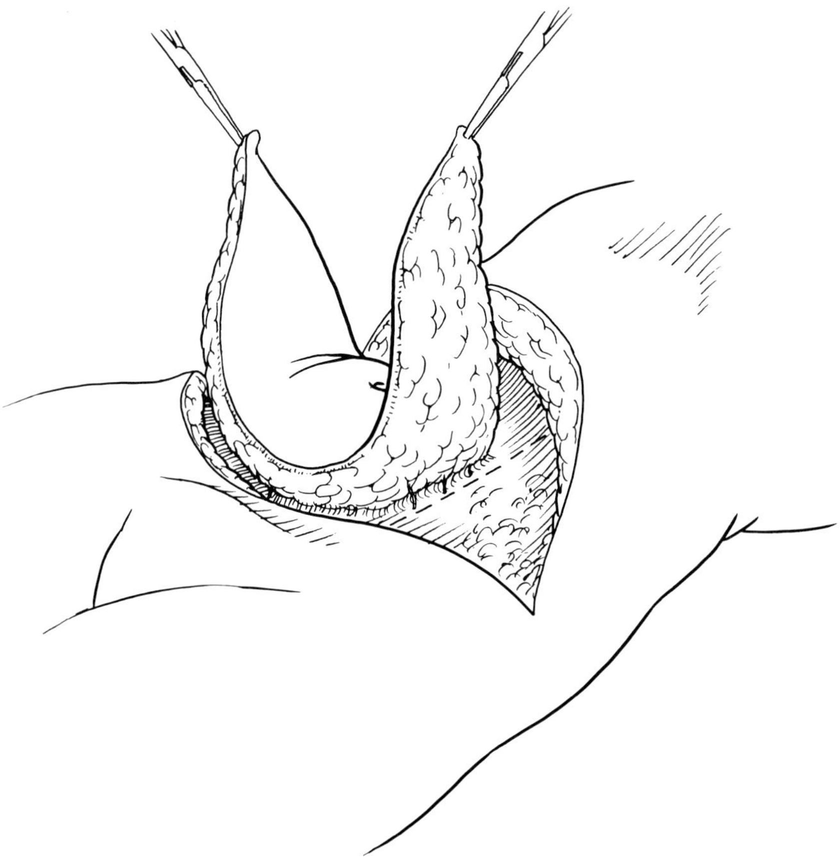

FIGURE 11.14 The skin and fat are mobilized from the deep fascia, working lateral to medial, and carrying the dissection just across the linea alba on the medial side and about 1 cm onto the rectus fascia on the lateral (ipsilateral) side. The dotted line corresponds to the lateral border of the left rectus abdominis muscle. Care is taken to preserve any large perforating vessels coming out of the rectus fascia medial to this 1-cm cuff. The tissues directly overlying the muscle are thus left undisturbed.

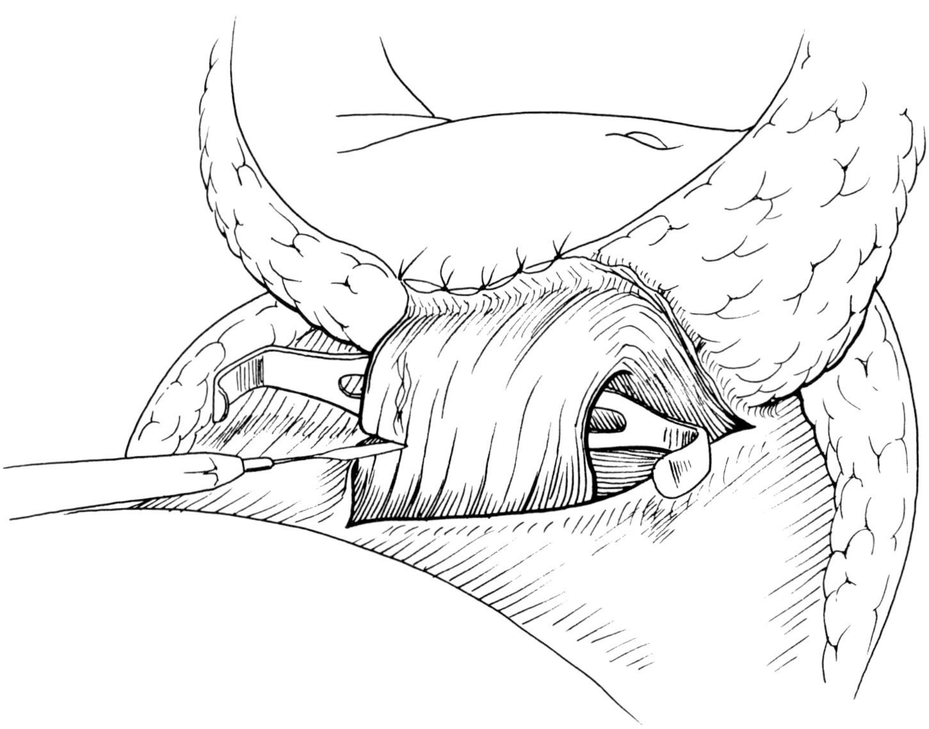

FIGURE 11.15 The rectus fascia is entered below the flap (in the suprapubic area) and the rectus abdominis muscle encircled with blunt (finger) dissection. The skin is secured to the rectus fascia with a few sutures to prevent shearing of the musculocutaneous perforating vessels during the later mobilization. The muscle is divided with the cutting cautery.

separated from the fascia during the mobilization, shearing off perforators to the skin in the process. The rectus muscle just above the pubis is now exposed. With blunt dissection, the index finger is used to encircle the muscle and an Army-Navy retractor is passed beneath it. The muscle is divided with the cutting cautery a few centimeters from its origin on the pubic bone (Figure 11.15). The muscle cephalad to this can be easily mobilized with finger dissection from the transversalis fascia, and as this is done, the intact anterior rectus fascia on either side of the muscle is incised. It is important to leave behind a centimeter or so cuff of anterior fascia on both the medial and lateral sides. This will be used for later fascial closure. Laterally, early in the lower dissection, the deep inferior epigastric artery and vein are encountered, entering the rectus muscle from the inferolateral deep aspect (Figure 11.16). These vessels are ligated and the dissection continued.

At a convenient point, perhaps halfway up during the lower dissection, attention is turned to the upper arc of the flap. The fascia (which is already exposed) is incised in a longitudinal (cephalad) direction about 2 cm from the medial edge of the rectus muscle, and the incision is carried up over the costal margin on the superficial aspect of the muscle. A tongue of fascia is left with the muscle, again in the shape of a V (only this time, an inverted V), and the dermis is sewn to the fascia with a few interrupted sutures. The dissection can now be carried caudally from this point, again leaving a cuff of medial and lateral anterior fascia behind. As the dissection proceeds, the umbilicus is approached, and the dissection is carefully carried around it. From underneath, the dermis of the umbilicus is exposed all the way around the umbilicus, leaving a thin layer of fat on the dermis. An index finger placed within the umbilicus can help this dissection

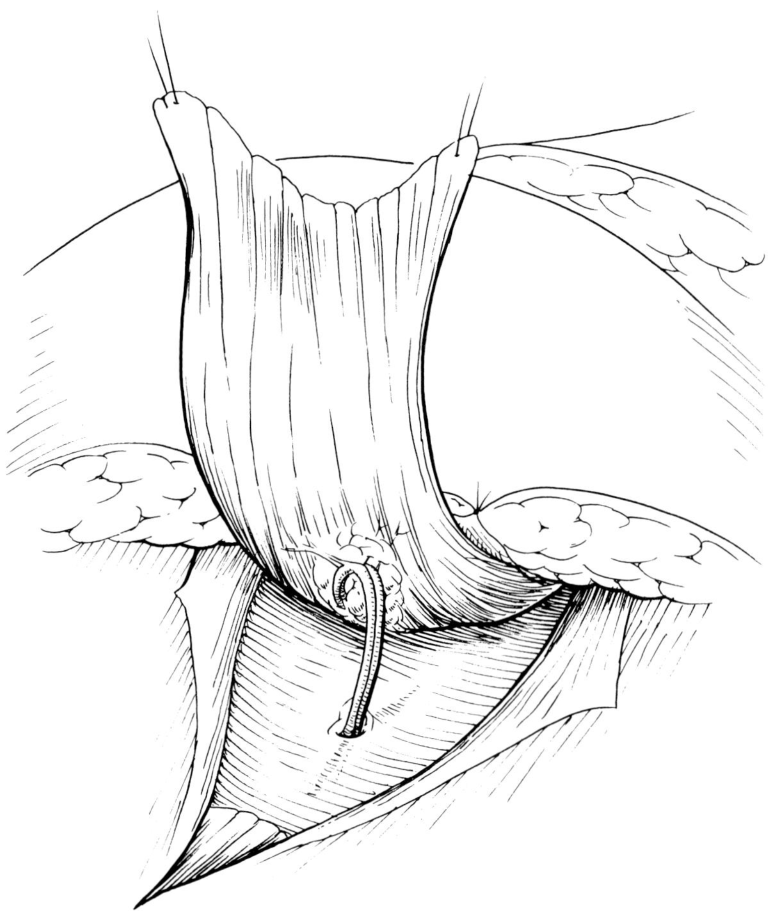

FIGURE 11.16 As the loose, submuscular attachments are divided, the dissection proceeds cephalad, and the deep inferior epigastric vessels are encountered. These vessels are ligated since the blood supply to the superiorly based flap is from the superior epigastric vessels.

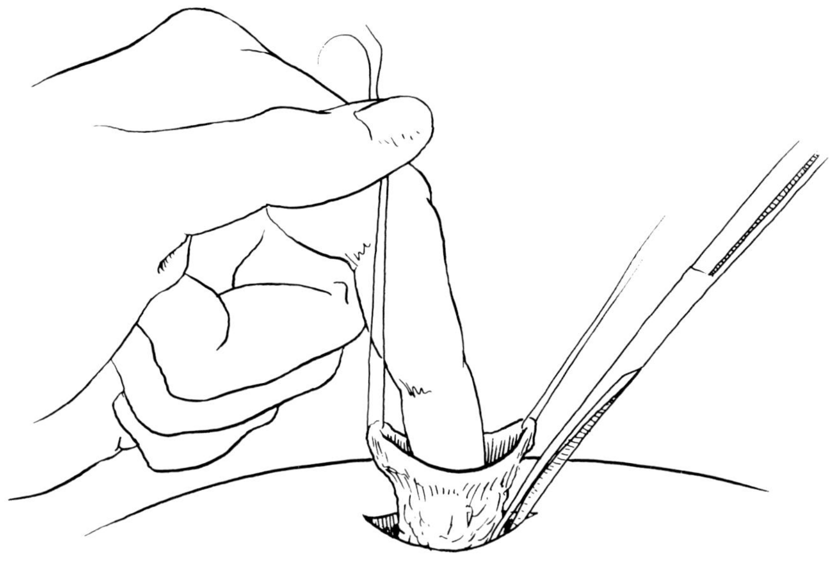

FIGURE 11.17 An index finger placed in the umbilicus helps the dissection. Care is taken to preserve a layer of fat on the dermis in order to ensure blood supply to the umbilicus.

(Figure 11.17). The skin of umbilicus is circumcised, leaving an approximate 2-cm-diameter umbilicus attached to the deep fascia. The flap is freed from the umbilicus and the dissection is continued from both cephalad and caudal directions, liberating the muscle and leaving the fascial cuff behind (Figures 11.18 and 11.19).

As the costal margin is approached, the dissection proceeds ever more cautiously, and a search is made for the superior epigastric arterial pedicle. This small vessel and its accompanying vein enter the muscle on its deep and medial aspect, approximately 5 cm from the midline and 5 cm caudal to the costal margin (Figure 11.20). Blunt, small Metzenbaum scissors can be of value here, as they gently spread the tissues and cut only what is transparent. Also in this region, the tendinous inscriptions of the muscle form tightly bound and adherent bands that must be sharply and carefully freed from the deep aspect of the muscle and from the medial and lateral fascial cuffs.

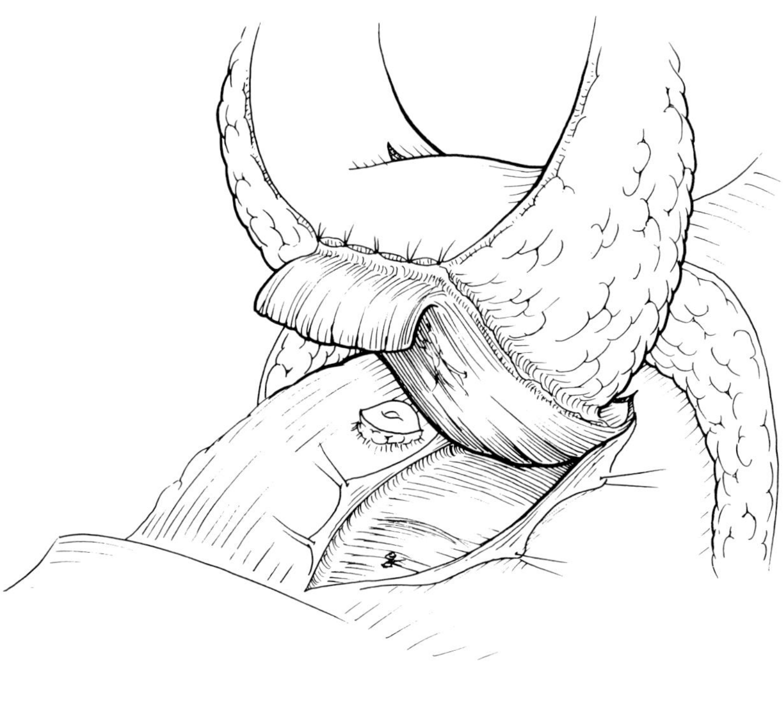

FIGURE 11.18 The dissection proceeds, leaving cuffs of medial and lateral rectus fascia for use in later abdominal wall closure. The tissues overlying the rectus muscle and beneath the skin flap are left intact.

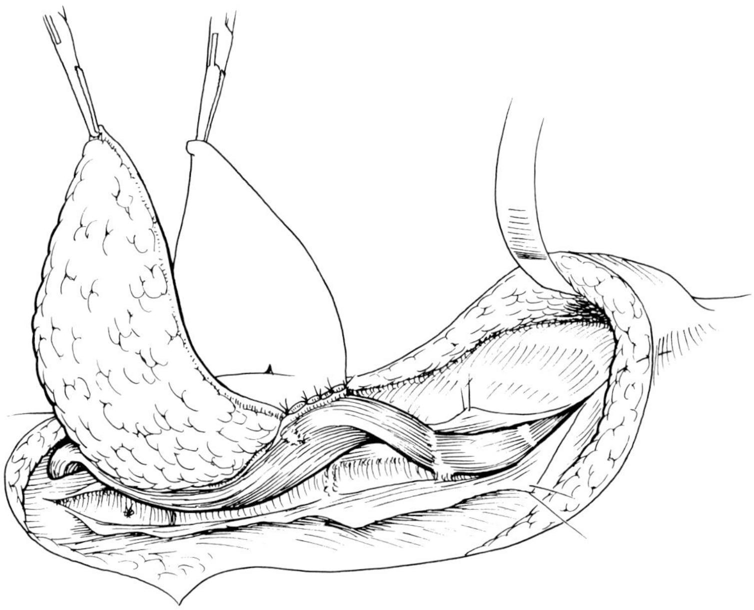

FIGURE 11.19 The muscle is mobilized over the costal margin, incising the anterior rectus fascia in the direction of the chest wall defect. This fascia, over the superficial aspect of the muscle, is opened widely to prevent kinking of the vascular pedicle when the flap is transposed to the chest wall. A tongue of anterior fascia is left intact to provide blood supply to the skin portion of the flap.

After the pedicle is located, it is kept under a protective eye while the muscle is serially freed from its cephalad insertions on the rib cartilages. The flap is almost completely mobilized at this point, and attention is turned to bringing it to the defect in the chest wall.

A large subcutaneous tunnel from the stalk of the flap (vascular pedicle) to the defect is established. This pathway is liberally enlarged until it easily admits the clenched fist of the surgeon (Figure 11.21).

The flap should be easily delivered through the tunnel, and after the defect has later been suitably prepared, it is brought into its new location at the recipient site (Figure 11.22). There should be absolutely no tension on the pedicle. It may be temporarily brought to rest in an upside-down attitude over the proposed chest wall defect while the abdominal closure is being accomplished.

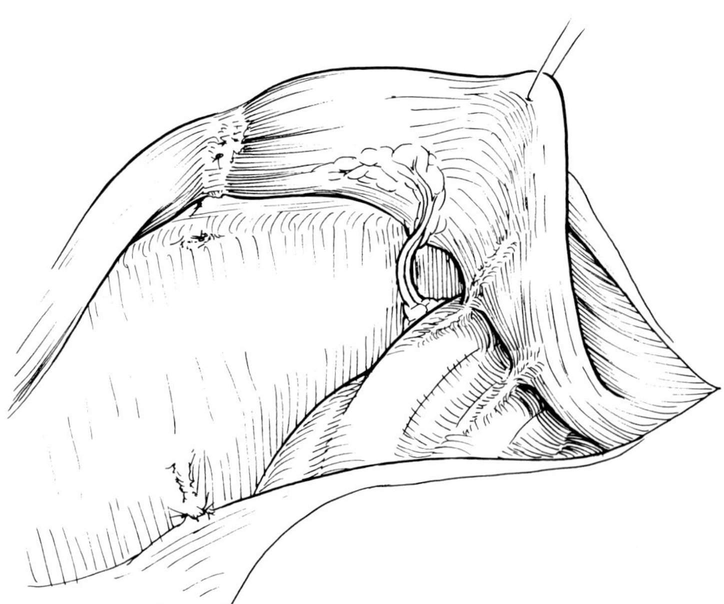

FIGURE 11.20 As the costal margin is approached, extreme care is taken to avoid injury to the superior epigastric pedicle, which enters the muscle on the deep aspect.

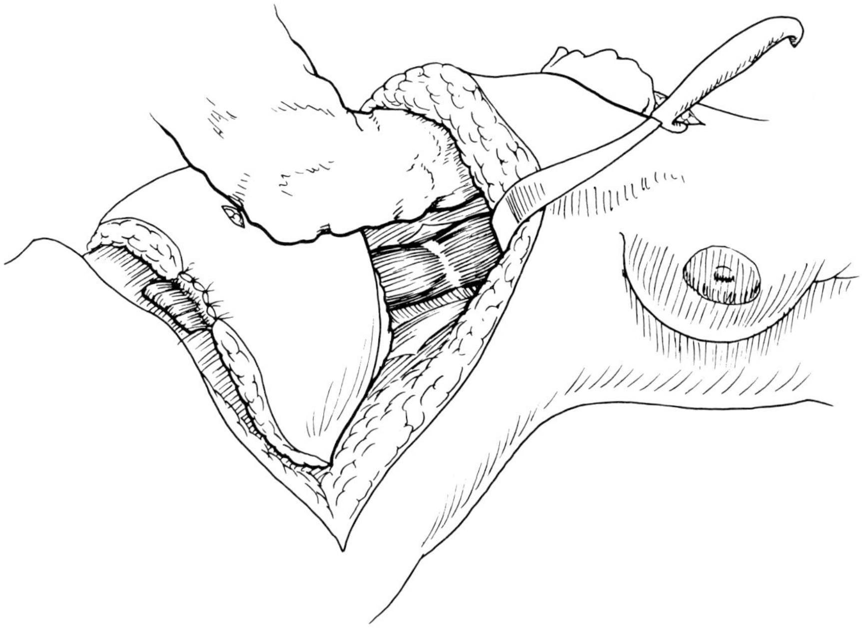

FIGURE 11.21 A wide subcutaneous tunnel is established from the area of the superior epigastric pedicle to the area of the chest wall defect. It should easily transmit the surgeon's clenched fist.

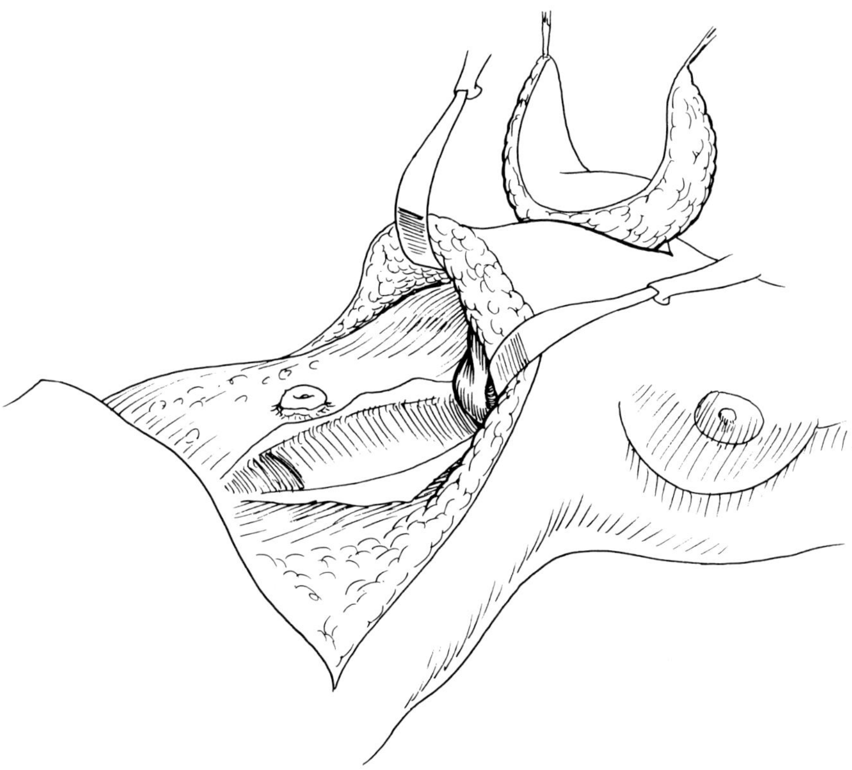

FIGURE 11.22 After the chest wall defect has been suitably prepared, the flap is delivered through the tunnel. There should be absolutely no tension on the pedicle. Care is taken to avoid twisting the pedicle as well. The flap should fill the defect loosely. There is, of necessity, a gentle twist of the muscle as it enters the tunnel. The surgeon must orient the flap so that this is minimized and in no way constricts the pedicle.

After irrigation, hemostasis is checked over the abdominal region, and the fascial cuffs are brought together with a running 0-prolene suture. Generous bites on the fascia are taken (Figure 11.23). If there is excessive tension, it is reinforced with synthetic mesh. A contralateral longitudinal relaxing incision can also be employed and fascial plications can be used to bring the umbilicus to the midline.

The patient is then brought to a sitting position with the knees bent, and the midline of the abdominal skin flap is sutured to the midline suprapubic skin. The approximation should be accomplished with only a minimum of tension. The new location of the

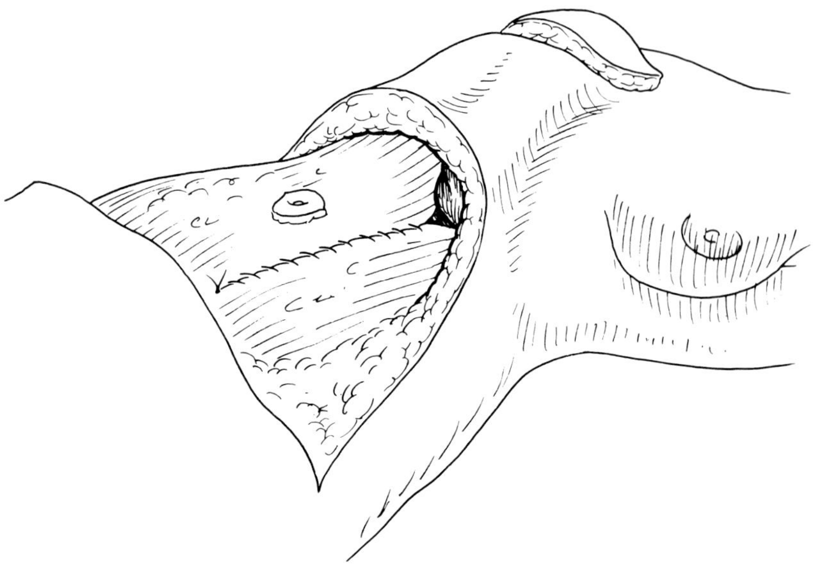

FIGURE 11.23 The fascial defect is closed with an interrupted or running monofilament suture. If tension is present, the closure is reinforced with a strip of synthetic mesh.

umbilicus is now marked on the abdominal skin. The patient is eased to a semi-Fowler position and the superior borders of the iliac crests are marked. These lateral markings are then connected across the semi-taut abdominal skin. The midpoint of the line is also marked, and as the surgeon reaches under the flap, the umbilicus is palpated. The tip of a tonsil clamp is used to tent upward on the flap at the location of the umbilicus, and this maneuver serves to confirm the proposed new location at the intersection of the new markings (Figure 11.24). A 2-cm horizontal (transverse) incision is made in the skin over the umbilicus, and the umbilicus is brought through this new aperture. It is helpful to place a suture at 6 o'clock and at 12 o'clock in the umbilicus and bring it through the aperture with tension on the suture (Figure 11.25). This also ensures that the umbilicus

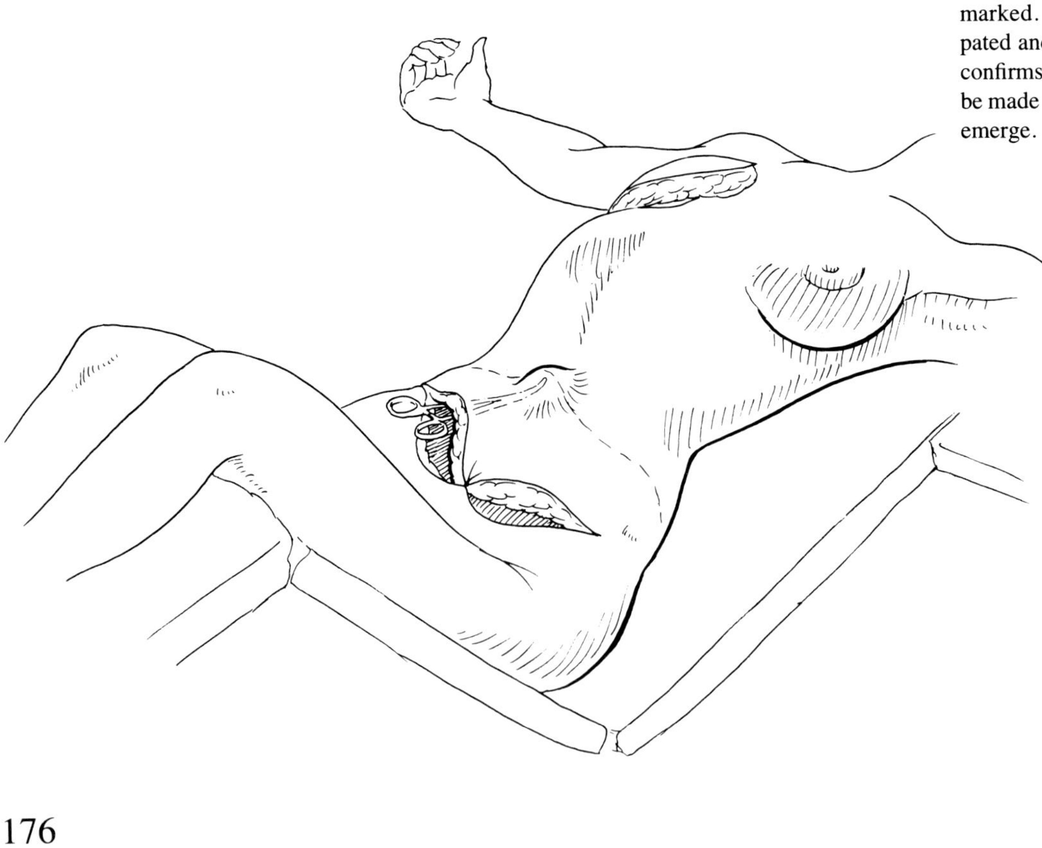

FIGURE 11.24 Locating and positioning the umbilicus is shown. The patient is bent at the waist and the knees raised. The midpoint of the abdominal flap is approximated to the midpoint of the lower flap. The superior iliac crests are palpated and joined with a line that passes across the midabdomen, which is also marked. The umbilicus is palpated and the tip of a long clamp confirms where the incision will be made to allow the umbilicus to emerge.

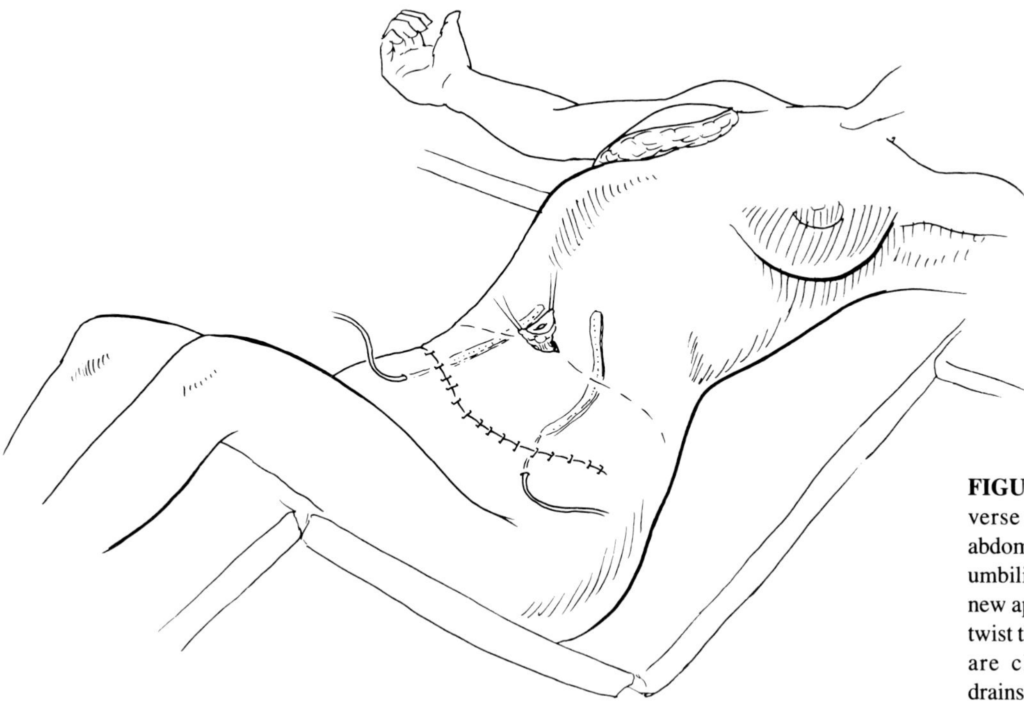

FIGURE 11.25 A 2-cm transverse incision is made in the abdominal skin and fat, and the umbilicus is drawn through the new aperture. Care is taken not to twist the umbilicus. The incisions are closed over soft suction drains.

does not twist as it goes through and in so doing strangulate its blood supply. The umbilicus is fixed to the abdominal skin with a series of fine interrupted sutures and the rest of the abdominal wound closed over two suction drains (Figure 11.25).

Attention is returned to the defect in the chest wall. After excision of the chest wall, the skeletal layer is reconstructed as necessary (see Chapter 5), and the flap is tailored to fit into the defect with no tension. The muscle layer is approximated to the fascial layer of the defect with interrupted absorbable sutures, and the skin layers are joined with skin staples after trimming the areas with lesser blood flow (Figure 11.2).

Mobilization of the Vertical Musculocutaneous Flap

This option is more reliable than the transverse flap since it incorporates the rectus muscle with a strip of skin and fat that directly overlies the muscle itself. Therefore, the musculocutaneous perforators directly arborize into the entire skin segment. It is mobilized in an identical fashion as the transverse flap, except that a vertical ellipse of skin and subcutaneous tissue is left undisturbed over the anterior fascia. During the planning phase, it is determined that a longitudinal flap is desirable in reconstructing the defect. It may be useful for sternal defects where removal of skin and deep tissues have left a sizable cavitary gap. The defect is measured and a corresponding ellipse (or other suitable skin island) is marked over the selected rectus abdominis muscle. Again, it must be certain that the internal thoracic artery to the rectus is intact before this flap is used. This vessel may be ablated if the sternal defect is large, and an alternative flap must then be used. After the arc of rotation is checked and the dimensions of the defect are measured, the final pattern is marked.

The skin and soft tissues are incised down to the anterior rectus fascia, with the umbilicus avoided and the incision beveled away from the skin segment of the flap (Figure 11.26). The fascia is incised over the suprapubic region, and the rectus muscle is isolated and divided (Figure 11.15).

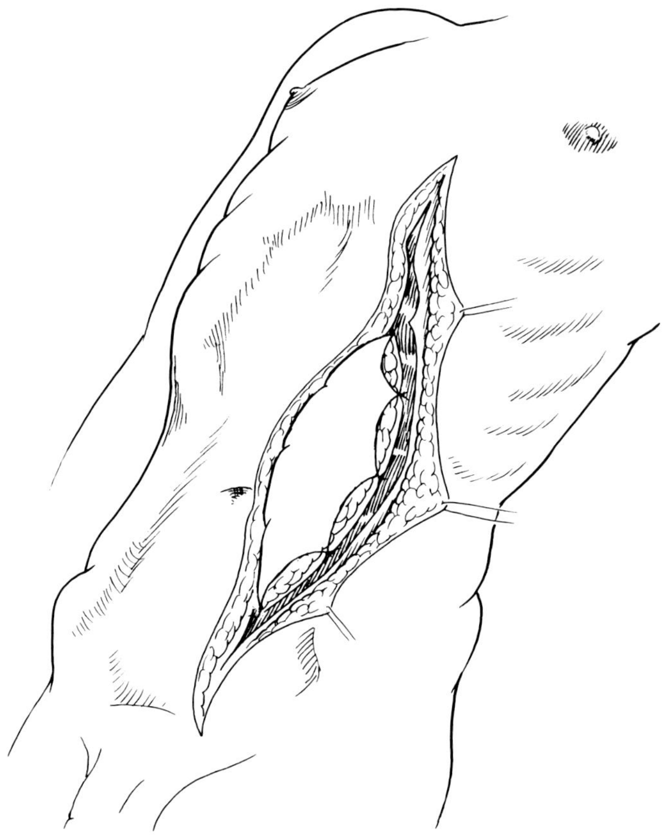

FIGURE 11.26 The vertical rectus abdominis musculocutaneous flap is shown. The previously measured and marked incision is entered and the fat beveled away from the skin segment. The dermis is fixed to the fascia with several sutures to avoid shearing of the perforators. The anterior rectus sheath is entered as described.

The dermis of the skin segment is sutured to the fascia so that the muscle and skin are mobilized as a unit, and the dissection commences in a cephalad direction. The flap is mobilized as described in this chapter, leaving a 1-cm cuff of rectus fascia both medially and laterally (for later closure of the rectus donor defect). The flap is fully mobilized, with the vascular pedicle carefully preserved, and is transposed into the defect. Care is taken not to twist the pedicle or expose it to any tension (Figure 11.27).

The fascial closure is accomplished as described, and the umbilicus, which remains in situ, is slightly moved toward the donor side. The skin is closed in routine fashion. The flap is sutured into the recipient bed as noted for the transverse rectus flap, and care is taken to protect the pedicle at all times. The skin closure is likewise as described.

Mobilization of the Rectus Muscle Alone

This option is often used for sternal defects in which skin has not been removed (e.g., after debridement for osteomyelitis). A vertical midline incision, circumventing the umbilicus, is deepened to the linea alba. The skin and subcutaneous fat are mobilized away from the fascia laterally and the fascia over the selected rectus muscle opened longitudinally. The muscle is isolated in the suprapubic region and divided (Figure 11.15). It is then mobilized as described, taking care to preserve the vascular pedicle.

The muscle is swung into the defect without torsion or tension on the pedicle. The rectus fascia is closed with large, monofilament sutures, and the abdominal skin closed. The muscle flap is positioned in the sternal cavity and secured with several absorbable sutures. The skin is closed over the muscle in routine fashion.

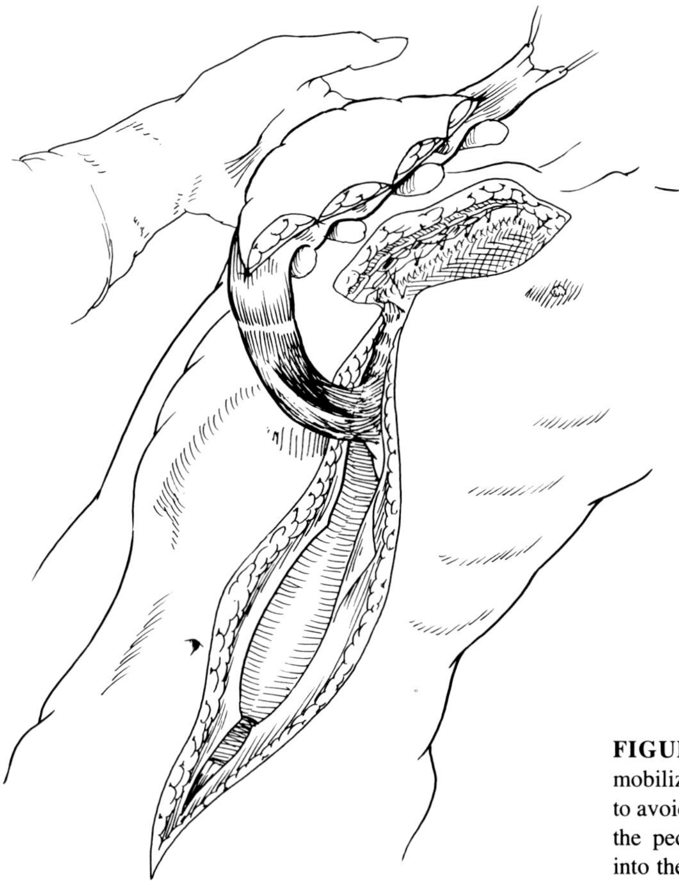

FIGURE 11.27 The flap is mobilized as described, with care to avoid any tension or torsion on the pedicle. The flap should fit into the defect loosely.

Disadvantages

There is risk of incisional hernia at the fascial level after this procedure. This can be decreased by incorporating a synthetic mesh to reinforce the abdominal fascial closure if any undue tension is noted. Weakness in sitting up has been noted but is usually well compensated for after a few weeks. Certainly this can be a more serious problem in young, active individuals, especially athletes. It is more debilitating if both rectus abdominis muscles are harvested, but this is also transient in most cases.

ILLUSTRATIVE CASE

Ten years ago, this 54-year-old female was treated for infiltrating ductal carcinoma with a radical mastectomy and postoperative radiotherapy. She subsequently developed local recurrence with osteoradionecrosis of the ribs. This resulted in a deep progressive ulceration with extension to the pleura. Involvement of the adjacent rib cartilages and bone made it necessary to perform a wide full-thickness excision of the chest wall. Reconstruction with a contralateral transverse rectus musculocutaneous flap is planned (Figure 11.28).

The defect extends from the midsternum to the midaxillary line. Chest tubes are inserted and prolene mesh is used for additional support. A large transverse flap is mobilized (Figure 11.29) and transposed into the defect (Figure 11.30).

The abdomen is closed over soft suction drains, and the areas with the poorest blood supply are trimmed from the flap. It is loosely sewn into the defect without any tension on the pedicle (Figure 11.31).

The patient did well for 1½ years until she succumbed from disseminated breast cancer.

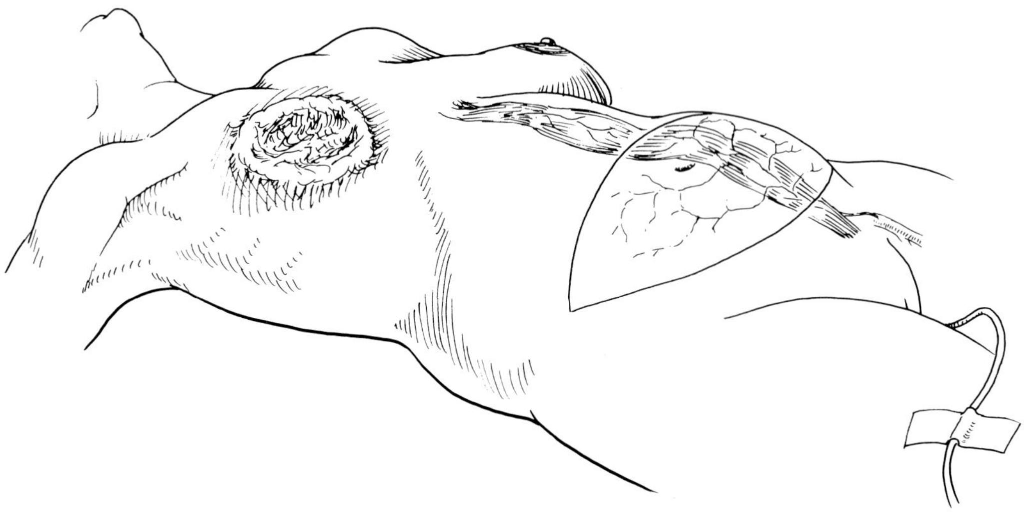

FIGURE 11.28 The patient has recurrent breast cancer and radionecrosis of the chest wall. A full thickness excision and reconstruction with a contralateral transverse rectus abdominis musculocutaneous flap are planned. The Foley catheter and other monitoring lines have been inserted. The flap is outlined.

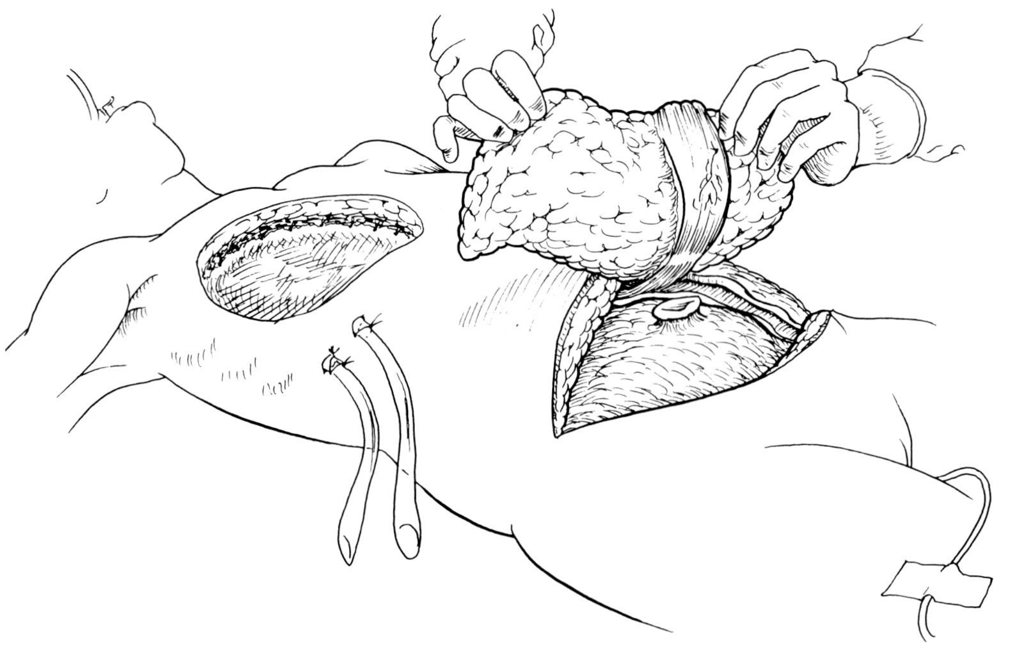

FIGURE 11.29 The full-thickness excision results in a substantial defect. Chest tubes are inserted and prolene mesh sewn to the musculoskeletal layer. A large contralateral transverse rectus abdominis musculocutaneous flap is mobilized.

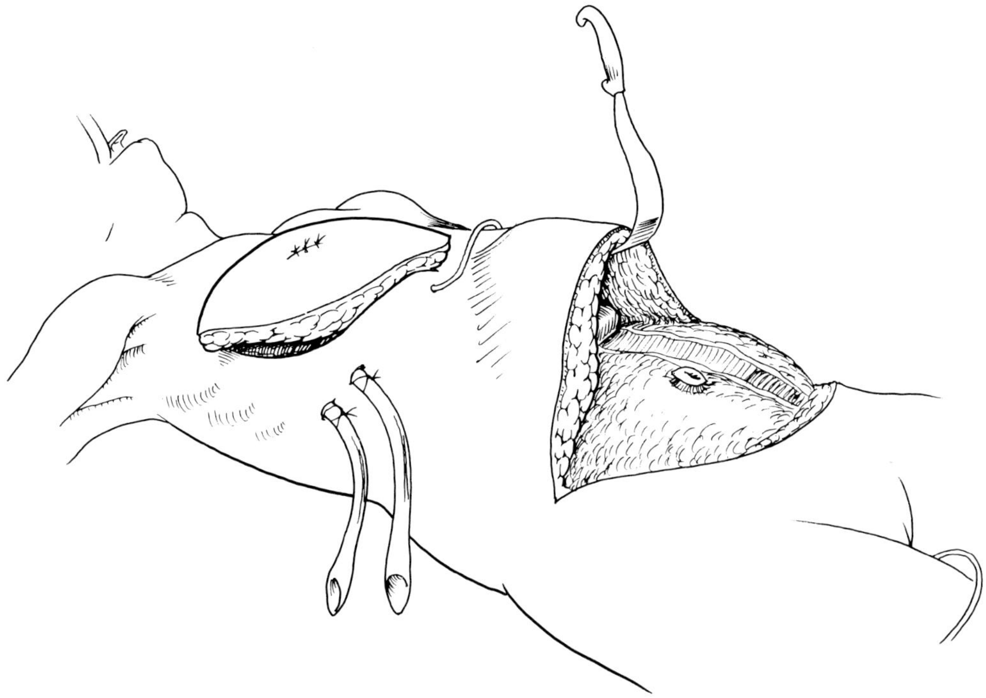

FIGURE 11.30 The flap is transposed to the chest and easily fits into the defect. There is no tension on the pedicle or on the closure of the defect.

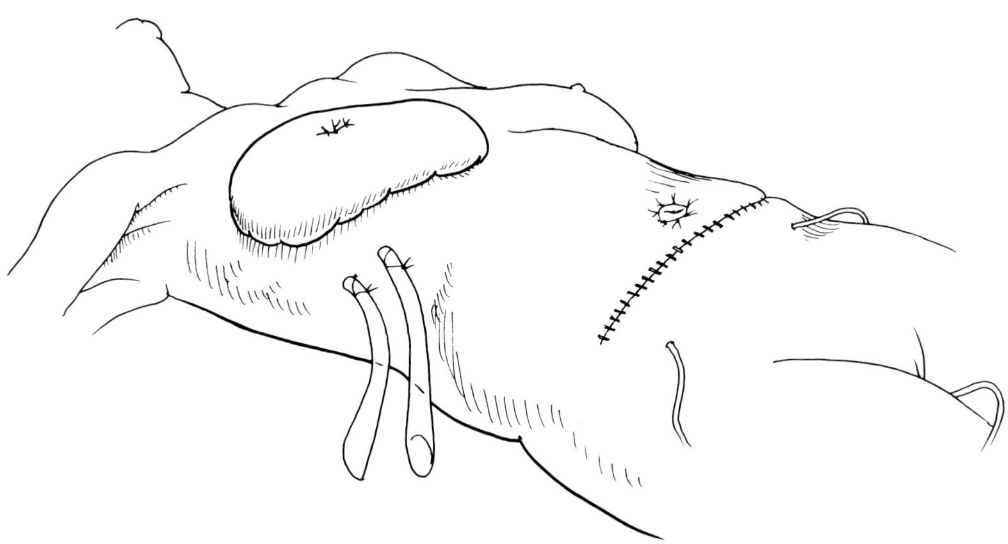

FIGURE 11.31 The areas with the poorest blood supply are trimmed from the flap, which is loosely sewn into the defect. The incisions are closed in routine fashion. This patient survived 1½ years before she succumbed to disseminated metastases.

12

The Trapezius Muscle and Musculocutaneous Flaps

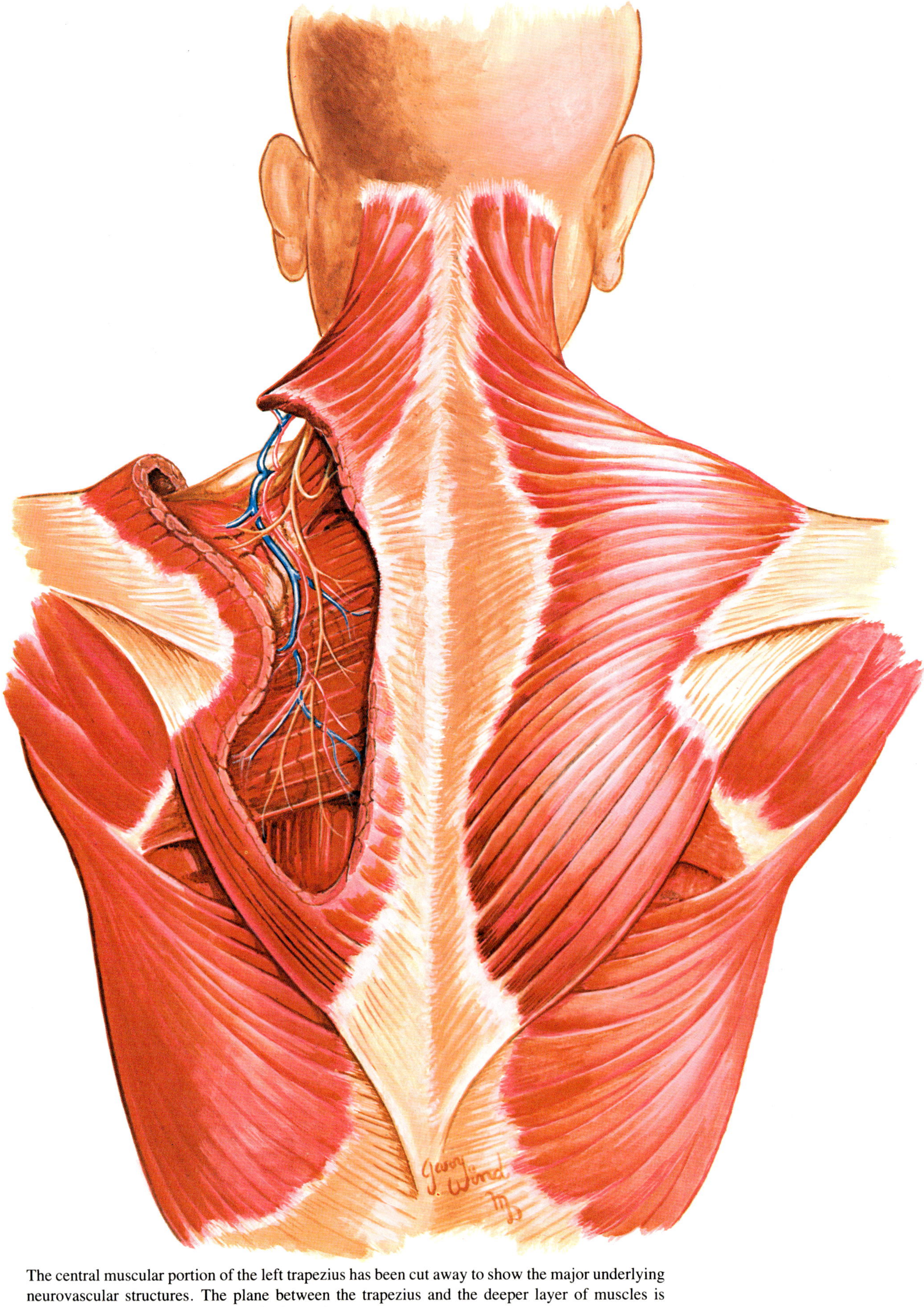

The central muscular portion of the left trapezius has been cut away to show the major underlying neurovascular structures. The plane between the trapezius and the deeper layer of muscles is opened as the lower trapezius flap is elevated.

Anatomy

The trapezius arises by a broad aponeurosis from the medial one-third of the superior nuchal line and external occipital protuberance, thence caudally from the ligamentum nuchae and from the spinous processes and supraspinous ligaments of C7 through T12 (Plate 12.1). The fibers converge and insert in a line along the lateral one-third of the clavicle, across the acromion and down the spine of the scapula. The fanlike arrangement of fibers allows segmental action to move the scapula in several directions as described next. The cephalad and caudad extremities of the origin may occasionally be reduced, and there may be some variation in the extent of clavicular attachment.

The investing layer of deep fascia splits to enclose the trapezius muscle. On the superficial surface of the muscle, the fascia is firmly adherent to the muscle and to the overlying superficial fascia of the back. Deep to the muscle, the fascia contains fatty deposits surrounding vascular channels. A clear fascial cleft separates this deep layer from underlying structures.

The arterial supply to the trapezius originates in the thyrocervical branch of the subclavian. The vessel to the trapezius traverses the caudal limit of the posterior triangle of the neck superficial to the trunks of the brachial plexus to reach the cephalad margin of the muscle. When this vessel also gives rise to a descending branch to the deep muscles of the upper back, it is called the *superficial branch* of the transverse cervical artery. About 50% of the time, this deep vessel arises independently, and the vessel from the thyrocervical trunk to the trapezius is called the *superficial cervical artery*. In either case, the vessel reaching the undersurface of the trapezius divides into major ascending and descending branches that supply the corresponding areas of the muscle. The venous drainage of the trapezius follows the pattern of the arterial supply and forms a unified vascular pedicle.

The trapezius is innervated by the spinal accessory nerve and branches of the ventral primary divisions of cervical nerves 3 and 4. After penetrating and innervating the sternocleidomastoid, the nerve diagonally crosses the posterior cervical triangle to reach the trapezius along with the vascular pedicle.

Acting in unison, the fibers of the trapezius rotate the scapula to elevate the shoulder in full abduction of the arm. The upper fibers are primarily responsible for this elevation and brace the shoulders against downward traction. These rotating fibers also play a role in rotating the head and drawing it backward. The middle fibers adduct the scapulae toward the vertebral column. The lower fibers depress the scapula and help brace the arms against upward force. Shoulder movements involve several different groups of muscles, and the absence of the lower trapezius (the portion most useful for transposition and reconstruction) does not significantly impair function.

General Characteristics

This flap is most useful for midline defects of the upper posterior thorax as well as cervical spinal and occipital wounds. It can be effectively mobilized without loss of shoulder function, as long as the upper portion of the muscle and the spinal accessory nerve are preserved. If used as a combined muscle-skin flap (musculocutaneous flap), it can safely carry a large segment of overlying skin with it.

Functionally and aesthetically, the trapezius muscle can be divided into two parts: (1) an upper and (2) a lower. The upper portion runs like a strip from the base of the neck laterally toward the acromion and forms the superior border of the neck as it joins the shoulder. It is the most functional portion of the muscle and must be preserved. Although it can be elevated and utilized for reconstructive purposes (such as intraoral resurfacing), problems related to the resulting donor site have led us to prefer other options. These problems were weakness, pain and dysesthesias about the shoulder, and sensitivity over the skin graft (which is needed to resurface the donor site). Likewise, it is associated with aesthetic problems related to the shoulder defect.

The lower portion of the muscle, on the other hand, can be very useful; it does not leave the patient with such functional and aesthetic disability. Like other muscle flaps, it can provide richly vascularized tissue to compromised areas. It is reliable, easy to mobilize, and readily accepts skin grafts. It has a wide arc of coverage and can reach the upper occiput, opposite scapular spine, and midline areas cephalad to T12 (Figure 12.1).

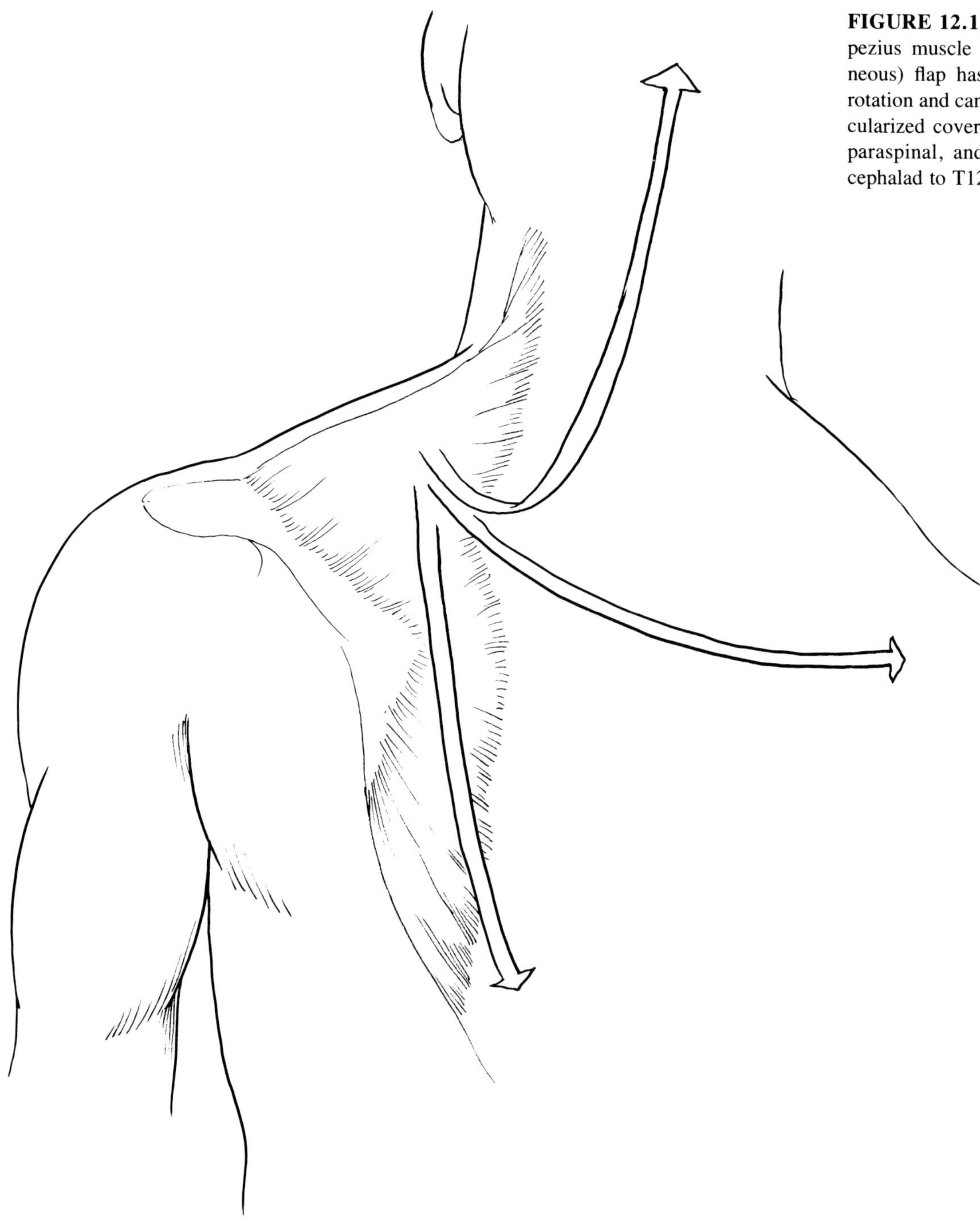

FIGURE 12.1 The lower trapezius muscle (or musculocutaneous) flap has a useful arc of rotation and can supply well-vascularized coverage for occipital, paraspinal, and midline defects cephalad to T12.

For cavitary defects of the upper midline spinal regions, it affords ample bulk to be used as a well-vascularized filler material. One of the most useful applications has been the chronic, nonhealing, postoperative wound of the cervicothoracic spinal area that has been compromised by adverse influences such as radiation or cerebrospinal fluid fistula (or both). Once the area is thoroughly debrided, the lower trapezius muscle flap can be rotated into the defect and a meshed, split-thickness skin graft applied to the surface of the muscle. If necessary, cerebrospinal fluid diversion (ventriculostomy) can be accomplished as a temporary measure until healing has occurred. In dealing with such wounds, the defect is cleansed as thoroughly as possible before flap coverage. A newly granulating recipient bed is the optimal surface for such a wound before flap rotation. As long as the upper trapezius is left intact and the spinal accessory nerve is uninjured, the patient should have no functional deficit.

It is possible to include a large segment of overlying skin with the flap. The problem with this alternative is that a skin graft must be used to close the donor site after removal of the flap. Also, such a flap can be excessively thick when situated over the shoulder or neck. For these reasons, it is sometimes best to use a muscle flap alone since this option is less bulky. If skin coverage is required, a split-thickness skin graft can be applied to the surface of the muscle after it is rotated into the defect. This method provides serviceable coverage, avoids a skin graft at the flap donor site, and gives a more natural contour.

Preoperative Planning

With the patient standing, the shoulders are elevated against the resistance of the surgeon's hands. This shrugging motion causes the muscle fibers to contract, allowing direct palpation of the muscle as well as an assessment of the comparative strength of the left and right sides. It is best to avoid the paralyzed muscle since the vascularity of such a flap is relatively unreliable. If the muscle contracts, it is suitable for use in reconstruction. As described, for each trapezius muscle there are two flaps: (1) the upper and (2) the lower. The lower flap is chosen for the reconstructive procedure. As with other flaps, the pivot point of the flap (the point that dictates and limits the range of the flap) is the vascular pedicle. The descending superficial transverse cervical artery runs along the deep aspect of the muscle and enters about 5–7 cm lateral to the midline at approximately the level of the spinous process of C7. The stationary end of the tape measure is placed at this point, and the opposite end is placed over the distal-most fibers of the muscle (Figure 12.2). This latter point is in the region of the spinous processes of T11 and T12.

One method of locating this point is to palpate and count spinous processes from the prominent C7 down to T12. The free end of the tape is then moved from this point (T12) to the prospective defect. It should cover the defect with room to spare (Figure 12.3). If used for complex cavitary defects of the cervicothoracic spinal region, it should fit loosely into the defect so that the muscle tissue completely fills the cavity. Before such closure, however, the defect must be thoroughly debrided and cleansed.

The Lower Trapezius Musculocutaneous Flap

The muscle-skin flap is described first, although the muscle-alone flap (described in the next section) is usually the initial choice for most defects. If a combined muscle-skin unit is to be used, the dimensions of the defect are accurately measured. A corresponding segment of skin overlying the trapezius muscle is marked to coincide with the measurements of the defect to be closed. In the operating room (or preferably the evening before the operation), a pattern can be made with paper (such as the paper in

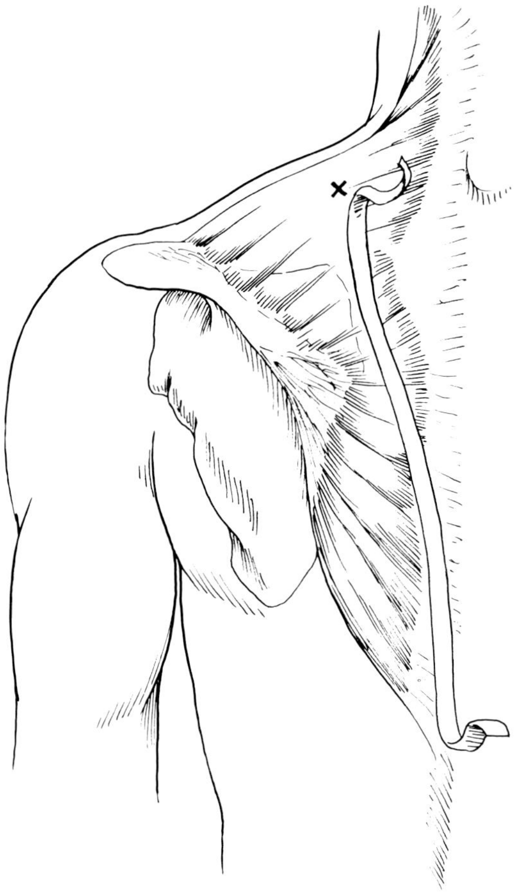

FIGURE 12.2 The tape measure is used to confirm that the arc of rotation of the flap will be sufficient to reconstruct the defect. One end of the tape is positioned over the vascular pedicle (approximately 5–7 cm lateral to the prominent spine of C7) marked X. The other end is placed over the distal-most trapezius muscle fibers (in the vicinity of T12).

FIGURE 12.3 The pedicle end of the tape is kept stationary while the free end is rotated up over the defect. It should cover the defect with room to spare.

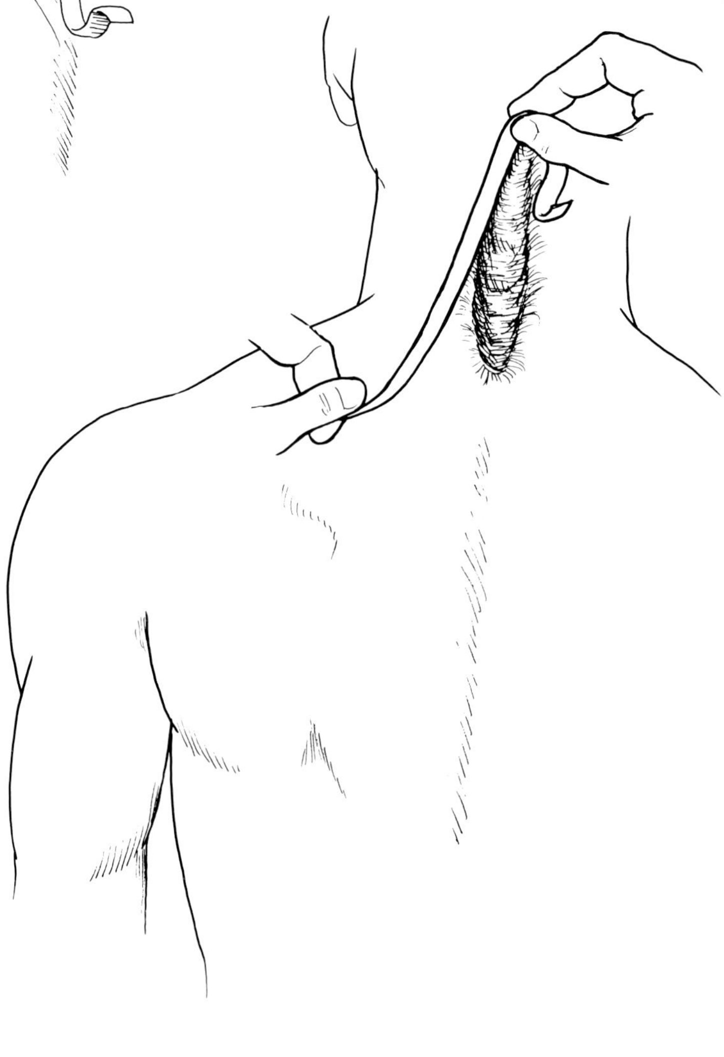

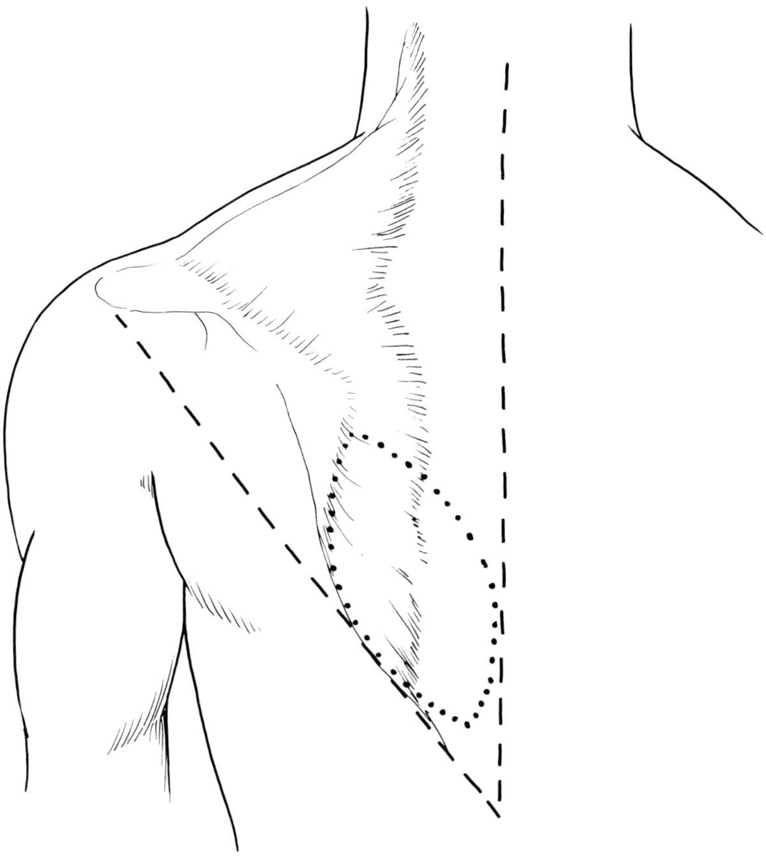

FIGURE 12.4 The borders of the lower trapezius correspond roughly to a line from the acromion to T12, which joins another line along the spinal column (dashed lines). The skin island, which derives its blood supply from the underlying muscle, should be within these borders (dotted line).

which surgeon's gloves are wrapped) or a hand towel. This pattern is trimmed so that it fits the defect with a few millimeters to spare in all directions. It must fit loosely in the defect so that a floppy closure is ensured with no tension whatsoever. The pattern is then brought to the skin overlying the muscle and the flap planned so that it will easily fit into the defect after it is rotated up to its final position. After the final measurements are made, the tape measure is then used to confirm them (Figures 12.2 and 12.3). The skin segment is marked over the trapezius muscle with brilliant green dye. (This dye is usually not washed off during skin preparation like other dyes.)

To make certain that the skin island overlies the muscle, the borders of the muscle are also determined. From the acromion to the spinous process of T12, a line is drawn. Another line, along the midaxis of the spinal column, is drawn. The skin island should be within these boundaries in order to utilize the territory most reliable in the vascular supply (Figure 12.4). It can, however, be extended several centimeters beyond the muscular borders. If an extended flap is used (i.e., a flap that employs a skin island exceeding the borders of the muscle), then this flap can be raised in a staged fashion. With this method, the entire flap is raised (e.g., during the preliminary debridement of the wound) and then returned to its original location without being moved to the defect. After 3 to 4 days, and before the flap is rotated into its final destination, any nonviable portion will have demarcated and can be excised before final transposition of the flap.

The skin island should be in the range of 8 cm in width and at least a similar dimension in length. This increases the likelihood that it will include a major branch from the muscle to the overlying skin. The larger the skin segment overlying the muscle, the greater the possibility that it will survive since it will then be more likely to include one of the skin perforators from the underlying muscle. It is these perforators that ensure its vitality. These steps may be done in the operating room but are best done preoperatively.

Mobilization of the Flap

After general endotracheal anesthesia, the patient is turned to the lateral decubitus or prone position. The head, neck, posterior thorax, buttocks (in the event that a skin graft may be needed), and upper arms are prepared and the drapes stapled to the skin. If a contaminated cervicothoracic wound is to be closed, and if it has been thoroughly cleansed by multiple debridement procedures, the flap is harvested first and the flap donor area closed before uncovering the contaminated area. If this course is selected, the operative area is prepared, and an absorbent sterile (cotton) sponge is placed into the prepared (yet contaminated) wound. A sterile rubber glove is placed over the sponge and stapled to the skin, isolating the wound from the rest of the prepared area. The operative field is quickly reprepared with antiseptic solution, and a betadine-impregnated plastic adherent drape is draped over the entire field. The skin island is then remarked and remeasured to confirm the preoperative plan. The skin island is incised and the incision continued in the midline down to the trapezius fascia. The dermis is secured to the fascia with several interrupted sutures (Figure 12.5). This is done to ensure that the skin and muscle will be moved as a unit and to avoid shearing the all-important cutaneous perforators (the sutures are removed before the final skin closure is done and after the flap has been rotated into position).

Next, the skin and subcutaneous fat outside the skin island are dissected free from the fascia of the trapezius muscle; this, in effect, uncovers the entire muscle except for the skin island. At this point, the trapezius muscle is visible above the spine of the scapula. It is usually unnecessary to mobilize the soft tissues further in this area. The lower trapezius flap can easily be liberated from the attachments to the scapular spine without dissecting near the nape of the neck. In this way, injury to the accessory nerve is prevented.

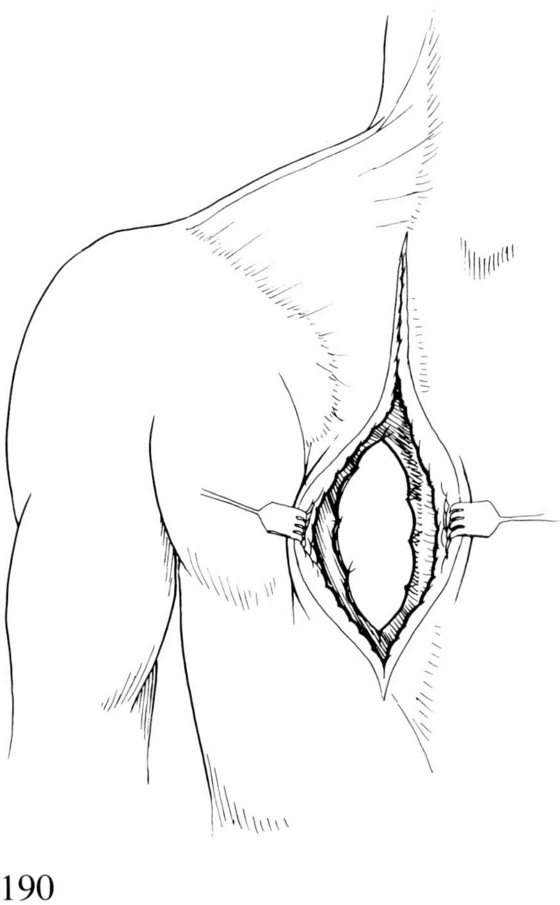

FIGURE 12.5 The skin is incised, beveling the fat away from the skin island and proceeding to the trapezius fascia. Several dermal-fascial sutures are placed along the edges of the skin island to prevent shearing of the musculocutaneous perforating vessels during mobilization of the flap.

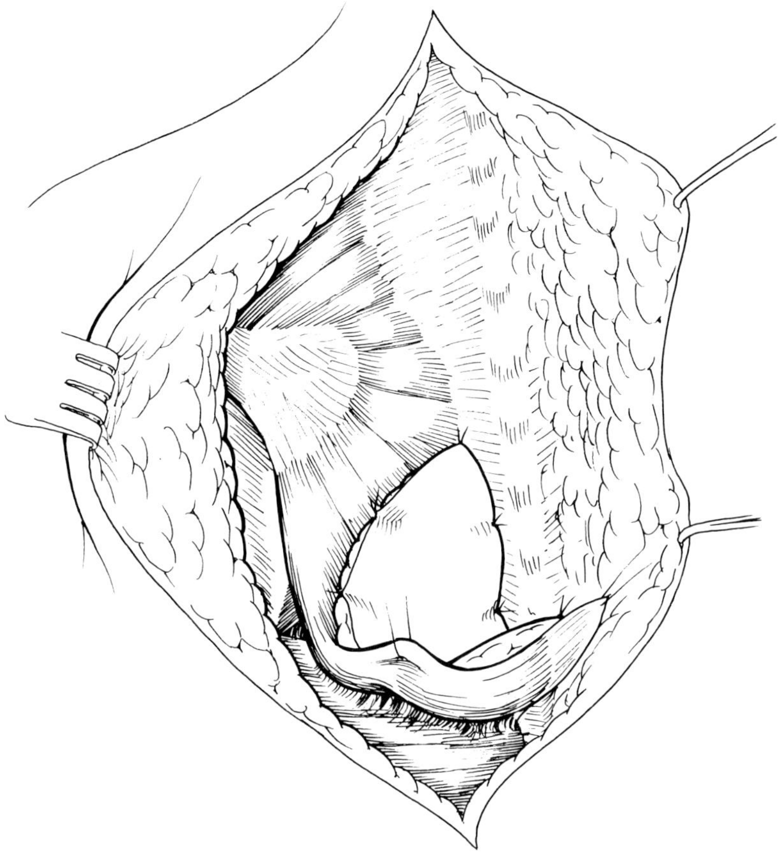

FIGURE 12.6 A plane is established beneath the trapezius muscle, and the dissection continued over the latissimus and paraspinous muscles. The origin of the muscle on the spinous processes of the vertebrae is sharply incised.

After the muscle is uncovered, attention is turned to the caudal portion of the muscle and its attachments to the spinous processes. Starting along the lateral border of the muscle, the thin fascia connecting it to the latissimus dorsi muscle is entered and a plane is established beneath the trapezius muscle (Figure 12.6). The muscle is carefully separated from the paraspinous muscles, proceeding laterally to medially and moving closer to the spinous processes. As the muscle is dissected free, its origin along the spinous processes is sharply incised. The muscle is gradually liberated from the underlying fascia, working cephalad and taking care to avoid injury to the undersurface of the muscle and its vascular pedicle. After the spine of the scapula has been reached, the range of the flap increases with each centimeter that it is freed from this spine (Figure 12.7). After dissection from the scapular spine, the flap is rotated into position, and if necessary, the dissection is carried further cephalad to ensure a tension-free closure (Figure 12.8). Once this is achieved, attention is turned to closure of the donor defect.

The skin and subcutaneous fat are mobilized laterally and inferiorly to close the defect remaining after harvesting of the skin island. If tension exists, a split-thickness skin graft is applied to the donor defect. The remaining portion of the incision is closed, and the previously covered spinal defect is now opened. After another cleansing of the defect, the muscle-skin flap is rotated into the wound and should fit comfortably within the depths of the defect without tension. The muscle is sutured to the depths of the defect with interrupted absorbable sutures. After this layer is secured, the previously placed absorbable sutures from skin to fascia (on the flap) are removed. This liberates the skin for closure. The skin is stapled and no dressing is necessary (Figure 12.9). A coating of antibacterial ointment is applied over all incisions, and this is maintained regularly during the postoperative period to prevent encrustation of the wound.

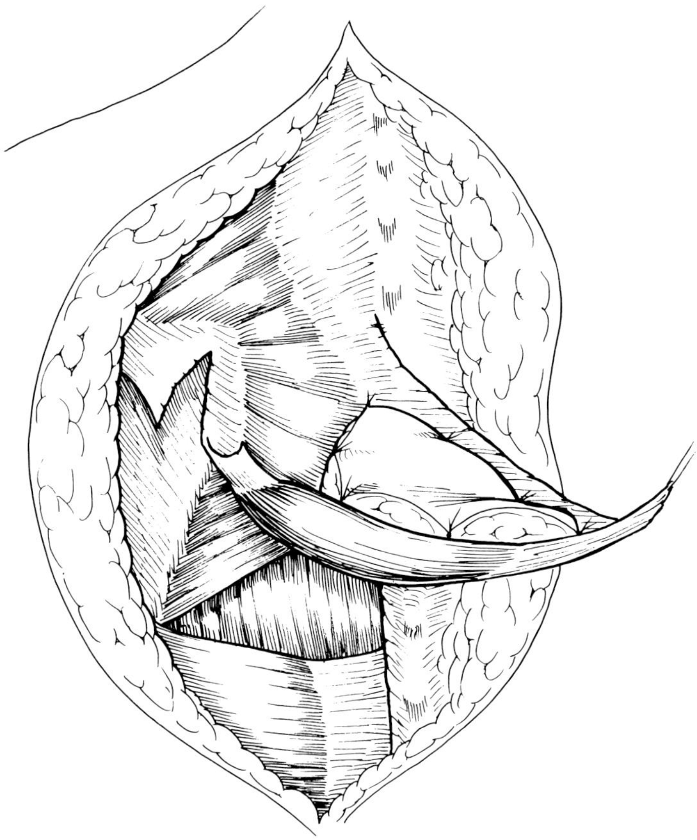

FIGURE 12.7 The submuscular dissection continues cephalad, and the trapezius is sharply liberated from the lateral spine of the scapula and the midline vertebral spines.

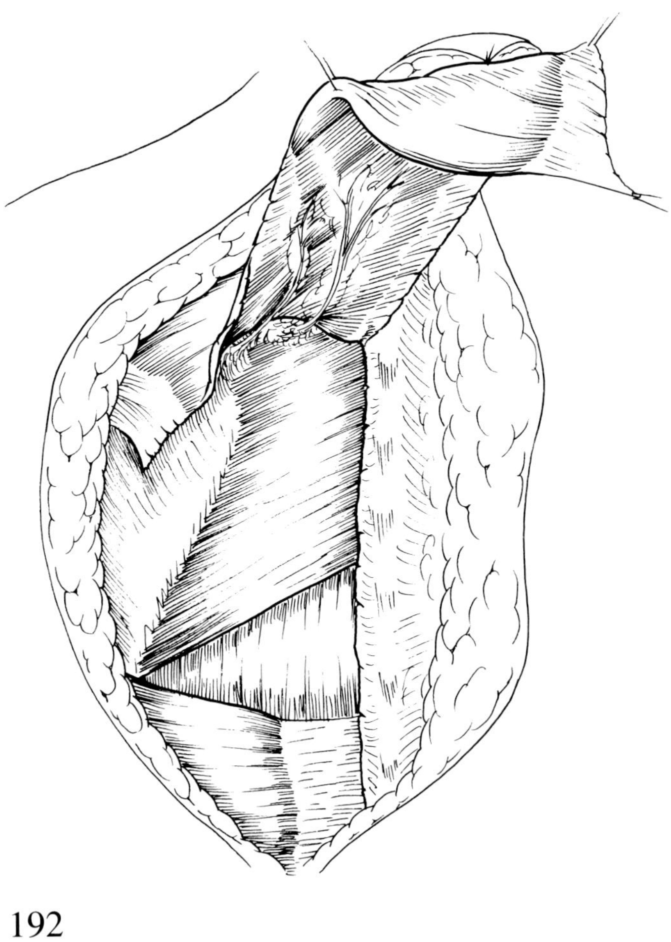

FIGURE 12.8 As the muscle is freed from the scapular spine, it becomes easier to rotate it up toward the defect. It is usually unnecessary to mobilize the flap much further than this, and such additional dissection may jeopardize the accessory nerve. Care is also taken not to injure the vascular pedicle, which enters the deep aspect of the muscle.

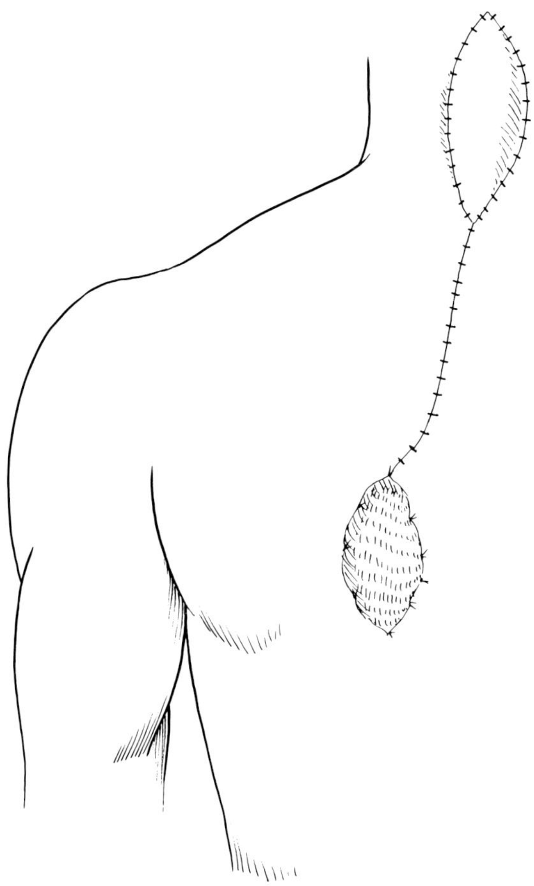

FIGURE 12.9 The dermofascial sutures are removed and the skin closed with fine sutures or staples.

The Lower Trapezius Muscle Flap

The principles and techniques as outlined also apply to the mobilization of the muscle flap alone. This flap is often the first choice since it avoids a skin graft over the donor site and usually gives a better contour than the combined muscle-skin flap (see the following example).

The major difference in harvesting the muscle alone is that the midline incision is used to uncover the muscle and the surgeon does not have to preserve a skin island. The dissection is faster since the skin and subcutaneous fat are quickly mobilized from the fascia overlying the trapezius and attention is rapidly turned to mobilizing the muscle from its origins. After the muscle is free, it is rotated up into the defect and sutured into position.

Again, the closure is loose and floppy. If skin coverage is required, a split-thickness skin graft, meshed 1.5 to 1 and applied unexpanded, is placed on the muscle and secured with fine, absorbable sutures. It is kept moist with saline-soaked gauze sponges for 3 days to allow the interstitial areas to epithelialize from the grafted skin. Since it is applied unexpanded, it should heal as a sheet. Yet it will fit the contours of the muscle well and withstand contamination from the wound much more readily than a sheet of skin; the meshing allows any drainage to flow through the interstitial openings. Sheet grafts tend to suppurate and lift off the recipient bed when such drainage is not possible. Any time a contaminated wound is present, meshing should be considered. The contour of such a technique is usually superior to that provided by the combined muscle-skin flap. Either option, however, can supply durable tissue that is able to heal securely and withstand postoperative radiotherapy.

ILLUSTRATIVE CASE

This 25-year-old male underwent incomplete resection of an astrocytoma involving the upper spinal cord and lower brain stem. High-dose postoperative radiotherapy was administered, and before this therapy was completed, the wound broke open. Multiple efforts at debridement and delayed closure failed, and the cavity deepened until the dura was exposed (Figure 12.10). A durable closure was needed in order to continue therapy and prevent intradural extension of the cavity (with resulting cerebrospinal fluid fistula or meningitis).

After a thorough cleansing of the wound, a lower trapezius muscle flap was harvested through a midline incision (Figure 12.11). The flap was quickly mobilized

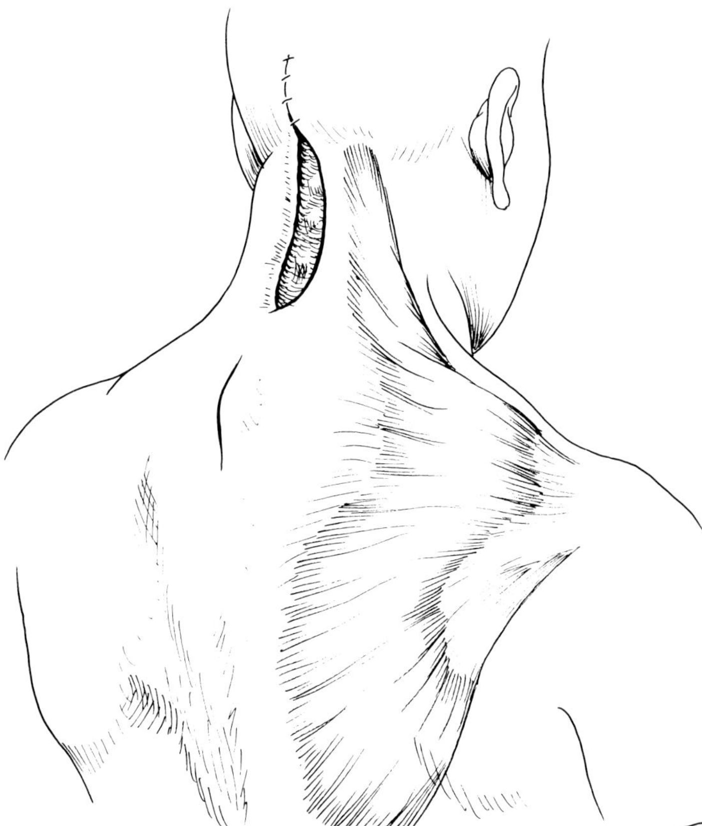

FIGURE 12.10 The patient has a deep posterior cervical wound, compromised by malignancy, radiation therapy, and infection. The cavity extends to the dura. This compromised wound needs healthy tissue in order to heal. The first choice is a well-vascularized muscle flap.

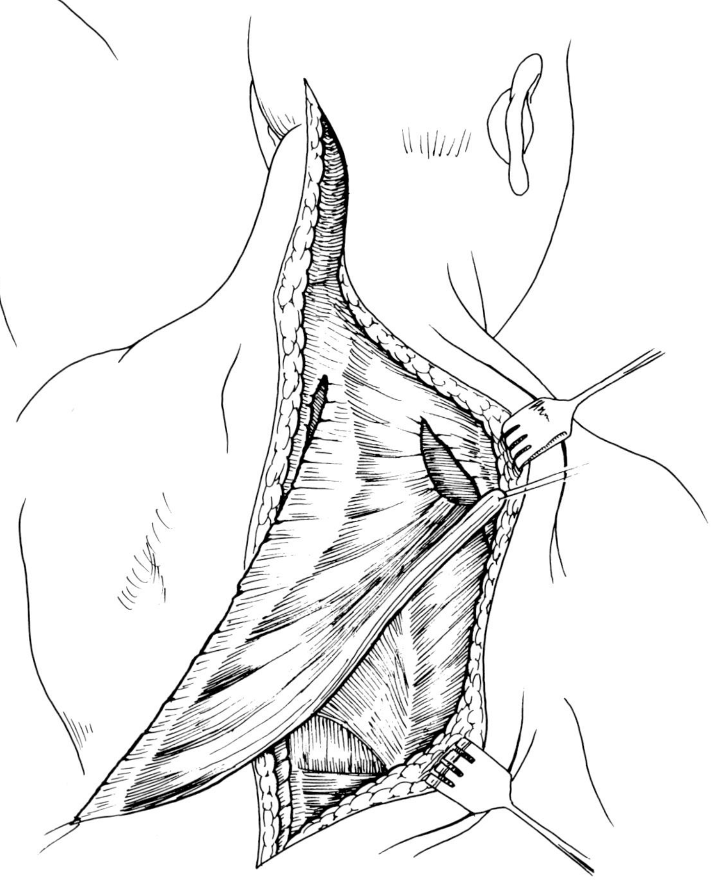

FIGURE 12.11 After a thorough cleansing of the defect, a lower trapezius muscle flap is harvested through a midline incision.

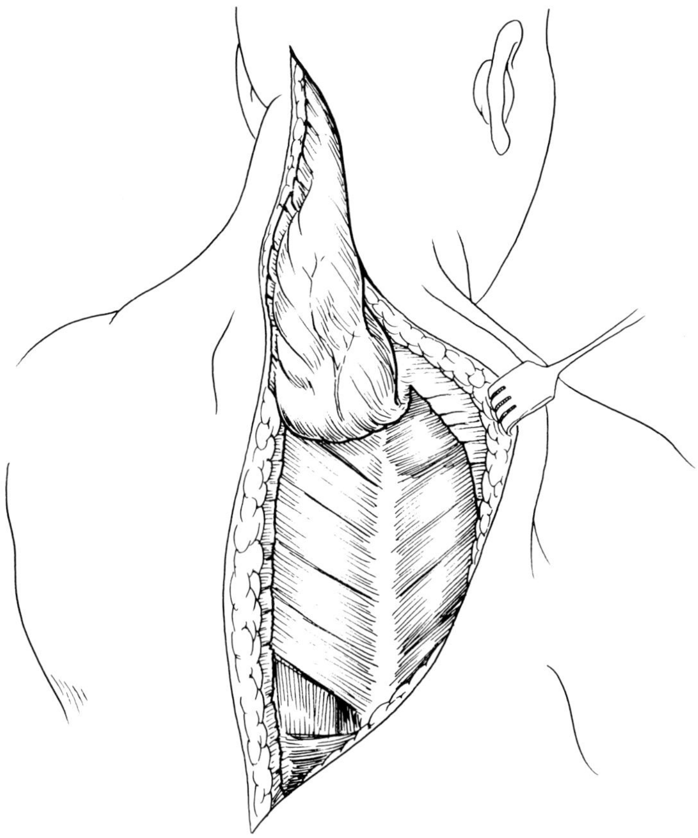

FIGURE 12.12 The flap is mobilized, taking care to protect the vascular pedicle, and rotated into the defect. It provides healthy, well-vascularized muscle tissue to this compromised wound.

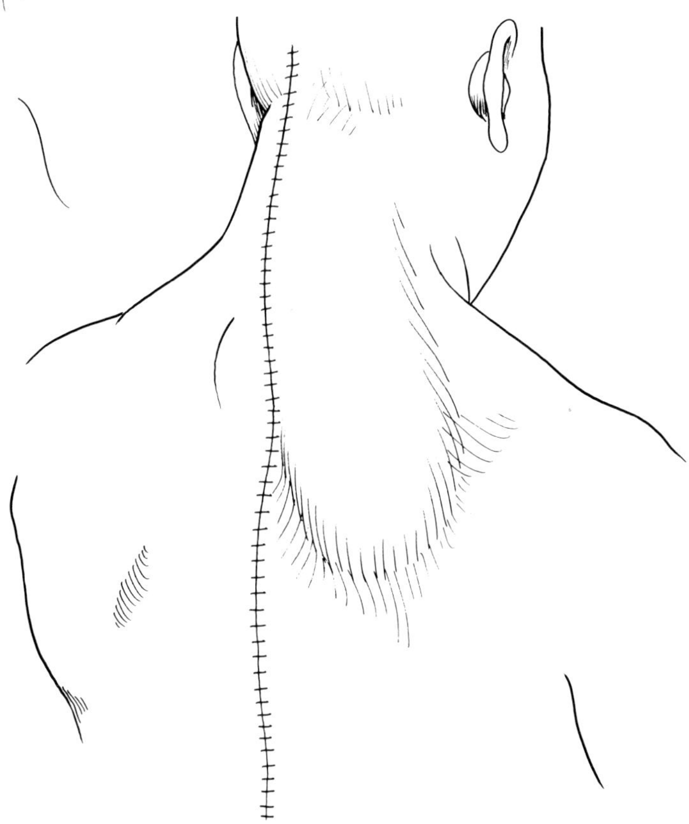

FIGURE 12.13 The skin is easily closed over the defect and muscle flap. The wound healed, and the patient completed the prescribed course of radiation therapy.

and easily filled the cavitary defect (Figure 12.12). Since there was no skin defect, the skin was closed over the muscle (Figure 12.13). The wound healed uneventfully. The patient completed his oncologic therapy and continues to do well 2 years later, with excellent upper trapezius function.

Reference

Seyfer A, Joseph A: Use of trapezius muscle for closure of complicated upper spinal defects. *Neurosurg* 1984;14:341.

SECTION III

Special Problems

13

Reconstruction of the Breast Following Mastectomy

Each year, even in the present era of limited resections and radiation therapy, a great number of women undergo mastectomy for malignant disease. The mastectomy may, in fact, follow radiotherapy or its complications. Although many of these women seem to accept the ensuing deformity readily, a growing patient population desire so-called breast reconstruction. Information on such procedures is often requested from the primary physician, in some cases even before the mastectomy. Although the operation may certainly be of benefit to some individuals, it is important that physicians dealing with mastectomy patients be acquainted with the limitations as well. This chapter outlines the principles of breast reconstruction, along with certain criteria for the selection of such patients. Some of the current techniques are presented along with examples of their use in mastectomy patients. The disadvantages of each technique are also discussed.

Indications

The capricious nature of breast cancer warrants caution when assigning a patient prognosis. One is never completely certain of eradication of the tumor, even with so-called favorable lesions and even after many disease-free years. Patients with Stage I (International Classification) or Stage A (Columbia Classification) are certainly acceptable candidates. If it is felt that local control has been achieved, even if the patient is not in one of these categories, then reconstruction may also be considered. It may be difficult to decide which of these latter patients should be recommended for the operation. The case for reconstructive surgery is that the patient will benefit from an improved quality of life. Of course, this is a subjective consideration and must be tempered with known parameters that make a patient a good or a bad surgical risk. Another factor is whether a woman should be denied the satisfaction of breast reconstruction in the face of a less-than-ideal prognosis.

Contraindications include those with inflammatory (anaplastic) carcinoma and those with aggressive lesions having extensive axillary involvement. These conditions compromise the prospect of local control of the tumor and make it risky to operate where active malignant tissue may be present. Radiotherapy is a relative contraindication but can usually be dealt with safely.

There are other reasons for proceeding with caution. Patients who have unrealistic expectations or who are under unusual emotional distress are poor candidates. If they desire the surgery because someone else wants it, they will usually be dissatisfied with the result, and it becomes a waste of time for all concerned. Also, one should not embark on a long chain of staged operations that would keep the patient out of the mainstream of life for extended periods.

Timing

Although immediate reconstruction can be an attractive option in some cases, there are also advantages to waiting. A 2- to 3-month interval accomplishes several things.

First, it allows accurate staging of the tumor (through histologic examination of all nodal tissue). Such analysis gives an indication of the risk of local recurrence and the need for further oncologic therapy before going ahead with the reconstruction. The team approach is also helpful, and the surgeon should work closely with the primary physician as well as the oncologists in determining the timing of the reconstructive effort. Certain modes of therapy can permanently alter the picture. As implied, local radiotherapy adds complexities to any reconstruction and, depending on the local requirements and conditions of the soft tissues, may necessitate recruitment of regional or distant flaps for a safe reconstruction.

Second, the waiting period allows the patient more time to come to grips with the physical changes and emotional turmoil that always accompany the mastectomy. This is tempered with the knowledge that, in some cases, immediate reconstruction may ameliorate this stress. Whichever course is selected, the patient must receive ample support from family and physician and must recognize that she can function well despite her loss. She may decide that she doesn't want any additional surgery and is perfectly content with an external prosthesis. This interval also reveals to her the extent of the mastectomy deformity and may enable her to appreciate the imperfect results offered by reconstruction.

Third, this period allows for consultation among primary surgeon, patient, and plastic surgeon so that all may become aware of any potential problems. It affords an opportunity for in-depth counseling so that the patient understands the time involved in a full reconstructive effort. For the patient with apparent local control but with an unfavorable prognosis, these considerations also apply. However, as implied, one must be more careful in this setting to weigh the potential benefit versus the time spent by the patient away from her family (and life in general) due to additional surgery and convalescence. If the decision is made to go ahead with reconstruction in such a patient, an effort should be made to minimize the number of operations and hospitalizations.

Finally, this period allows for healing and tissue equilibrium to return so that local tissues are soft and pliable. Immediate reconstruction (with a submuscular prosthesis insertion or flap procedure performed at the time of the mastectomy) can also be a positive influence in the recovery of certain patients. The one mode or the other must be tailored to fit each patient's needs.

General Principles

Architecturally, the goal of breast reconstruction is the fabrication of a soft, conical mound, with natural texture and symmetry, surmounted by a pigmented nipple-areolar complex. Symmetry is of great importance, and comparison with the remaining breast gives the surgeon an idea of the challenge that lies ahead. Unfortunately, it is always difficult to fabricate a breast-substitute that will satisfactorily match the unaffected side. In fact, it is usually easier to modify the intact breast to match the reconstructed side.

The surgeon is thus presented with an important early decision as to what to do with the remaining breast. Some women make this decision relatively easy by demanding another mastectomy as prophylaxis against cancer. Indeed, this is a good option for some since it also provides a symmetrical starting point for the reconstructive effort. The prospect of multicentricity and incipient carcinoma must also be considered in this remaining breast, and it may be wise to consider mastectomy in selected cases. A strong family history of breast cancer or a pervasive fear of cancer may dictate this course of action.

Other alternatives (to be performed on the remaining breast after the reconstruction) include reduction in size to match the reconstructed side, augmentation (enlargement) with a silicone prosthesis, or mastopexy (uplift of ptotic tissues) (Figure 13.1A and B). Obviously, each of these alternatives depends on the size and shape of the breast and what must be accomplished to reach the desired symmetry.

The patient's motives and goals must coincide with the realistic capabilities of the surgeon. In this regard, the surgeon must know what truly bothers the patient the most about her deformity. Is it the infraclavicular hollowing after her radical mastectomy? Or is it the inability to pursue athletic activities due to the external prosthesis? Sometimes just providing an internal gel prosthesis (i.e., insertion of a submuscular implant) satisfies the patient's goal. Other patients may desire a full restorative effort.

In planning a reconstruction, the progression is from the simplest to the more complex procedure. If it is possible to utilize local tissues, they should be used rather

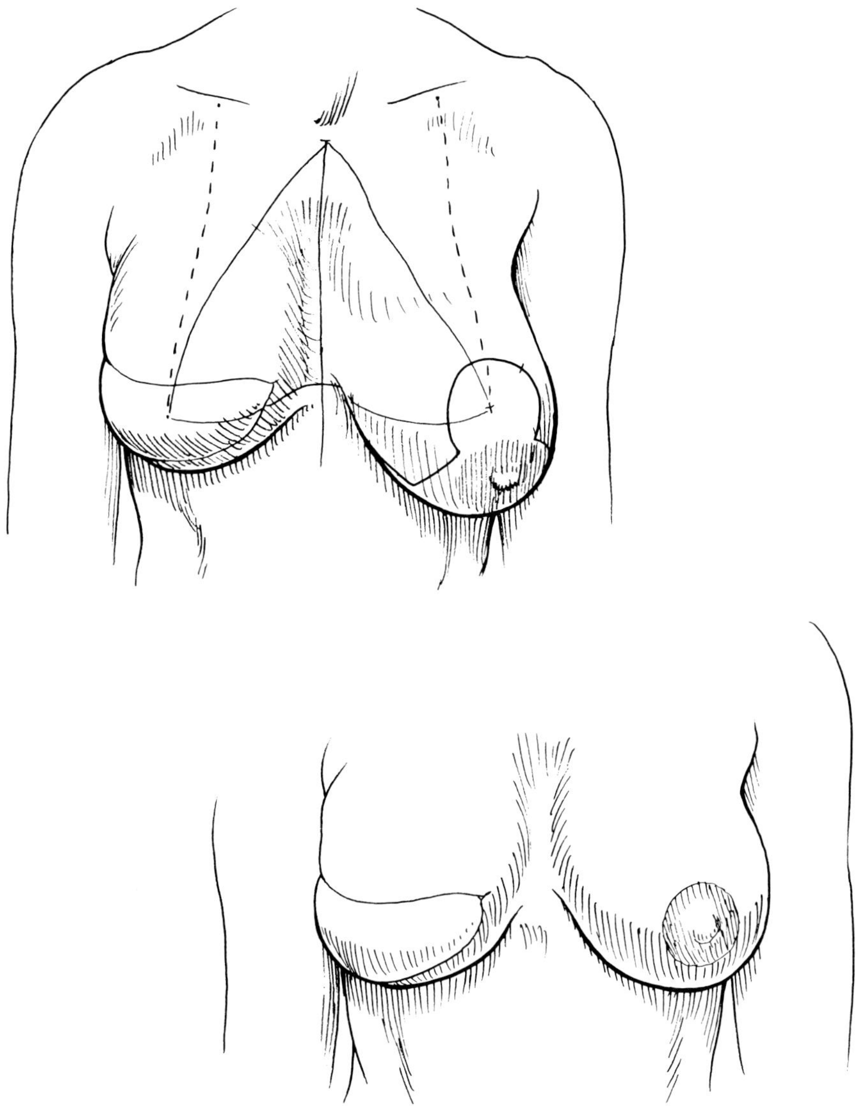

FIGURE 13.1A This patient has had a right-sided latissimus dorsi musculocutaneous flap to restore a modified radical mastectomy defect. To attain symmetry, a left-sided mastopexy (uplift) is planned and the measurements and markings have been drawn (upper illustration).

FIGURE 13.1B (Lower illustration) The mastopexy has been performed, and sufficient time has elapsed for postoperative changes to have been completed. There is now a more symmetrical fullness medially as well as an overall elevation of ptotic tissues. The patient can now be considered for nipple-areolar reconstruction.

than compromising another area with the use of distant or free flaps. All too often, however, not enough local tissue is available for a reasonable mound. One maneuver that may help to assess the need for more tissue is to have the patient place her hand behind her head. This stretches the skin and can readily reveal the problem of placing a prosthesis under such taut muscle and skin. Some of the more common methods of breast reconstruction are now presented, along with the advantages and disadvantages of each technique. This is not meant to be an exhaustive discussion but rather a presentation of some of the current and reliable techniques.

Prosthesis and Local Tissue

The simplest method of reconstruction is the insertion of a soft silicone gel prosthesis beneath a local musculofascial envelope. The advantages of this approach are that it is usually a quick procedure and does not add additional scars. The old scar is used to gain access to the submuscular plane. Of course, there is no such plane if the pectoralis muscle has been removed. Therefore, it is not applicable to those who have had a radical mastectomy.

The disadvantages are that the pocket can seldom be made ample enough to allow the insertion of a large enough prosthesis to match the opposite breast; this results in a smaller, flattened reconstructed mound that tends to ride higher than the normal breast (due to muscle forces). The scar capsule that forms around the prosthesis also makes a number of these breasts firm to the touch. In addition, it is difficult to restore an effective inframammary fold.

Planning

The ideal patient for a prosthesis is the patient who has an intact pectoralis major muscle, along with loose skin and subcutaneous fat. Such a patient has natural infraclavicular and anterior axillary fold regions, which should flow smoothly into the newly fabricated submuscular mound. With the patient standing, the inframammary crease is marked so that it matches the opposite side. Usually, a transverse scar is present and affords good access to the submuscular plane without making new incisions.

Technique

The old incision is entered and the pectoralis muscle is split in the direction of its fibers. The submuscular space is entered and a generous pocket is established beneath the pectoralis major, serratus anterior, and rectus abdominis fascia. This can usually be accomplished through blunt, finger dissection (Figure 13.2). Medially, the lower pectoralis attachments along the sternum are detached. The pocket is usually made 2–3 cm lower than the opposite inframammary crease in anticipation of upward migration of the prosthesis. A silicone gel prosthesis (as large as will comfortably fit and as close in size to the other breast as possible) is placed in the pocket (Figure 13.3), and the muscle layer is closed. The skin is closed with fine sutures or skin staples.

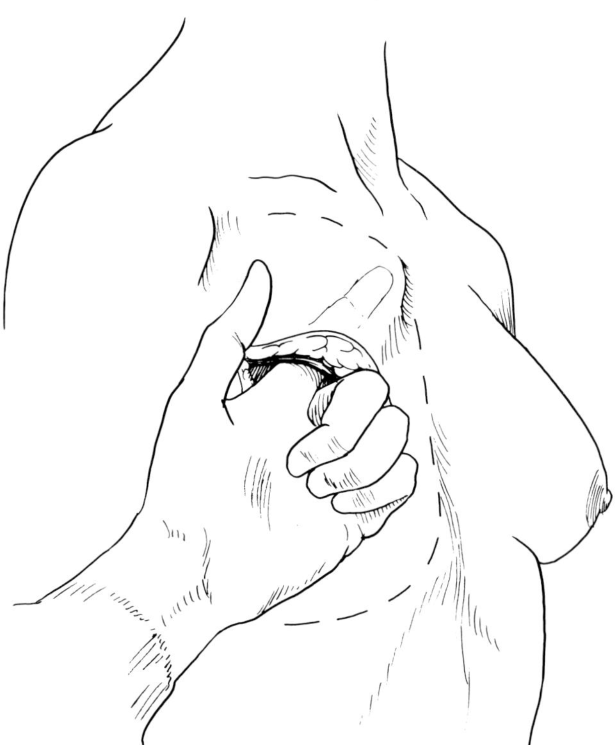

FIGURE 13.2 A generous pocket is established beneath the pectoralis major muscle, freeing the sternal attachments and carrying the dissection 2–3 centimeters below the inframammary crease.

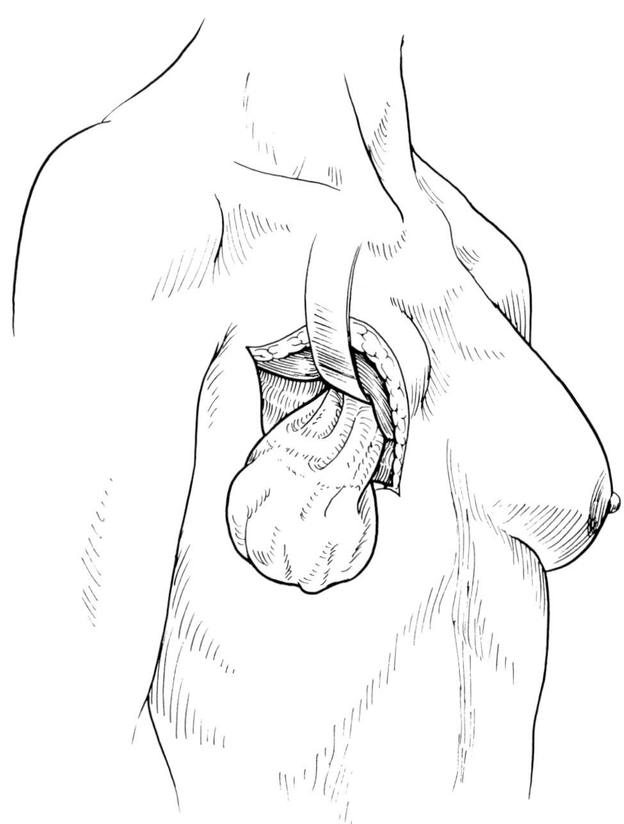

FIGURE 13.3 The submuscular reconstruction is completed with the insertion of a soft, silicone gel prosthesis into a generous submuscular pocket in order to reconstitute the breast mound. The original mastectomy incision has been reentered so that no new incisions are made.

Postoperatively, an effort is made to keep the prosthesis in the lower confines of the pocket, since muscle tone and contractile forces tend to push it upward. This is helped by not allowing the patient to wear a brassiere for several weeks after the operation, since such apparel seems to push the prosthesis upward. If it remains in a high-riding position, it may be impossible to reposition the prosthesis without revisional surgery. If the patient requires a larger pocket before insertion of a prosthesis, consideration can be given to using a soft-tissue expander to stretch out the skin and subjacent layers.

Tissue Expansion Followed by Prosthesis

With this method, a pocket is fabricated under the muscle and subcutaneous layers in the same manner as described, after which an inflatable silicone prosthesis is inserted into the space. The expander has a one-way valve through which saline can be serially injected (over a period of weeks) in order to fill it to a predetermined level (Figure 13.4). This allows the pocket to easily accept a larger prosthesis. Later, when the pocket has been totally expanded (to approximately one and one-half times the size of the final prosthesis), the balloon is removed and a smaller prosthesis is inserted.

The problems with this technique are that it is often uncomfortable (skin stretching); it requires serial clinic visits to obtain a large expansion; the patient must tolerate the large expansion for a period of time before a smaller prosthesis is ultimately inserted; and there is shrinkage of the pocket with time after the smaller prosthesis is inserted. Capsular contractures (firmness) also occur with this method, as with any method that uses prosthetic materials.

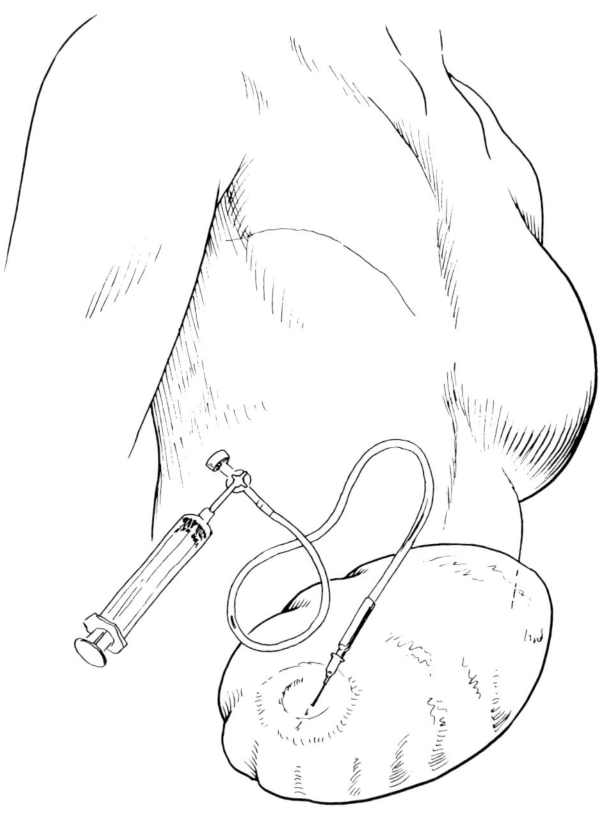

FIGURE 13.4 A tissue expander can be used to stretch the soft tissues in preparation for insertion of a silicone gel breast prosthesis. The pocket for the tissue expander is fabricated beneath the musculofascial envelope after entering the old incision. Over a period of weeks, the volume is increased by injecting saline into the balloon expander's one-way valve, which is palpable under the skin. Here, the expander is shown outside the body for illustrative purposes.

Flap Reconstruction

If it is decided that more soft tissues are needed to reconstruct the breast, the two leading options are the transverse rectus abdominis musculocutaneous (TRAM) flap and the latissimus dorsi musculocutaneous flap. These methods provide more skin and tissue bulk from which a breast mound can be fabricated.

The Transverse Rectus Abdominis Musculocutaneous Flap

The transverse rectus abdominis musculocutaneous flap is applicable to the radical mastectomy defect as well as that of the modified radical mastectomy. It is economical of tissue; that is, it uses the loose, often-unwanted lower abdominal skin and fat and moves them to a location where skin and fat are sorely needed. The flap is reliable and gives an excellent texture and color match since it consists primarily of skin and fat from the ventral torso. A prosthesis is usually not required since the flap affords excellent bulk and can be used to fill out the subclavicular region after a radical mastectomy. Problems include the length of operation necessary to harvest the flap, the potential for lower abdominal hernias, a continued deficiency of the axillary fold in radical mastectomy reconstruction, and the fact that it is not as hardy as the latissimus flap. If selected for immediate reconstruction, the plastic surgery team should begin the mobilization of this flap at the same time as the mastectomy is being performed. This saves hours of anesthesia time for the patient.

Planning

This operation is the best available for the patient who has had the pectoralis major muscle removed (radical mastectomy), but it can also give an excellent restoration to those who still retain the muscle. The patient should have sufficient lower abdominal skin and fat to make a reasonable breast mound, and the fat should be thick. Loose skin with little underlying fat is not only inadequate but may be unreliable from a vascular standpoint. Therefore, thin patients are poor candidates. Likewise, those whose fat hangs in a loose panniculus or apron are poor selections since the blood supply to such tissues also is unreliable. Cigarette smokers are poor candidates both from a vasospastic aspect (and possible flap necrosis) and for the prolonged anesthesia time required for the operation. The best candidate for the operation is one who has thick, but somewhat adherent, subcutaneous fat but whose tissue can be grasped easily by the examiner. Likewise, the abdominal soft tissues must have sufficient laxity so that the defect can be closed after the removal of this segment of skin and fat.

The preoperative markings are made exactly as described in Chapter 11. One must be extremely cautious about old scars and avoid doing this flap if the superior pedicle is at risk due to a previous operation (such as cholecystectomy or coronary bypass in which the internal mammary artery has been used to revascularize the heart). Areas on the contralateral side of a midline scar are also at risk.

The inframammary crease is marked about 1 cm higher in anticipation of the downward pull of the transverse abdominal closure. The costal margins are marked, as well as the rectus abdominis muscle on the opposite side of the mastectomy defect. With the patient standing, a large ellipse is marked (see Figures 11.5–11.8 from Chapter 11). A mental picture is formulated as to how the flap will fit into the defect. It is best to plan the rotation of the flap so that the areas with the best blood supply fill the upper and middle portions of the reconstructed breast. The areas with the lesser blood supply are excised (see Figure 11.2 from Chapter 11 and Figure 13.12). The rectus muscle forms a gentle twist as it is brought up to the defect (Figures 13.13, 13.14).

Technique

The technique for harvesting the contralateral transverse rectus abdominis musculocutaneous flap is described in Chapter 11 and fully illustrated at the end of this chapter. The method is exactly the same except for the dissection over the chest wall and the insetting of the flap as a breast.

After the flap is harvested, attention is turned to the chest, and the mastectomy incision is reopened widely. See Figure 13.7 for planning the incision after a radical mastectomy. The following steps are illustrated in the example at the end of this chapter. The flap is oriented so that the abdominal skin and fat fill the deficit left by the mastectomy. This requires the temporary positioning of the abdominal flap under the reopened breast skin. The flap is stapled into a selected position to assess optimum aesthetic results. Attaining this goal usually necessitates unstapling and restapling until the best position is attained, with care to avoid any tension on the pedicle of the flap. After a final orientation is selected, a marking pen is used to outline the skin that will be removed or trimmed from the flap. The staples are then removed and the marked areas are excised. It may be best, in some cases, to de-epithelialize portions of the abdominal skin since this preserves bulk, yet allows closure of the chest skin over these areas. An effort is made to trim the less reliable regions of the abdominal flap since these may undergo necrosis postoperatively. After the final design is established, the pedicle is assessed to ensure total lack of tension, and the skin and deeper tissues are closed in layers. The inferior margin of the flap is usually situated at the inframammary fold of the reconstructed breast. This allows the breast to assume a more natural shape, especially when the patient is upright, and the soft tissues are free to hang softly over this edge (so-called natural ptosis).

The Latissimus Dorsi Musculocutaneous Flap

This flap is best for reconstructing the modified radical mastectomy defect in which the pectoralis major muscle remains intact. It can also be of value in the patient without this muscle (radical mastectomy defect). In this instance, it is used to fill out the infraclavicular hollowing and to augment the anterior axillary fold either alone or in preparation for a later rectus abdominis breast reconstruction.

The flap is not well suited in patients who are obese since the excessive thickness of the flank skin and fat on these women does not fit well with the thinner flaps of the anterior chest wall. Such latissimus flaps have a step-off on the reconstructed breast at the interface between the thicker and thinner elements. This step-off can be difficult to camouflage for some patients.

In using this flap, an effort is made to place the skin segment on the muscle so that it will be situated in the lower quadrants of the reconstructed breast. In this way the scars are hidden by the brassiere. Such positioning also gives a more aesthetic fullness in the upper quadrants, especially when a prosthesis is used to augment the reconstructed area. A prosthesis is, in fact, usually necessary to give enough fullness to the breast mound after the flap is in position.

Planning

The preoperative assessment is made exactly as outlined in Chapter 8. The previous mastectomy scar is ignored and a diagonal or lower quadrant incision is planned and marked so that the skin portion of the latissimus flap will fit into the lower outer quadrant region of the new breast (Figures 13.5 and 13.6). With a hand towel, a skin island is mapped out and transposed anteriorly as shown in Chapter 8 (Figures 8.8–8.9). This is checked several times to ensure that the optimum use of the muscle and its skin

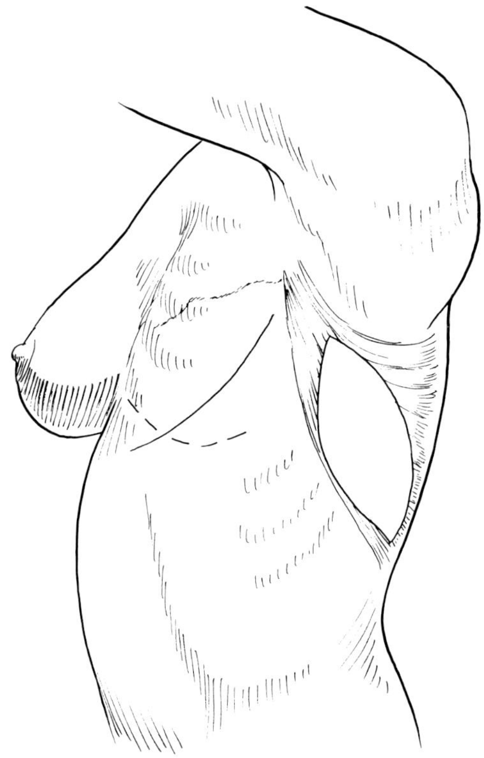

FIGURE 13.5 In planning for the use of the latissimus in breast reconstruction, the skin island is marked on the muscle so that it will eventually be situated in the lower outer quadrant of the newly fabricated breast. This will hide the scars within the brassiere and give a more natural contour. The old mastectomy scar is ignored and a diagonal incision (solid line) is planned. The inframammary crease is also marked (dashed line).

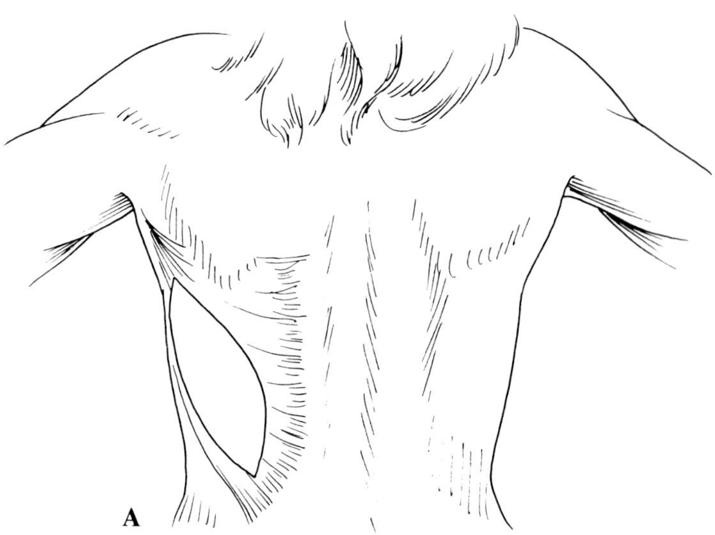

A

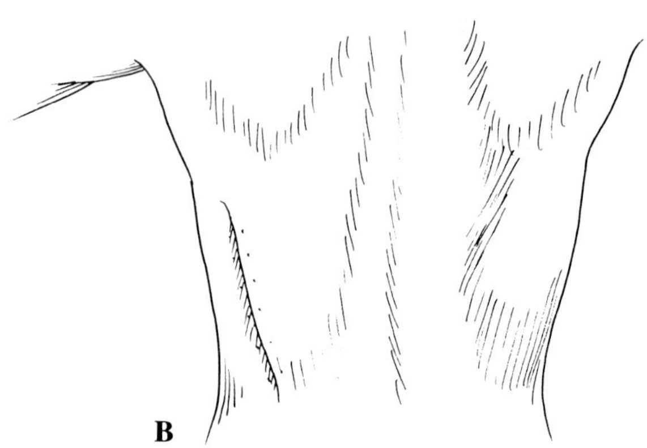

B

FIGURE 13.6 The skin island has been marked and is usually 6–8 cm wide by 10–12 cm in length. The diagonal orientation allows the skin to fit easily into the lower outer quadrant of the newly fabricated breast mound on the anterior chest wall (A). This hides the flap within the brassiere and also allows the posterior incision to be concealed, even in low-cut apparel (B).

island are being made in fashioning a breast mound. A mental note is made regarding the size prosthesis that may be required to augment the latissimus flap. This estimate is largely a matter of experience, but nonsterile prosthesis samples can be used preoperatively to arrive at a working volume. They are placed on the chest wall and in the brassiere to estimate anticipated volume.

Technique

The flap is harvested exactly as described in Chapter 8. After the flap is mobilized up to the thoracodorsal vascular pedicle, attention is turned to the anterior chest, and the previously marked incision is opened. The incision is deepened to the plane beneath the pectoralis major muscle, and the submuscular pocket is enlarged. To achieve the necessary medial extent of the pocket, it may be necessary to liberate a portion of the pectoralis origin along the caudal sternum. A generous subcutaneous pocket is established inferiorly, reaching about 2 cm below the inframammary crease. This is done to allow for any cephalad migration of the prosthesis postoperatively. A wide subcutaneous tunnel is made through the axilla to allow anterior transposition of the latissimus, and the musculocutaneous unit is brought forward (Figure 13.7). There should be absolutely no tension on the vascular pedicle. If it is tight, it is returned to the back and the flap is further liberated with the pedicle under direct vision. It should fit loosely into its new position.

The border of the latissimus is sewn to the inferolateral edge of the pectoralis major muscle and inferiorly to the deep fascia of the serratus anterior and rectus abdominis. A soft, silicone gel prosthesis (300–400 cc more or less, depending on the preoperative estimate of the thoracic cage and the opposite breast) is inserted under the latissimus muscle, and the free edge of the latissimus is attached to the fascia along the lateral thorax with a few interrupted sutures. This prevents posterior migration of the prosthesis

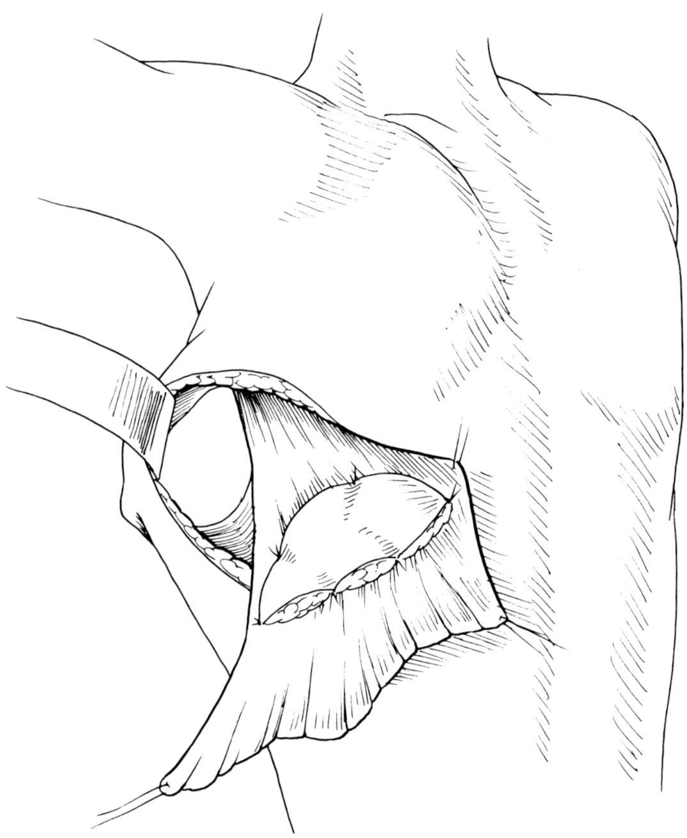

FIGURE 13.7 The latissimus dorsi musculocutaneous flap has been mobilized and is ready for transfer through the axillary subcutaneous tunnel and onto the anterior chest wall.

to the axilla or through the axillary tunnel to the back. The skin island is joined with the anterior chest wall skin with fine sutures or skin staples, and Bacitracin Ointment is applied as a dressing.

The Problem of the Anterior Axillary Fold

Unfortunately, when dealing with a deformity in which the pectoralis muscle has been removed (radical mastectomy), it is extremely difficult to reconstitute a normal-appearing anterior axillary fold. Yet this is important since the unrestored defect is so noticeable. The infraclavicular hollowing, although ameliorated by a good rectus abdominis flap, can also present a challenge (Figure 13.8).

Custom-made, soft, silicone gel prostheses can be made to fill the defect. However, these are usually unsatisfactory since their edges are noticeable under the skin. They are also subject to migration even when sutured to periosteum or covered with a velour backing.

Another alternative has been to move the insertion of the latissimus dorsi muscle anteriorly and fix it to the humerus. This is done after the standard latissimus breast reconstruction. It too has not been totally satisfactory since the fold is not well restored.

A promising alternative is to use the latissimus to fill the infraclavicular hollowing by suturing it to the manubrium and along the clavicle. It can be folded and sutured to the coracoid process, or a de-epithelialized skin segment can be fixed to this process with permanent sutures. Later, a rectus abdominis musculocutaneous flap can be used to reconstitute the breast mound. This alternative has been used successfully in good-risk, selected patients.

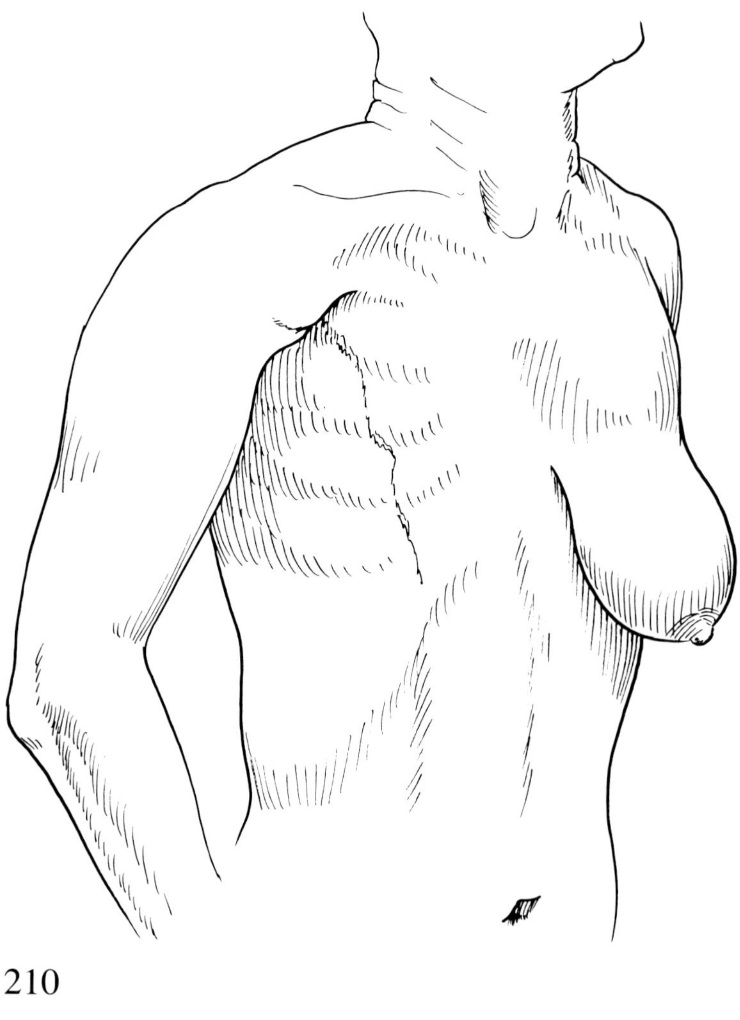

FIGURE 13.8 The radical mastectomy deformity, with infraclavicular hollowing and the absence of an anterior axillary fold, is exceedingly difficult to reconstruct. Alternatives include custom-made prosthesis, latissimus dorsi flap with transfer of its insertion, rectus abdominis flap alone, or rectus-latissimus combination.

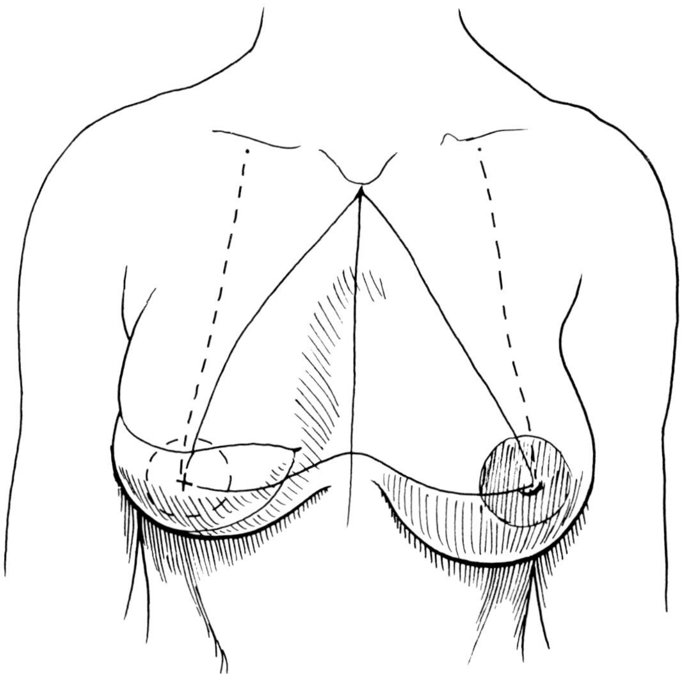

FIGURE 13.9 The patient has had a right-sided latissimus breast reconstruction and a left-sided mastopexy (uplift) for symmetry. She has been measured for nipple-areolar reconstruction. In this patient, the triangle measures 19 cm on each side.

Nipple-Areolar Reconstruction

After 6 to 8 weeks, the postoperative changes have receded sufficiently and the reconstructed tissues have settled enough to consider accurate nipple-areolar placement. This should be done only after both breasts are in optimum position (i.e., any procedure on the remaining breast to attain symmetry must have already been accomplished), and is usually done under local anesthesia. The notch-nipple distance should be in the range of 18–21 cm, and this distance should form each limb of a roughly equilateral triangle (Figure 13.9).

The nipple position is marked with the patient standing, and a 38- to 45-mm-diameter areola is centered on the mark, depending on the size of the normal nipple-areolar complex. A full-thickness, well-thinned skin graft is harvested from the extreme upper inner thigh and the donor site closed primarily (Figure 13.10A).

The previously marked new areolar area is de-epithelialized, and the skin graft from the thigh is sutured into the defect with fine sutures. A central, 1-cm-diameter circle is removed from the center of the graft, and a superficial disklike segment of the nipple from the remaining breast is removed. This nipple graft is sutured to the de-epithelialized breast skin at the center of the skin graft, ensuring good contact with the exposed dermis below (Figure 13.10B). Sometimes the nipple graft must be radically thinned to remove the lactiferous ducts. This, however, is important so that the dermal elements can rapidly acquire enough capillary ingrowth to survive. A glycerin-soaked cotton tie-over dressing is applied.

If both breasts have been removed, a nipple must be reconstructed from local tissues. A reliable option has been the four-flap technique. A cross, having 1-cm-wide limbs is designed, with the center in the previously marked 4.5-cm-diameter areola. With a 5-mm distance between the periphery of the areola and the end of each limb, the limbs are elevated from the dermis. The base of each limb is deepened into the subcutaneous fat so that the flaps are free of the dermis. The center of the cross is left undisturbed so that the limbs maintain their blood supply, and the limbs are then sewn together to form a nipple. A full-thickness skin graft from the thigh is applied around the nipple, as described, to restore the areola (Figure 13.11). The tie-over dressing is left in place for 5 to 7 days and an antibacterial ointment is applied to the graft to minimize scaling and encrustation.

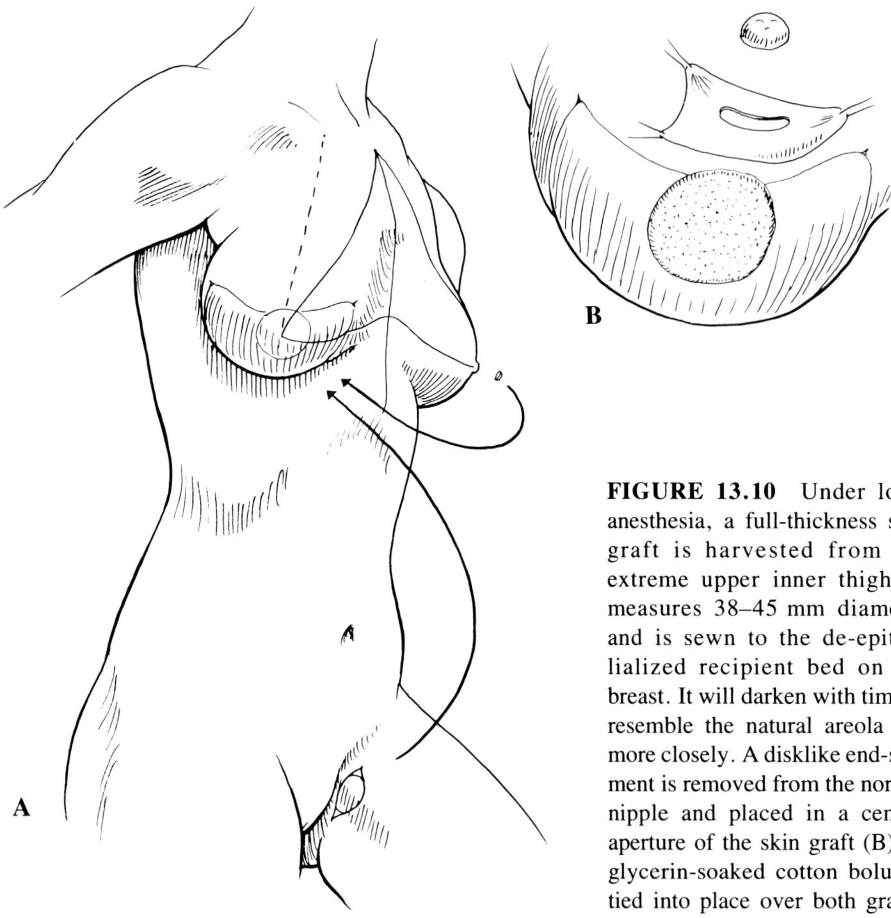

FIGURE 13.10 Under local anesthesia, a full-thickness skin graft is harvested from the extreme upper inner thigh. It measures 38–45 mm diameter and is sewn to the de-epithelialized recipient bed on the breast. It will darken with time to resemble the natural areola (A) more closely. A disklike end-segment is removed from the normal nipple and placed in a central aperture of the skin graft (B). A glycerin-soaked cotton bolus is tied into place over both grafts.

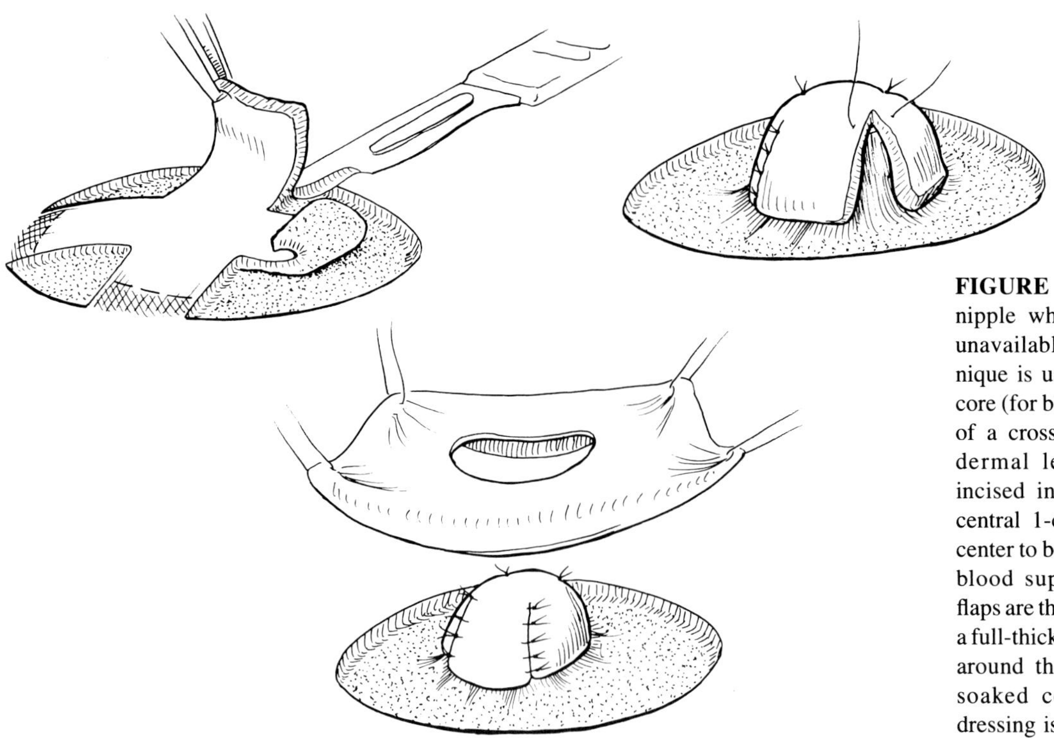

FIGURE 13.11 To restore a nipple when a donor nipple is unavailable, the four-flap technique is used. Leaving a central core (for blood supply), the limbs of a cross are elevated at deep dermal level. The dermis is incised into the fat around the central 1-cm core (to allow the center to be elevated), leaving the blood supply intact. The four flaps are then sutured together and a full-thickness skin graft lowered around the nipple. A glycerin-soaked cotton bolus tie-over dressing is applied.

ILLUSTRATIVE CASE

This 52-year-old female underwent a right radical mastectomy for infiltrating ductal carcinoma 10 years before the current admission. There were no lymph node metastases, and no additional therapy had been administered. The patient desired breast reconstruction. A contralateral rectus abdominis musculocutaneous flap is planned (Figure 13.12). The flap is mobilized as described in Chapter 11 and transposed to the chest wall defect after reopening the original incision (Figure 13.13). Care is taken to

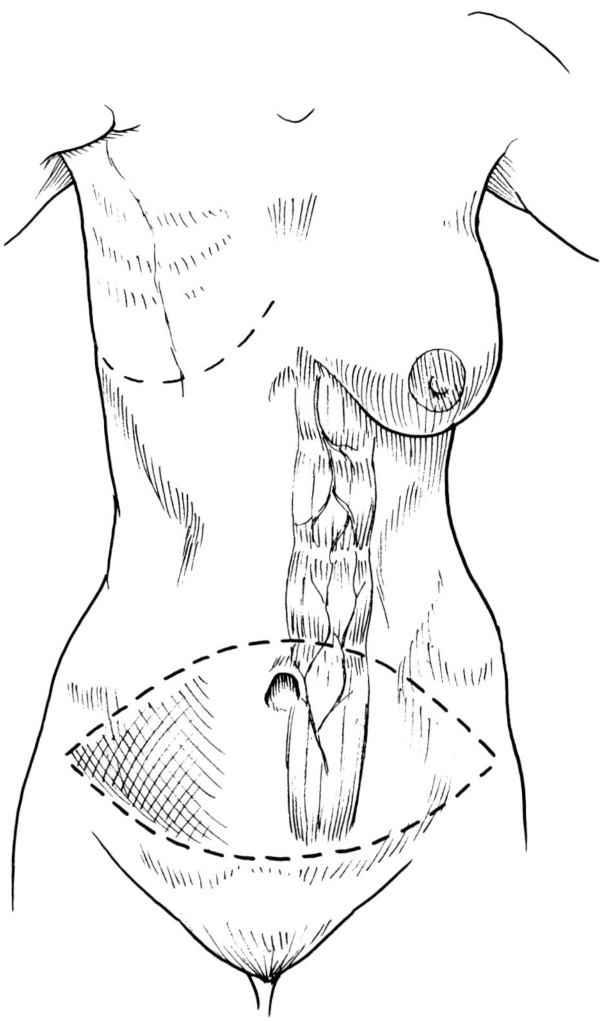

FIGURE 13.12 The patient is marked for a contralateral rectus abdominis flap. A generous ellipse is planned, and the area with the poorest blood supply corresponds to the crosshatched extremity of the ellipse. The dashed line represents the inframammary fold, and the healed Halsted incision is evident.

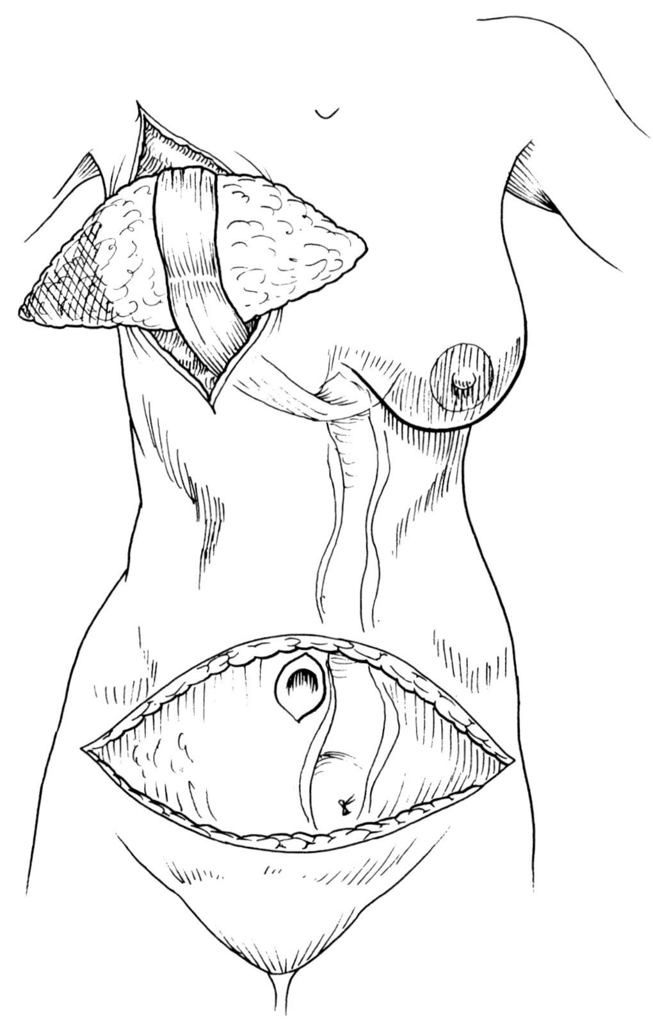

FIGURE 13.13 The rectus abdominis flap is mobilized and transferred to the chest wall defect. In this patient, the mastectomy incision has been reopened to accommodate the abdominal tissues. The crosshatched area is the area with the poorest blood supply. It will be excised. The umbilical aperture on the flap is closed from the underside of the flap to prevent skin indentation on the newly fabricated breast mound.

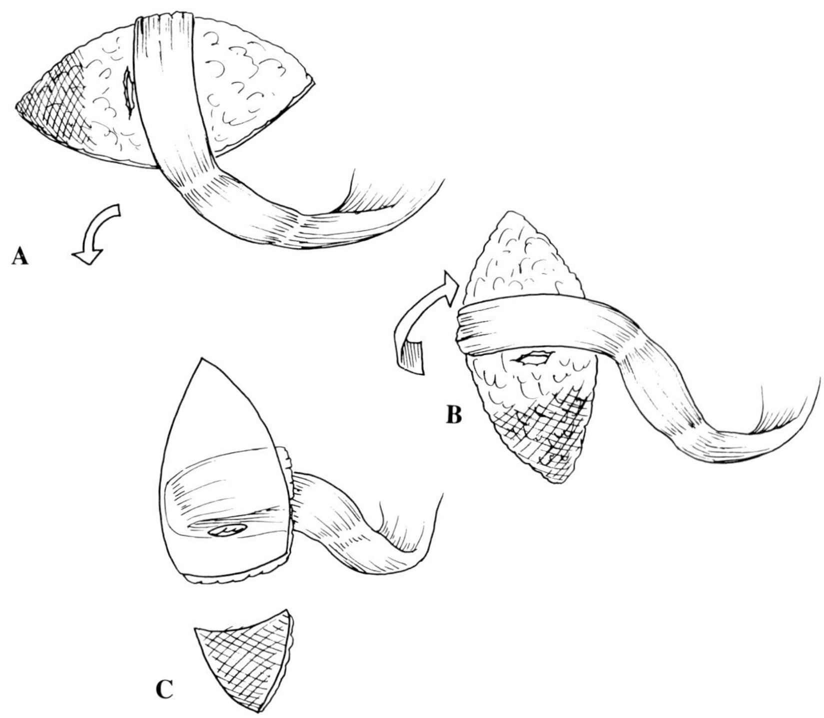

FIGURE 13.14 One method of insetting the rectus flap is illustrated. Care is taken to avoid any constraint or torsion on the pedicle. In this case, the flap is first transposed directly to the chest (A), rotated slightly counterclockwise so that the crosshatched area is inferior (B), and gently turned upward so that the skin surface is facing outward. The crosshatched area is excised (C). It represents the region with the poorest blood supply.

avoid tension or torsion of the vascular pedicle (Figure 13.14). The flap is tailored to the requirements of the deformity, with the goal of restoring a symmetrical breast mound and filling out both the infraclavicular deficit and the anterior axillary fold (Figures 13.15 through 13.18).

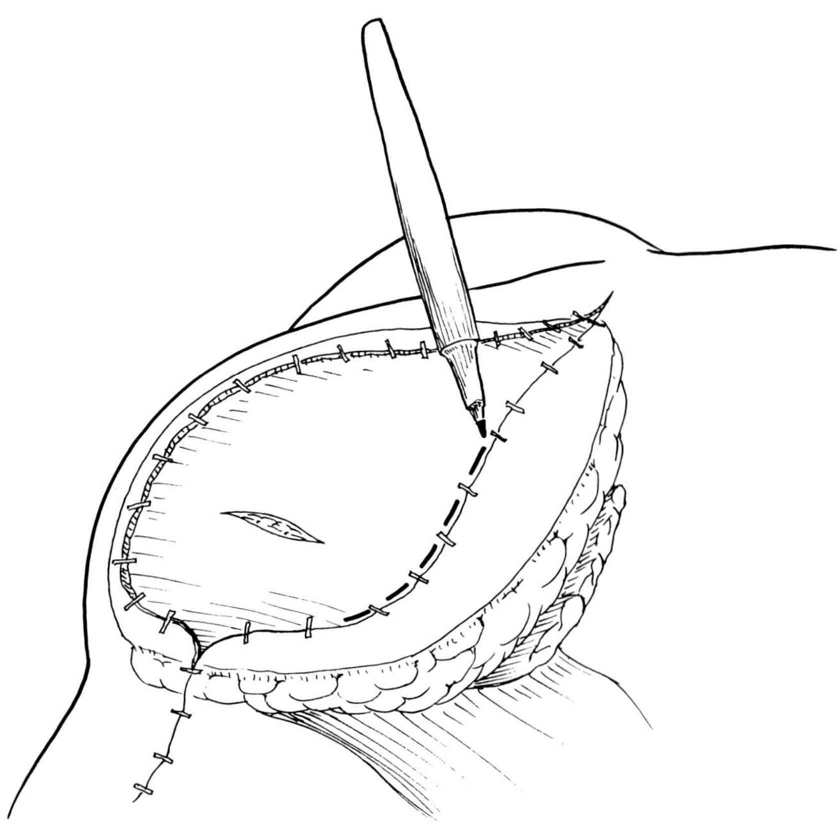

FIGURE 13.15 The flap is temporarily fixed into place so that it can be sculptured. The goal in this patient is to fill out the subclavicular space and to provide a natural-appearing breast mound. The flap is attached to the chest wall with temporary staples and the margins of overlapping chest skin marked on the abdominal skin.

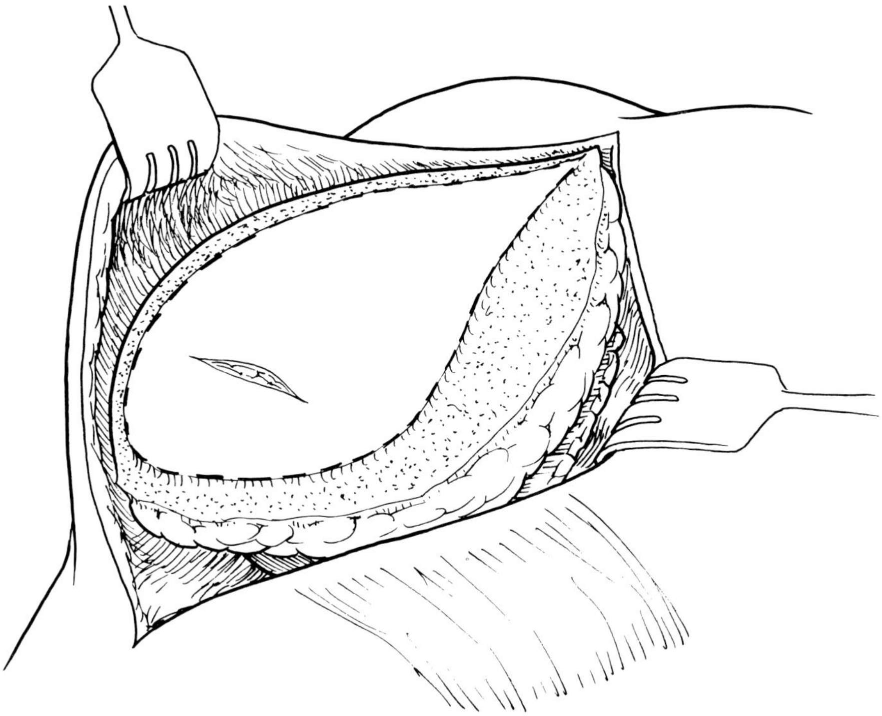

FIGURE 13.16 The staples are removed and the abdominal skin (which was covered by overlapping chest skin) is de-epithelialized, leaving the dermis to provide more soft tissue bulk. The apex of this dermis is fixed to the clavicle with nonabsorbable monofilament sutures.

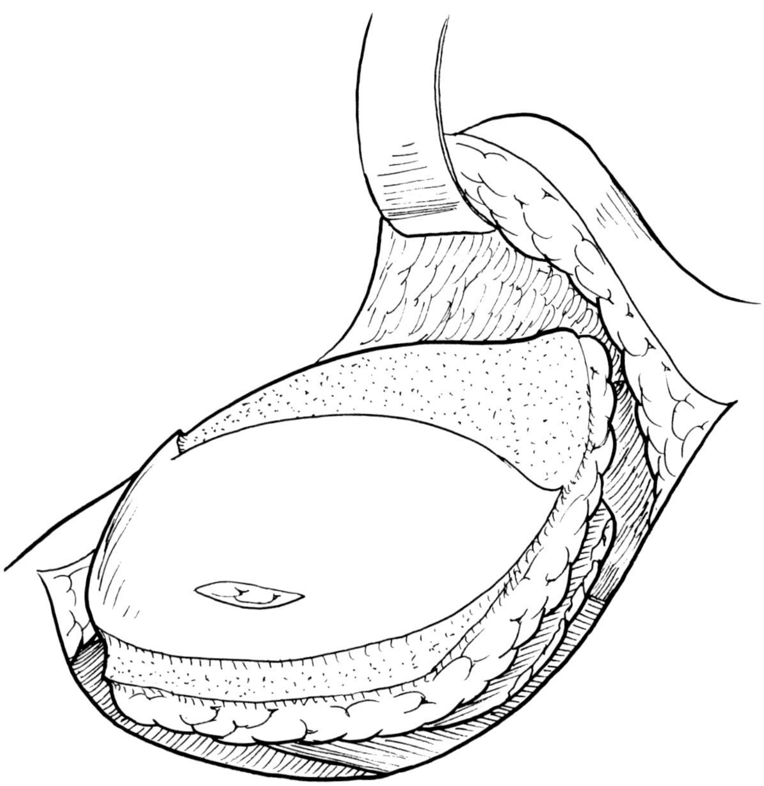

FIGURE 13.17 In this alternative design (often used in reconstructing the modified mastectomy defect), a transverse chest wall incision is used. This incision is made at the new inframammary crease, and some of the skin between this incision and the old mastectomy incision may be discarded to make room for the flap. The abdominal skin is sculptured as described.

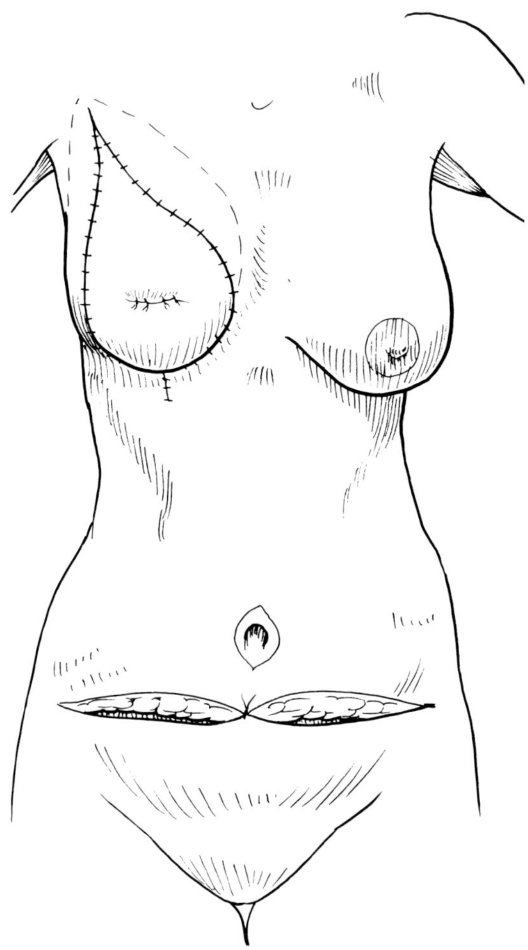

FIGURE 13.18 After the breast has been tailored, the skin incisions are closed with fine sutures.

14

Tracheoesophageal and Bronchopleural/ Cutaneous Fistulas

Tracheoesophageal Fistula (Acquired)

Tracheoesophageal fistulas are challenging because they invariably involve damaged tissues that have a diminished capacity to heal and that are subject to the irritative effects of abnormally directed secretions (Figure 14.1). Certain steps are usually required to prepare the patient for a reconstruction that will endure.

In this chapter, the general principles for evaluating acquired tracheoesophageal fistulas are discussed along with methods of dividing the fistula and restoring the continuity of the esophagus and the tracheobronchial tree. As a rule, the underlying pathologic process that gave rise to the fistula must be controlled, strong nutritional support must be instituted, and healthy tissues must be interposed between the repaired enteric tract and the trachea if the repair is to be successful.

Evaluation of the Fistula

Several different processes are known to cause tracheoesophageal fistulas. By far, the most common is a malignancy arising in the alimentary tract or in the tracheobronchial tree. Fistulas caused by malignant lesions often are not amenable to reconstruction since the patient usually has a short life expectancy. In these patients, adequate palliation can be achieved through gastrointestinal diversion and feeding

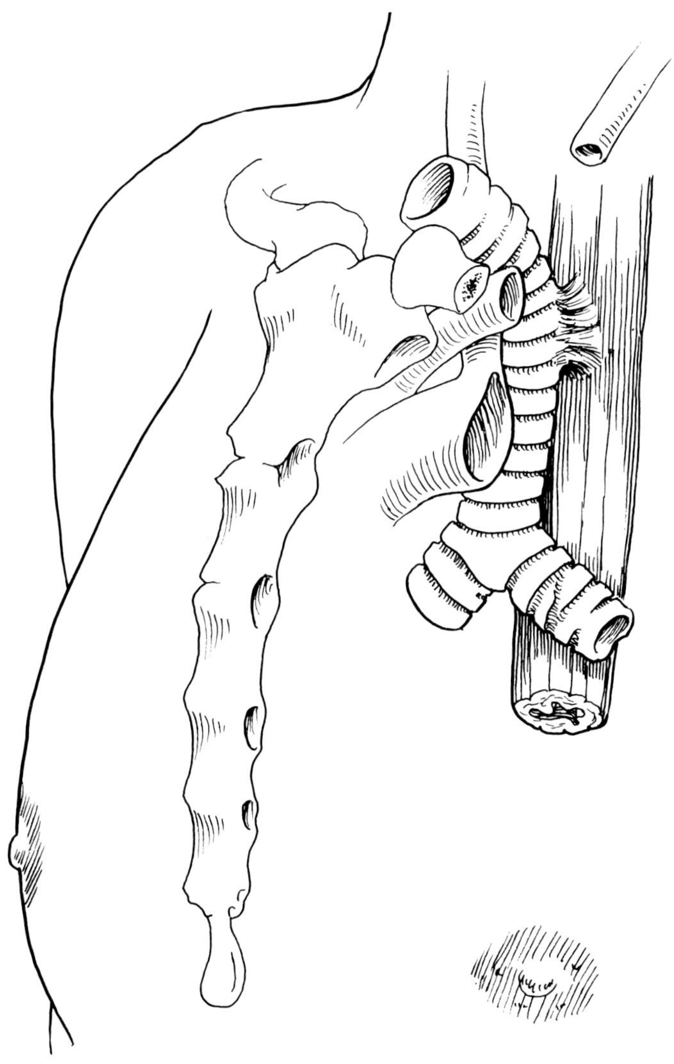

FIGURE 14.1 Tracheoesophageal fistula can be caused by both benign and malignant processes. They are often compromised by adverse influences and must be thoroughly evaluated. The repair consists of division of the abnormal connection, repair of the openings in the trachea and esophagus, and interposition of healthy muscle tissue. This fistula is located near major vascular structures and followed radiotherapy. It is causing a chronic aspiration pneumonitis.

stomas. Other types of acquired tracheoesophageal fistulas, however, are amenable to division, repair, and reconstruction. These include mediastinal and cervical fistulas arising from infection and disruption of suture lines in the interposed gastrointestinal tract; radiation necrosis of tissues between the trachea and the esophagus after treatment of a primary tumor; pressure necrosis from an endotracheal tube or intraesophageal stethoscope (or both); and certain localized cancers. The diagnostic workup should include localization of the fistula, assessment of underlying disease, and evaluation of associated infection.

One of the most important diagnostic modalities is endoscopy. Bronchoscopy should be performed both to localize the fistula and to obtain a good tissue sample. This latter can help to confirm or rule out a malignant process. Fiberoptic bronchoscopy can be used to assess the bronchial tree distal to the fistula for bronchiectasis, evidence of aspiration, or other injury. Esophagoscopy can be valuable in measuring the size of the defect as well as for obtaining additional tissue samples if there is a question of malignancy.

Certain radiographic tests can also be helpful. The most important of these x-ray examinations is an esophagogram. This must be performed with a contrast medium that is associated with minimal bronchial inflammation. Barium, even in its diluted forms, can cause severe bronchitis (and pneumonitis) and should be avoided if at all possible. Other agents that have equal contrast capabilities and cause less irritation to the tracheobronchial tree are available. Computerized tomography (CT) may help to detect the presence of mediastinal infection, assess for lymphadenopathy, and define the extent of the communication between the esophagus and the trachea. Bronchography is of limited value since it is less likely to outline the fistula well and requires considerable expertise to position the catheter for optimal visualization. This examination, however, may confirm the presence or absence of distal suppuration in the tracheobronchial tree. If the fistula communicates with the skin, a sinogram may be beneficial in evaluating the length of the sinus tract, as well as any associated abscess or false passage that communicates with the tracheobronchial tree or the enteric tract.

Nutritional Support

Before the operation to repair the fistula, the patient must be brought into optimal nutritional and medical condition, and any associated infection must be adequately drained. If infection is present, a preliminary exploration may be necessary to achieve drainage of the abscess. Drainage may be directed through the pleural space or through the mediastinum, depending on the location of the abscess and the preference of the surgeon. Drainage of the abscess and diversion of the enteric tract are usually necessary to achieve stabilization of the fistula. The esophagus can be diverted by a cervical esophagostomy. This controlled fistula is established by the standard marsupialization of the lateral wall of the esophagus to the skin in the region of the lower sternocleidomastoid muscle. This lateral fistula preserves esophageal function and length, yet diverts the flow of saliva away from the tracheoesophageal connection. At the same time, it may be necessary to provide for gastric decompression and the control of acid reflux. Both of these goals can be partially achieved by the establishment of a gastrostomy.

In some patients, continued reflux of gastric contents may require isolation of the esophagus. This can be accomplished by placing a band (such as an umbilical tape) around the distal esophagus. This assures that gastric contents do not enter the esophagus and continue the inflammation around the fistula or cause an aspiration pneumonitis.

Efficient use of the enteric tract while the patient is being prepared for the operation can be challenging. A feeding jejunostomy may be established independently or at the time of the gastrostomy. In such instances, a number 16 red rubber catheter (with additional holes cut in it) is placed in the jejunum at a convenient point about

15–18 inches distal to the ligament of Treitz. Using the Witzel technique, this jejunostomy is brought up to the anterior abdominal wall and fixed to the inner aspect of the parietal peritoneum with permanent sutures. (See Chapter 10, Figure 10.15.) The jejunostomy is used to feed the patient distal to the stomach so that no reflux can occur as a result of enteric supplements. In some patients, even the jejunostomy is not sufficient to attain a positive nitrogen balance. In these individuals, peripheral nutrition or total parenteral nutrition may be considered in order to ensure good nutritional support. Such support cannot be overemphasized and can mean the difference between success and failure.

Repair and Reconstruction

In general, the goals are to isolate the fistulous tract, divide it, and restore the walls of both the trachea and the esophagus. If possible, the reconstruction should also interpose healthy muscle tissue between the membranous trachea (where most fistulae occur) and the esophageal closure.

In approaching the lower cervical region, removal of the medial half of the clavicle as well as a portion of the adjacent manubrium can be helpful in avoiding injury to the innominate and subclavian vessels. This maneuver allows more room for accurate dissection and good exposure of the fistula (Figure 14.2). The tracheoesophageal groove is located and the fistula isolated. Before division, the position of the endotracheal tube is confirmed as well as its balloon (i.e., distal to the fistula) so that ventilation is securely maintained.

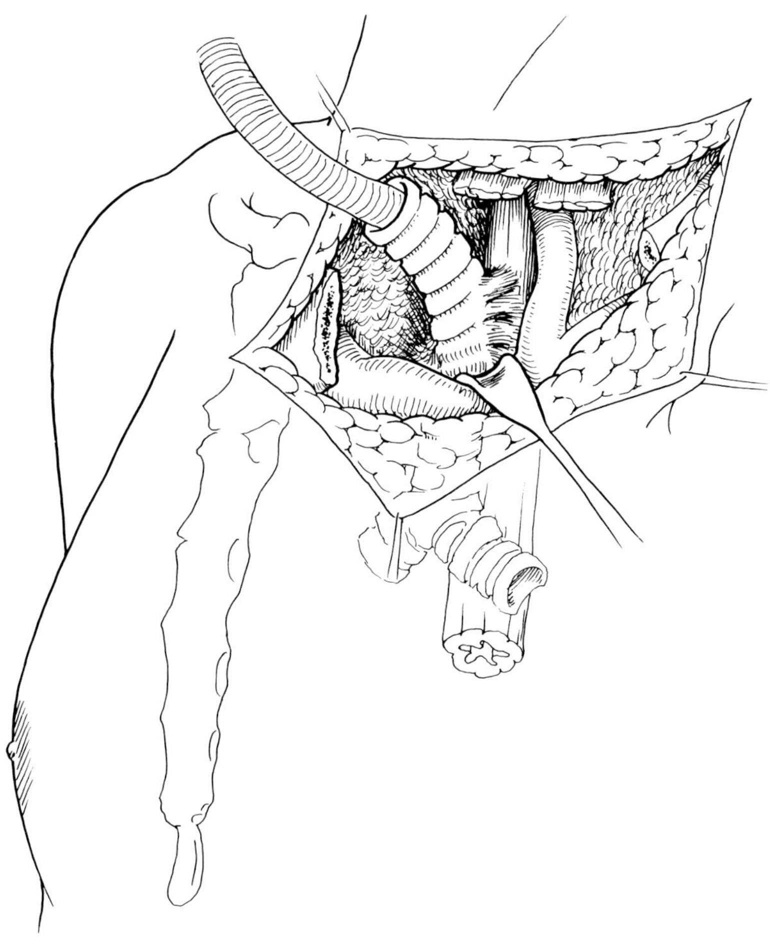

FIGURE 14.2 A large tracheoesophageal fistula secondary to radionecrosis (after laryngectomy) is shown. Segments of clavicle and manubrium have been removed to allow safe, wide dissection and exposure of the fistula.

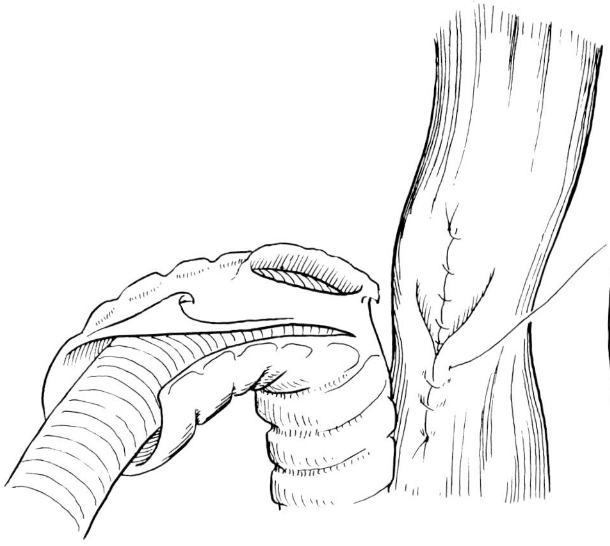

FIGURE 14.3 The esophageal opening is closed in two layers; the membranous trachea, being in poor condition, is removed.

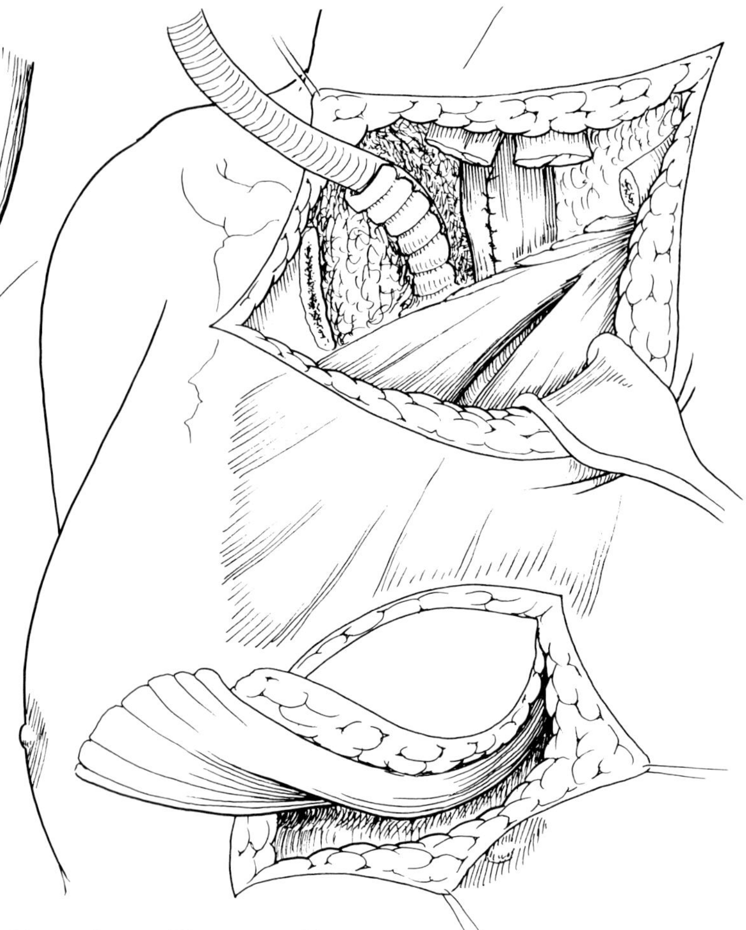

FIGURE 14.4 In the same case as the previous figures, the fistula has been divided and the esophagus repaired. A pectoralis major musculocutaneous flap is mobilized both to resurface the tracheal defect and to interpose healthy muscle between the repaired trachea and esophagus.

The fistula is divided and the esophagus is closed in two layers. The mucosal layer is closed with a fine, running absorbable suture. A second layer of running sutures is used to close the muscle layer (Figure 14.3). A cricothyroidotomy has been accomplished as part of the exposure, and this seems to help avoid functional problems related to esophageal motility and diverticula. The esophagus is assessed to assure that there is no stenosis associated with the closure. In such an event, consideration for the provision of epithelial lining must be made. This could involve anything from the microvascular interposition of free intestinal segments to major musculocutaneous flap operations. The preference would be a microsurgical free flap of interposed jejunum.

The second choice would be a pectoralis major musculocutaneous flap, with the skin segment providing the lining necessary to correct the stenotic segment of esophagus. The trachea may also have a mature (chronic) opening that is too large to close primarily. If the opening is small, one can consider the interposition of healthy muscle between the repaired esophagus and the trachea. Tiny holes such as these granulate with scar epithelium and close spontaneously. The danger of this is the subsequent formation of granulomas within the trachea, which can attain a size large enough to cause obstruction. Larger openings may require a skin graft on the interposed muscle, with the graft sewn to the edges of the tracheal hole (this is the preferred approach); tracheal resection, with removal of the damaged region; or establishment of a mediastinal tracheostomy below the level of the fistula (Figures 14.4 through 14.6).

For intrathoracic fistulae, the principles are the same: repair of the esophagus and tracheobronchial segments and interposition of healthy muscle or omental tissue. Such intrathoracic repair may require the transfer of serratus anterior, latissimus dorsi, omentum, or other healthy flap into the mediastinum to bolster the repaired area. It is necessary to resect portions of the upper ribs to allow the latissimus or serratus to enter the thorax without constraint on the vascular pedicle (Figure 14.7).

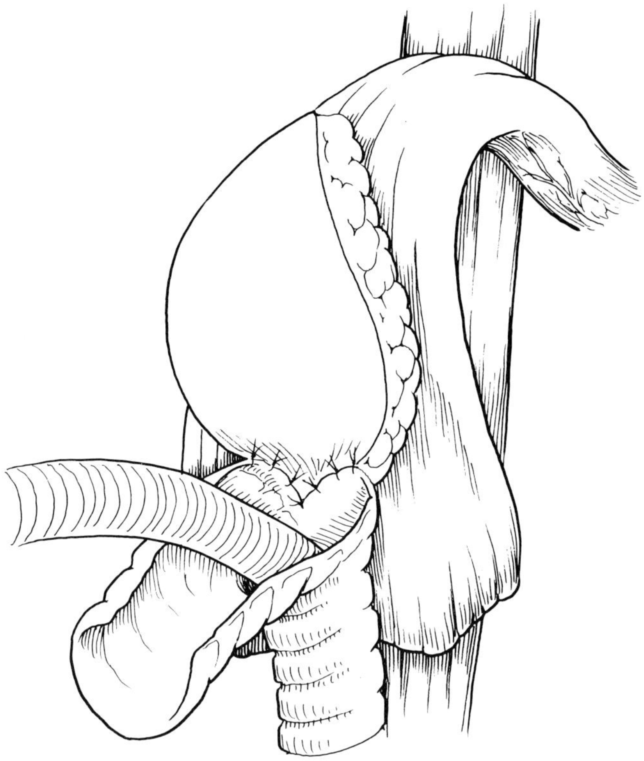

FIGURE 14.5 The skin segment of the flap is used to resurface the excised posterior trachea. The muscular portion of the flap is interposed between the esophagus and trachea at the location of the repair.

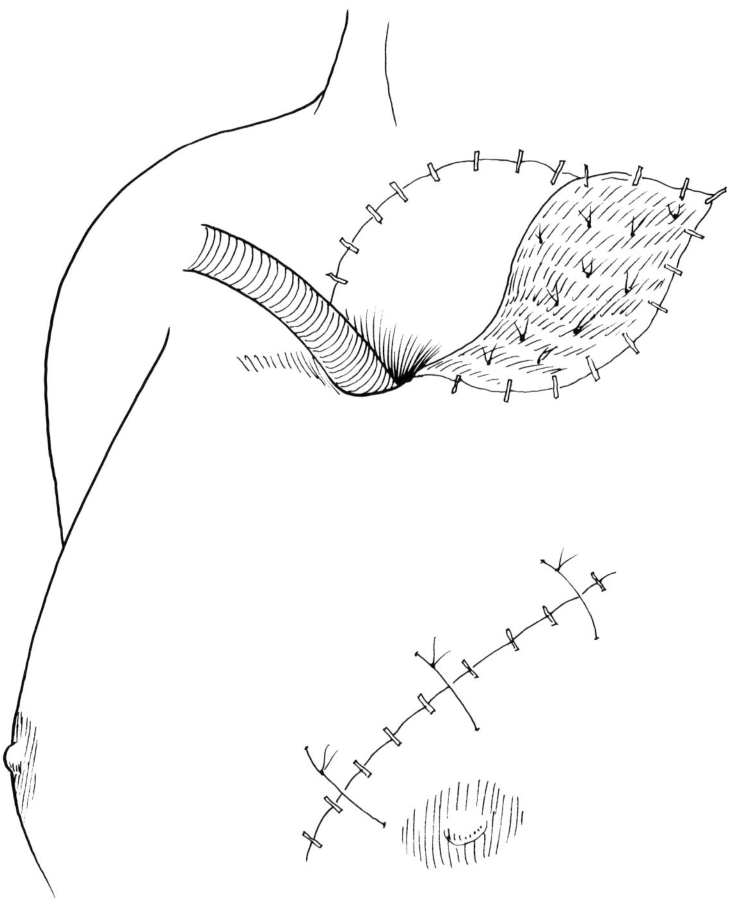

FIGURE 14.6 The airway is converted into a mediastinal tracheostomy, and the exposed portion of the muscle is covered with a meshed, split-thickness skin graft. The donor defect of the pectoralis flap is closed primarily.

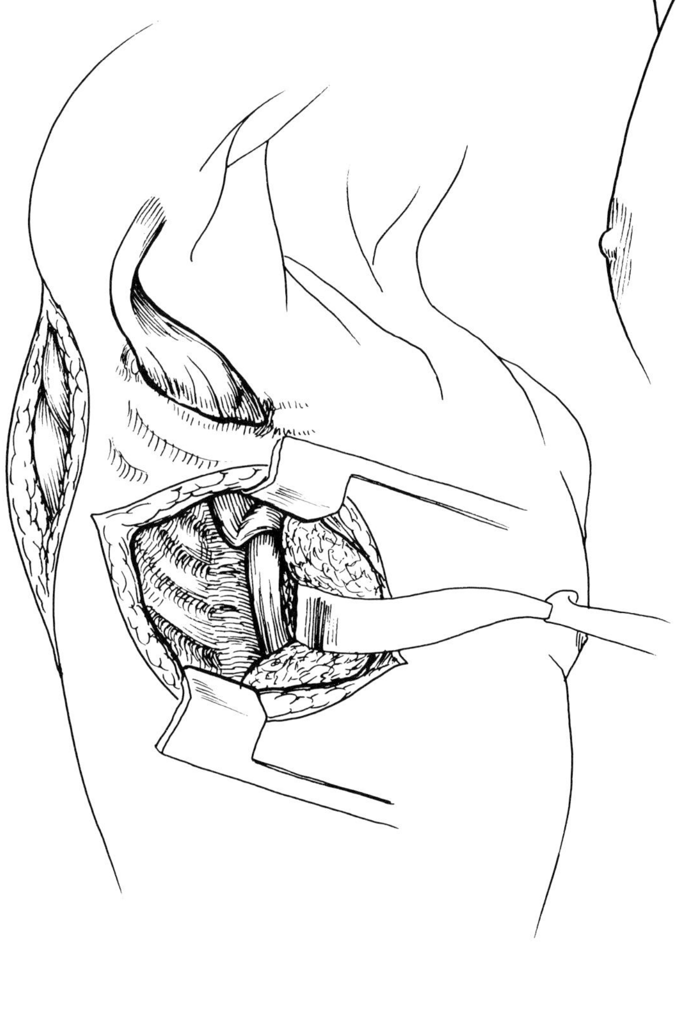

FIGURE 14.7 Intrathoracic transfer of a latissimus muscle flap is accomplished in order to interpose healthy tissue between the repaired trachea and the esophagus. Segments of the upper ribs are removed to allow the flap to enter the thorax without constraint on the pedicle.

Bronchopleural and Bronchopleurocutaneous Fistula

Bronchopleural fistula is an abnormal connection between the tracheobronchial tree and the pleural space. Its extension to the skin surface (and thus the external environment) represents a bronchopleurocutaneous fistula. These lesions can be difficult to treat successfully and often arise in tissues already compromised by adverse influences.

Common etiological factors include residual malignant tissue at the bronchial suture line, infection (especially after aspiration pneumonia or lung abscess), and ischemic necrosis of the bronchial stump. These factors, along with the pressure differential across the bronchial closure, can result in a local dehiscence and a continuous stream of air across the bronchial opening and into the pleural space. This is heralded by an increase in the bubbling from the chest tubes that cannot be traced to external disruption of the sealed drainage system.

The air leak does not allow the disrupted tissues to coapt and to seal the communication, and the channel becomes established. Depending on the size of the defect, the process can be self-limiting and may allow the pleural seal to reestablish itself around the fistula. On the other hand, the fistula may be subject to local factors that enlarge or prolong the process, resulting in a chronic opening along the chest tube tract.

It is important both to establish the etiology of the fistula and to correct any immediate threat to the patient's life. Acutely, efforts are directed at fully expanding the lung through strong suction (via large-bore chest tubes) and at maintaining adequate gas exchange. Once the patient's ventilation is stabilized and the fistula is no longer a source of respiratory embarrassment, time can be taken to assess the process more thoroughly.

Often the cause of the fistula is already known and lengthy investigatory steps are bypassed. Such may be the case, for example, with a posttraumatic fistula. In this instance, aggressive debridement and drainage may be required and extensive preoperative studies may not be necessary at all. However, certain procedures may be helpful in other circumstances.

Bronchoscopy may be done to assess the conditions around the fistula and to rule out the presence of residual infection or tumor. Both healthy and diseased areas within the tracheobronchial tree are carefully noted, and any suspicious region is biopsied. Appropriate cultures can also be obtained. If a cavity is present, it too can be investigated through the bronchoscope.

Bronchography can be helpful in evaluating the contour of the airways. A sinogram through the chest tube can delineate the extent of the cavitary defect, and thoracoscopy can be of value in assessing the bronchial opening from the external aspect. These studies, of course, must be individualized according to the needs of the patient. Further details are beyond the scope of this atlas.

Treatment

The immediate concern is reestablishment of effective ventilation, with the goal of fully expanding the lung. The suction on the chest tubes is turned up, and the visceral and parietal pleurae are given the opportunity to adhere around the tubes. If successful, adhesions form over the next week and the lung remains inflated. The fistula is then converted to a tube tract that, if clear of necrotic tissue, closes by secondary intention. If the lung fails to expand, any loculated areas of pus must be eradicated. These areas may be radiographically confirmed as air-fluid levels. Repeat thoracotomy is performed, the loculated areas opened and debrided, and large-bore chest tubes used to maintain postoperative drainage. If such treatment fails to obliterate the cavity, consideration is given to a procedure to close this nonfunctional space (described in next section).

Throughout this process, the surgeon must ensure that the patient's tidal volume is not depleted by loss of air through the suction apparatus. With a high-volume fistula, arteriovenous shunting may supervene, with a gradual and insidious decline in the patient's effective ventilation. Likewise, especially in debilitated individuals, fatigue and exhaustion may occur and pose a serious threat to the patient's life. Under these circumstances, ventilatory assistance with a high-frequency or jet respirator may be necessary while control of the fistula is being established. As a corollary, nutritional support during this critical period must be maintained by whatever means necessary. This cannot be overemphasized and is consistent with standard general surgical principles.

The Air Leak

It is unusual for the air leak to remain open in the face of a well-debrided and granulating cavity. This is especially true if the patient is in good nutritional balance and has no evidence of tumor or infection (especially tuberculosis) at the bronchial stump. Healthy stumps usually contract, seal, and granulate in without treatment. If not, a healthy muscle flap can be used to obliterate the cavity and a small skin graft (the size of the bronchial opening) sewn on the muscle. This patch graft is then sewn to the edges of the bronchus as lining for the inside of the bronchus. This technique has been more reliable than a direct closure of the bronchus, which is usually in poor condition and friable.

The Empyema Cavity

With a large postempyema cavity, there are several options for management after this space has been thoroughly cleansed. These include healing by secondary intention, a marsupialization procedure, skin closure after instillation of antibiotic solution, and closure with flaps.

Healing by secondary intention can occur rapidly in young, otherwise healthy individuals. It can be a prolonged ordeal in others. The cavity is kept open and allowed to obliterate itself with granulation tissue, fibrosis, and contraction.

Marsupialization, or suturing the skin to the pleura around the entire external skin margin, is designed to facilitate healing by secondary intention. Usually, the eighth rib is removed as well. The technique matures the margins of the cavity so that skin closure will not occur until the deeper tissues have filled in (Figure 14.8). The Eloesser flap is a similar procedure, except that a superiorly based tongue of skin is sutured to the pleura after removal of a portion of the rib. This, too, matures the cavity to allow for a safe secondary course of healing (Figure 14.9). These procedures are usually employed to establish effective drainage of a difficult empyema.

Skin closure after filling the cavity with a neomycin solution (after Clagett) should be considered only if the bronchus is completely sealed. If the solution enters the tracheobronchial tree, it can cause a severe contact bronchitis. The goal is obliteration of the residual space with the fluid. However, to attain the seal, mobilization of retracted skin flaps is necessary, and there is a degree of tension along the closure. This is a distinct disadvantage.

Closure with flaps can be an attractive alternative. It is a one-stage operation; it supplies healthy, well-vascularized (and therefore infection-resistant) tissue to an area where it is needed; it can be used effectively even in large cavities.

The first choice is muscle tissue. The latissimus dorsi or serratus anterior can be mobilized on the thoracodorsal vascular pedicle and brought into the thorax directly. The muscle is sutured into place with absorbable sutures after a final (and thorough) debridement (Figure 14.10). Care is taken to ensure a safe, nonconstrictive route (usually subcutaneous) for the vascular pedicle. The skin at the margins of the cavity can usually be closed over the muscle. If not, a meshed skin graft can be applied to the surface of the muscle to provide epithelial coverage.

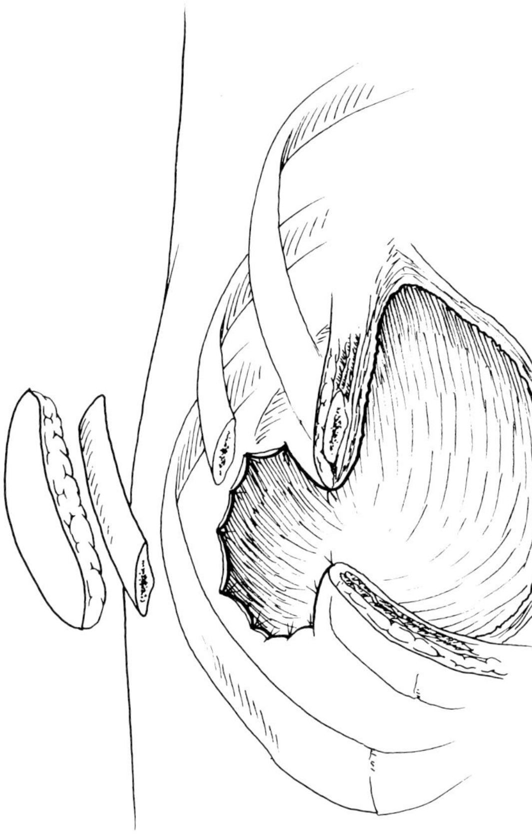

FIGURE 14.8 Marsupialization of the empyema cavity allows healing from the inside out. The cavity will gradually fill in with granulation tissue and close by contraction.

FIGURE 14.9 (A and B) The Eloesser flap keeps the skin open and facilitates the closure of the empyema cavity.

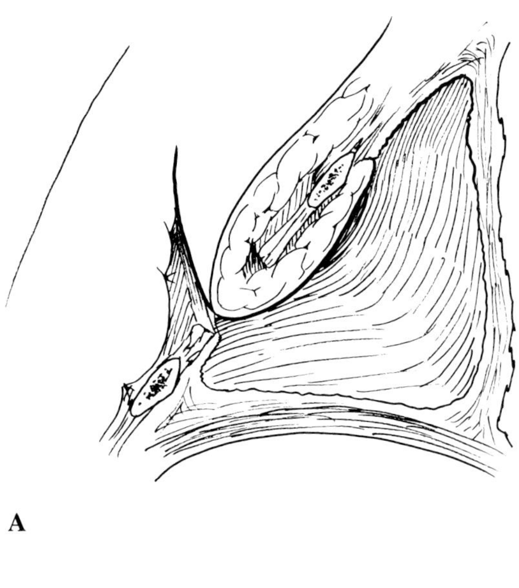

A

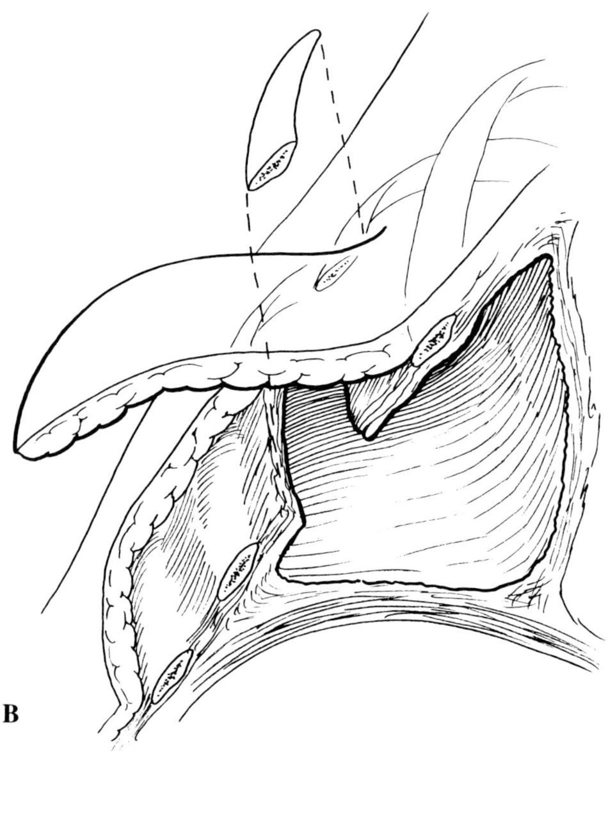

B

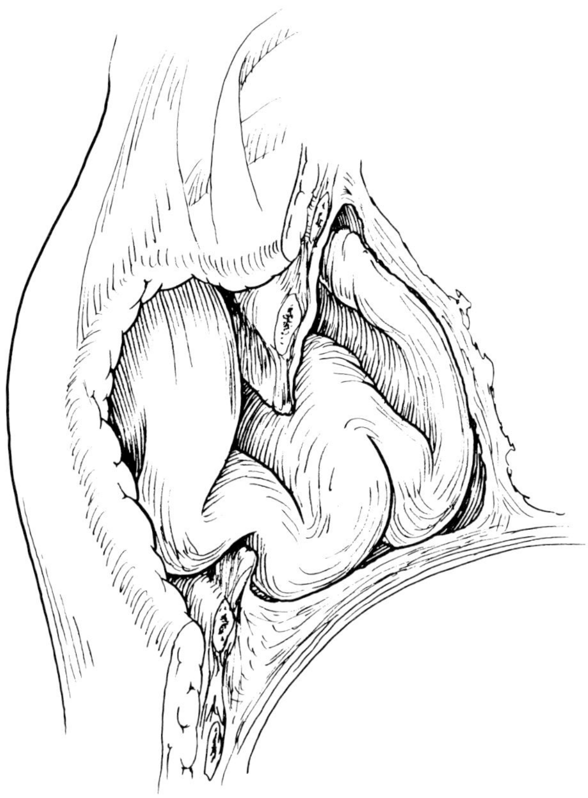

FIGURE 14.10 Filling the empyema cavity with muscle such as a latissimus flap is the procedure of choice. Care is taken to ensure a thorough cleansing of the cavity and a nonconstrictive route for the muscle flap.

With pneumonectomy cavities, or those closer to the diaphragm, the omentum can supply the tissue for cavitary obliteration. If the hemithorax and diaphragm are nonfunctional, the omentum can be routed through the diaphragm. If these elements are functioning, however, the safest route is through a subcutaneous tunnel and then into the cavity. This prevents the potential of herniation of abdominal contents through the diaphragm secondary to the negative intrathoracic pressure.

Both muscle flaps and the omentum are excellent for supplying healthy tissue to these cavities. They should be considered as the first choice in the restoration of such defects.

15

Congenital Defects: Poland's Syndrome, Pectus Deformities, and Sternal Clefts

An important concept in the assessment and treatment of chest wall anomalies is the wide spectrum of physical defects associated with each condition. Although the patient may have certain physical findings consistent with a well-described syndrome, the expression of that abnormality is often incomplete. For this reason, a detailed examination is performed to assess the extent of the defect, to detect other associated congenital problems, and to determine the prospects for a successful repair. The decision to reconstruct the defect depends on many factors, including the age and sex of the patient, the location and extent of the anomaly, condition of nearby structures (particularly musculoskeletal tissues), and, most importantly, the degree of functional or cosmetic disability. In this chapter, three anterior anomalies are discussed: Poland's syndrome, pectus deformities, and sternal clefts.

Poland's Syndrome

This well-described syndrome consists of the unilateral absence, partial or complete, of the pectoralis major muscle, the pectoralis minor muscle, costal cartilages 2, 3, and 4, and a wide variety of anomalies of the upper extremity (Figure 15.1). This constellation of defects also frequently includes unilateral mammary hypoplasia, in which the breast is undersized and the nipple-areolar complex is somewhat small and laterally displaced. The breast asymmetry is, of course, more noticeable in the female. In both sexes, the pattern of hair growth on the affected side of the chest and in the axilla may be disturbed. Ipsilateral brachysyndactyly is a component expressed as variable shortening of upper extremity elements and webbing of the digits.

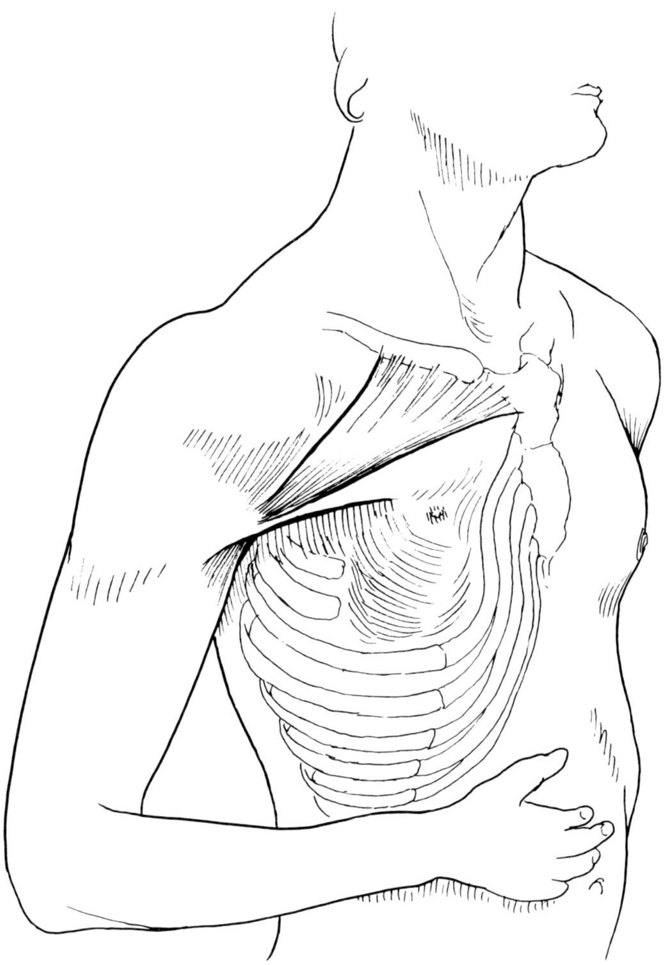

FIGURE 15.1 Poland's syndrome includes unilateral absence of the pectoral muscles, upper costal cartilages, mammary hypoplasia, and upper extremity anomalies.

Preoperative evaluation consists of a thorough history and physical examination as well as the standard PA and lateral chest radiographs to detect associated anomalies. Palpation usually reveals the extent of the anterior rib shortening, and rib films may show additional defects. Thorough muscle testing can reveal the presence (or absence) of portions of the pectoralis major muscle as well as the condition of the latissimus dorsi muscle (see Chapters 8 and 9) for potential use in reconstruction of the defect.

Preoperative Planning

The goal is to provide symmetry to the chest wall by restoring the soft tissue bulk that is absent. The patient may have a single area that bothers him or her more than others, and it is important to know his or her goals long before any contemplated operation. In this way, the surgeon can select realistic patients who thoroughly understand the limitations of any procedure that is planned. This philosophy is consistent with the nature of such surgery since it is primarily cosmetic.

As a general rule, the operation is postponed until most of the chest wall growth has taken place. This has usually occurred by the late teenage years, and this is also the time when the defect seems to assume increased importance in the patient's life.

In males, the absence of the pectoralis musculature may be a source of embarrassment when participating in sports. In females, the unilateral absence of the breast and underlying muscles cause an asymmetry that may be exceedingly difficult to conceal, even with a good external mammary prosthesis. The goal in males is the provision of sufficient subcutaneous bulk to simulate a pectoralis muscle. The goal in females is the provision of a natural-appearing, symmetrical breast mound. In both sexes, the reconstruction of an acceptable anterior axillary fold is a secondary, though important, goal.

The current, standard method of reconstruction involves the subcutaneous transposition of the ipsilateral latissimus dorsi muscle to the anterior chest wall. One advantage is its large, reliable, pedicled flap, which uses muscle tissue to fill in an area where the same type of tissue is missing. The scar is relatively hidden, and little, if any, strength deficit accrues to the patient. If more protection for the thoracic viscera is required, a synthetic mesh may be used prior to transposition of the flap (Figure 15.2). In the female, a soft, silicone gel prosthesis can be placed deep to the transposed muscle to restore the breast mound.

The disadvantage, in both sexes, is that it is difficult to obtain a natural-appearing anterior axillary fold. This is true even if the insertion of the latissimus muscle is moved to a new location on the humerus specifically to restore this fold. The normal fold is, of course, due to the spiraling fibers of the pectoralis major muscle. This complex design is difficult to simulate if it is missing.

Technique

The latissimus is harvested through an incision parallel to its anterolateral fibers and several centimeters dorsal to its anterior border. The incision is carried across the midaxillary region from posterior to anterior in order to provide access to the sternum and clavicle. The muscle is mobilized as described in Chapter 8, and the skin and subcutaneous tissues are dissected off the ribs over the upper, anterior chest wall. A generous tunnel is established through the axilla, and the muscle is transferred through this aperture to the anterior thorax (Figure 15.3). There must be no constraint on the thoracodorsal vascular bundle.

The distal portion of the muscle is folded on itself (with the free end deep) in order to provide more bulk medially and sutured in this configuration. It is then fixed to the periosteum of the sternum and along the inferior aspect of the clavicle with nonabsorbable sutures, such as clear nylon.

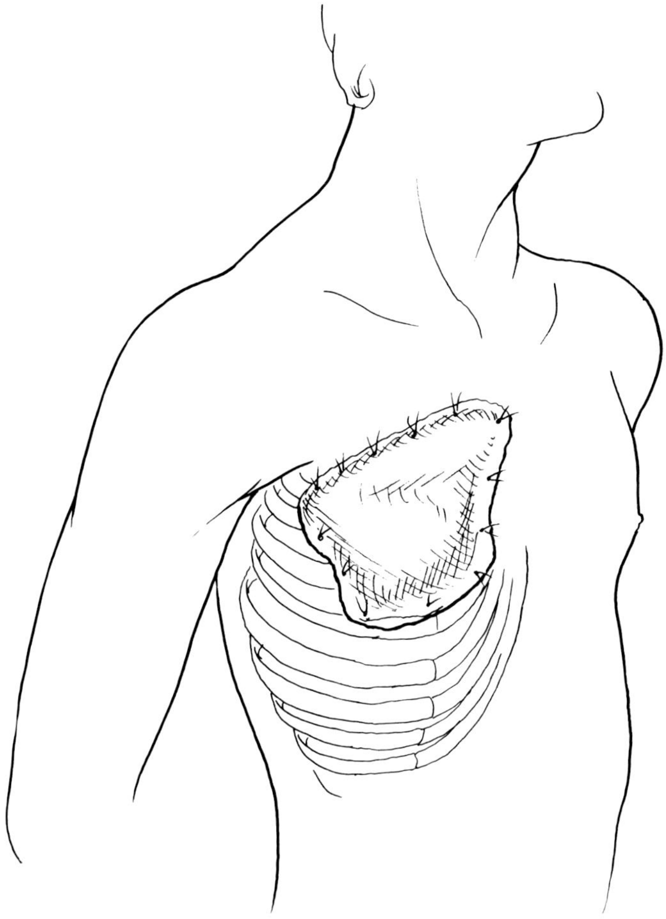

FIGURE 15.2 Synthetic mesh may be placed for added visceral protection.

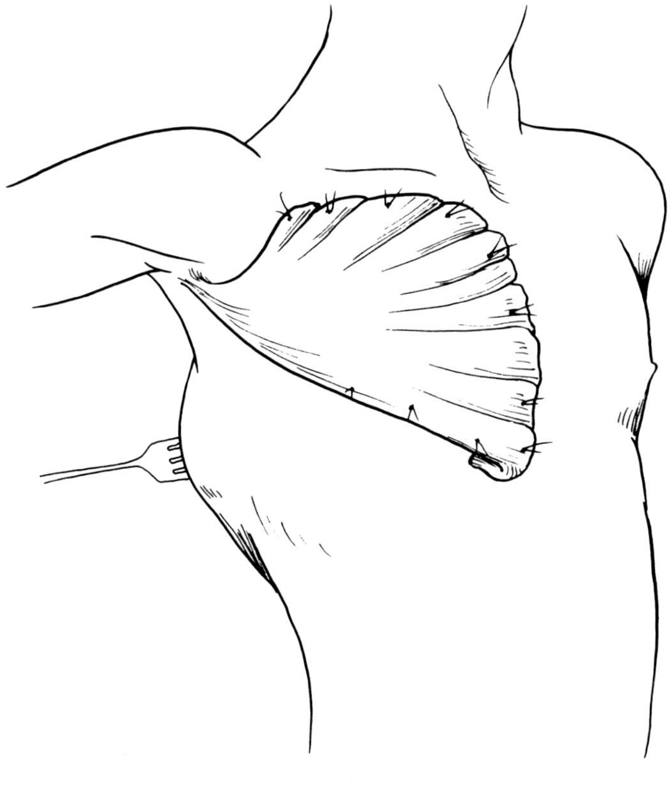

FIGURE 15.3 Correction of the chest wall defect of Poland's syndrome is accomplished with transposition of the ipsilateral latissimus dorsi muscle. The medial edge may be folded to simulate a more natural fullness.

In the female, a soft, silicone gel prosthesis is inserted beneath the muscle to simulate the breast mound. It is usually necessary to enlarge the submuscular space into the subcutaneous tissues over the lower anterior chest wall before inserting the mammary prosthesis. The pocket is extended 2–3 centimeters caudal to the level of the normal inframammary crease to allow for possible cephalad migration of the implant postoperatively. Prosthesis size may be estimated preoperatively by comparing prostheses to the size of the normal breast (see Chapter 13).

After the prosthesis has been inserted beneath the latissimus muscle, the lower edge of the muscle is sewn to the rib/serratus fascia to prevent the prosthesis from migrating posteriorly. The posterior skin incision is closed over a suction drain as described in Chapter 8.

The Anterior Axillary Fold

This area is difficult to construct effectively. If it continues to present a cosmetic problem to the patient after the latissimus muscle has been transferred, consideration may be given to detaching the insertion of the latissimus from the humerus and moving it anteriorly. It is then reattached to the humerus with an eye toward simulating the natural pectoralis major attachment. Care must be taken to avoid injury to the neurovascular bundle. It is helpful to suspend a portion of the muscle to the coracoid process in order to provide more subclavicular bulk. Custom-made prostheses, although seemingly an attractive alternative, are usually unsatisfactory over a period of time due to migration and noticeable contour irregularities.

Pectus Deformities

Pectus Excavatum

Pectus excavatum is an abnormality of the anterior chest wall manifested by a sunken sternum and varying degrees of ingrowth and incurving of the costal cartilages (Figure 15.4A). The depressed portion may also have a rotational component to it such that the sternum is facing toward one side or the other (usually to the right) (Figure 15.4B). In such instances, the breast toward which it is facing may also appear to be rotated inward and may be hypoplastic.

The incidence of the abnormality is about 8 per 1,000 individuals, and males predominate with a 2:1 or 3:1 ratio. The etiology of the malady is unknown. In this section, the general characteristics of the anomaly are discussed, along with our preferred method of reconstruction.

Preoperative Evaluation The child is usually brought to the physician because the mother notes a cosmetic deformity of the anterior chest wall. In most children this defect is noted shortly after birth, although in some it may become most noticeable during a period of rapid skeletal growth. A familial nature of the deformity has been observed, but a uniform pattern of occurrence within families is incomplete. For example, more than one parent or sibling may exhibit the deformity within a certain family, but in other probands, it occurs as an isolated case, with no known relatives having a similar problem.

The history reflects a spectrum of symptoms, depending on the magnitude of the defect. In patients with a mild contour irregularity, there is no demonstrable physiological derangement, either in cardiac output or in ventilatory capacity. However, with a marked deformity, the patient may have minimal exercise tolerance and a decrease in maximum inspiratory expansion due both to cardiac compression and to the fixed curvature of the anterior chest wall. Physiologic studies have shown that the defect is

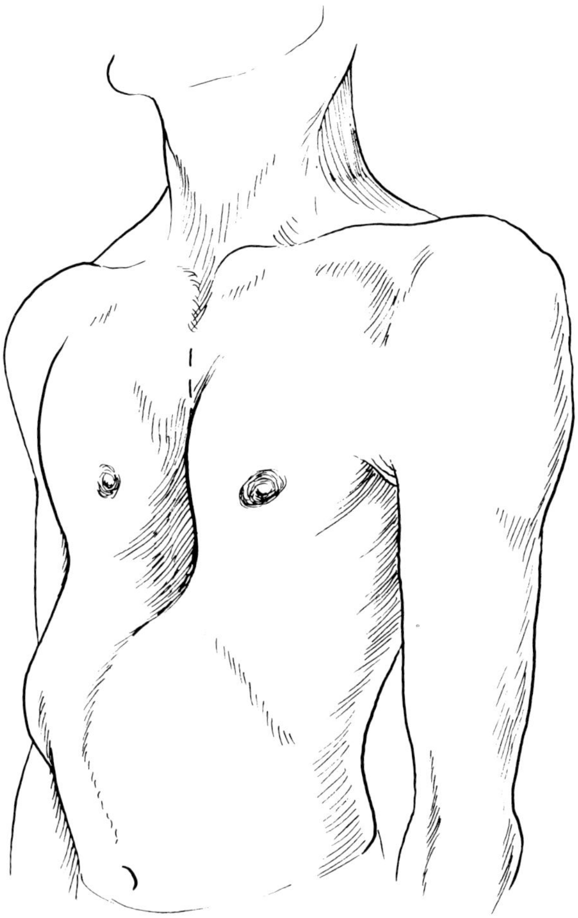

FIGURE 15.4A A pectus excavatum presents the appearance of a sunken chest wall, often with inward rotation and hypoplasia of one breast. The dashed line indicates the surgical incision.

FIGURE 15.4B The sternal depression and rotation along with the costal deformities are illustrated. The cross section shows how the heart can be compressed and displaced by the defect.

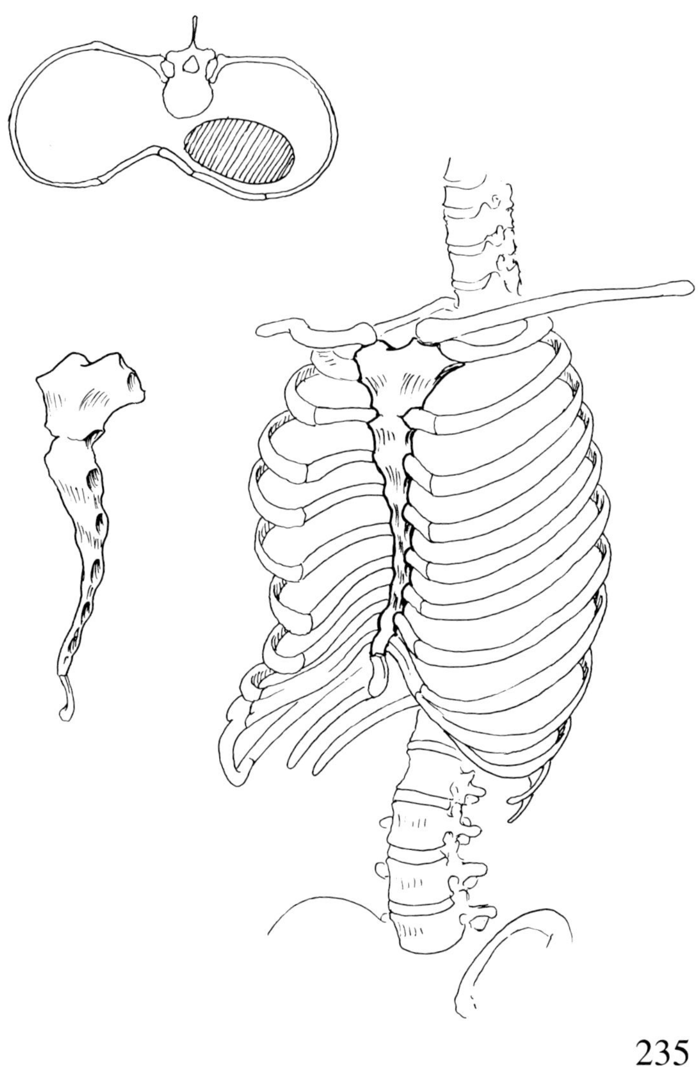

most compromising when the individual is exercising in the upright position. Such physiologic derangements are less likely to be detected if the patient is supine or recumbent, and this may be reflected in the symptoms. Some patients complain of being unable to keep up with their peers or to participate in athletics. Others have vague symptoms related to early fatigue.

On physical examination, the child often exhibits a slumped appearance, with rounding of the shoulders, a sunken chest, a protuberant abdomen, and the head tilted forward. The pot belly is most likely related to displacement of the thoracic viscera and a decrease in upward diaphragmatic excursion. This causes the upper abdominal viscera to be displaced somewhat inferiorly, causing the typical appearance. A few individuals show a wide, flat sternal depression, along with flaring of the costal margins. Depending on the displacement of the heart, the cardiac impulses may be further to the left than is normal.

Laboratory Studies The chest x-ray (PA projection) shows a somewhat enlarged cardiac silhouette, which is displaced to the left: the lateral view shows a depressed sternum. The computerized tomographic scan can be most helpful since it shows the actual displacement of the heart, the decrease in volume of the affected pleural space, and the relationships of the sternum to the malformed segments of the ribs.

Surgical Correction A myriad of operations have been proposed for the correction of this deformity. Probably the most popular has been that described by Ravitch in which the costal cartilages are excised and the sternum is reshaped. The following operation is a modification of that technique.

A vertical, midline incision is performed from the manubrium to the xiphoid process. The subcutaneous tissues are divided down to the sternum, and the costal cartilages on both sides are widely exposed by reflecting the pectoralis major muscles laterally. Once the cartilages (from the lower costal margins up to the second ribs) have been exposed, the perichondrium over each segment is incised along its midaxial line from the costochondral junction medially to the sternum. Transverse incisions are then made at each end of this opening, and the perichondrium is reflected circumferentially in all directions. The cartilage is then transected and totally excised, leaving a bed of perichondrium (Figure 15.5). The sternum is then bluntly separated from the areolar tissues on its posterior aspect by excising the xiphoid process, introducing a finger into the anterior mediastinal space, and sweeping the pleural reflections laterally. The second costal cartilages are transected at a 45° angle on both sides so that after the sternum is moved forward, the cartilaginous ends can be overlapped anteriorly and secured. Transverse sternal osteotomies are then performed as deemed necessary to reshape the bone.

Posterior osteotomies are favored by Ravitch. The ostomy used in our repair (as originally described by Robiseck and his associates) is on the anterior surface of the deformed sternum (Figure 15.6). The area of the sternum that curves inward is transected, and the sternum is elevated to the same plane as the manubrium. Three nonabsorbable sutures are placed to close the osteotomies. Each suture is tied down so that the deformed portion of the sternum is elevated into the proper plane. In some cases, a second anterior osteotomy may be necessary to achieve the desired correction. In those with a particularly severe concavity, a Steinmann pin is placed behind or through the body of the sternum and secured to the anterior surfaces of the ribs. The ends of the pin are bent into small loops and permanent sutures are placed through each loop and into the adjacent rib.

Once the sternal deformity has been corrected, a soft suction drain is placed beneath the sternum and brought out through a separate stab incision. The mobilized soft tissues are reapproximated in the midline and the skin closed (Figure 15.7).

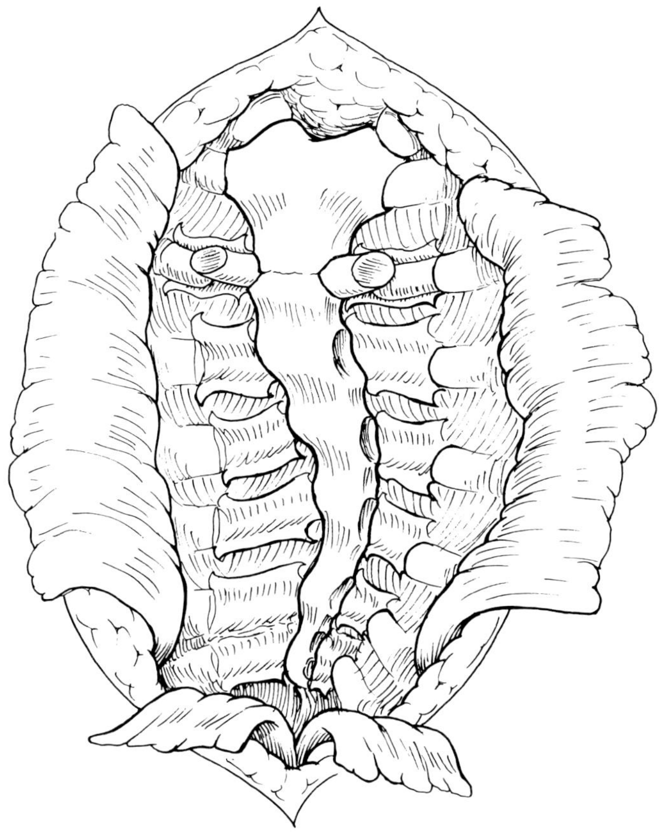

FIGURE 15.5 The pectoralis and rectus abdominis muscles are elevated and the costal cartilages below the second rib are excised. The second cartilages are transected at a 45° angle for anterior displacement (overlap).

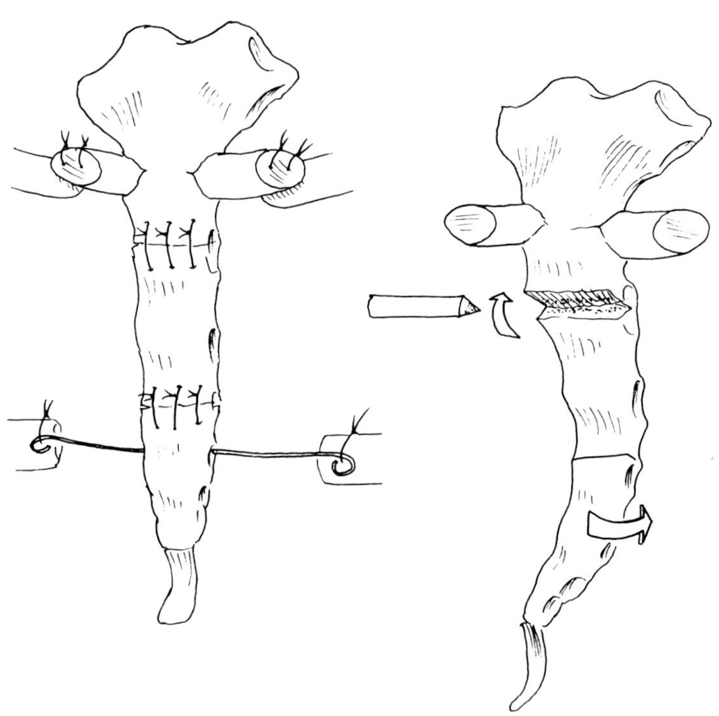

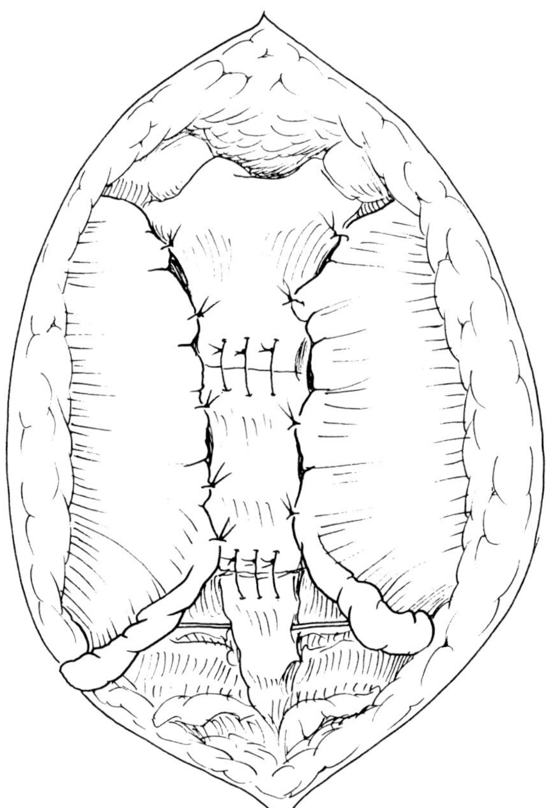

FIGURE 15.6 Anterior osteotomies are used to correct the curvature and rotational deformities as shown. A Steinmann pin may be used for severe deformities to elevate the lower segment. A closing wedge osteotomy is used for the upper segment.

FIGURE 15.7 The pectoralis muscles are sutured to the periosteum at the sternal borders and the incision is closed over a small suction drain.

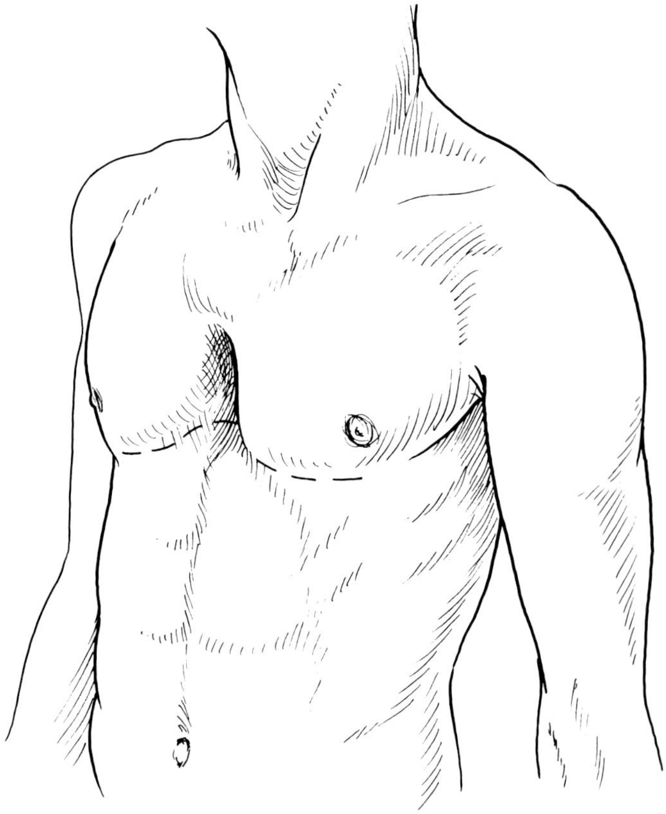

A

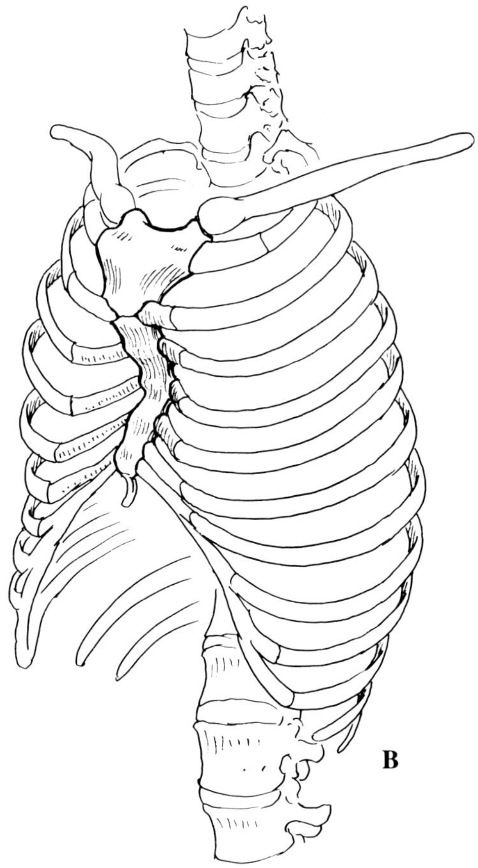

B

FIGURE 15.8A The pouter pigeon type of pectus carinatum is illustrated with the incision indicated by the dashed line.

FIGURE 15.8B The underlying bony defect consists of a typically Z-shaped sternum.

Pectus Carinatum

Pectus carinatum is an unusual deformity and is only about one-eighth as frequent as pectus excavatum. Two types are recognized. The first, as described by Ravitch, has been termed the *pouter pigeon breast* (Figure 15.8A). In this deformity, the sternum has a characteristic Z shape in the sagittal plane (Figure 15.8B). The midportion is depressed, while the manubrium and the lower portion of the gladiolus are curved anteriorly. In the second type, which is a true keel breast, the sternum seems to be arched far forward of the ribs (Figure 15.9A). However, it is not so much anteriorly displaced as the costal cartilages are depressed around it (Figure 15.9B). This depression is particularly notable in the third to the sixth costal cartilages, which are curved inward, making the sternum relatively prominent anteriorly. Both deformities are the result of abnormal ingrowth of the costal cartilages.

Preoperative Evaluation As with the excavatum anomaly, the patient is usually brought to the office by the mother because of the cosmetic deformity. Many are apparent from infancy; others, like pectus excavatum, become more prominent only during growth spurts. The penetrance and modes of inheritance are also similar to the excavatum defect. However, physiological effects due to the deformity are rare. Hence, most patients are asymptomatic.

In most instances, the physical findings are limited to the deformity of the sternum and the incurving of the adjacent costal cartilages. Palpation of the pouter pigeon breast shows the cartilages to be bent and the central portion of the sternum to be pressed inward. The manubrium and the distal portion of the gladiolus are prominent. Occasionally, there is an associated hypoplasia and inward rotation of one breast.

In the patient with a true keel breast, the sternum is anterior and appears quite prominent. The costal cartilages on both sides have grown inward and then have curved outward immediately adjacent to the sternum, almost as if someone had grasped the sternum and pinched hard on both sides of it. The sternum may be flattened yet

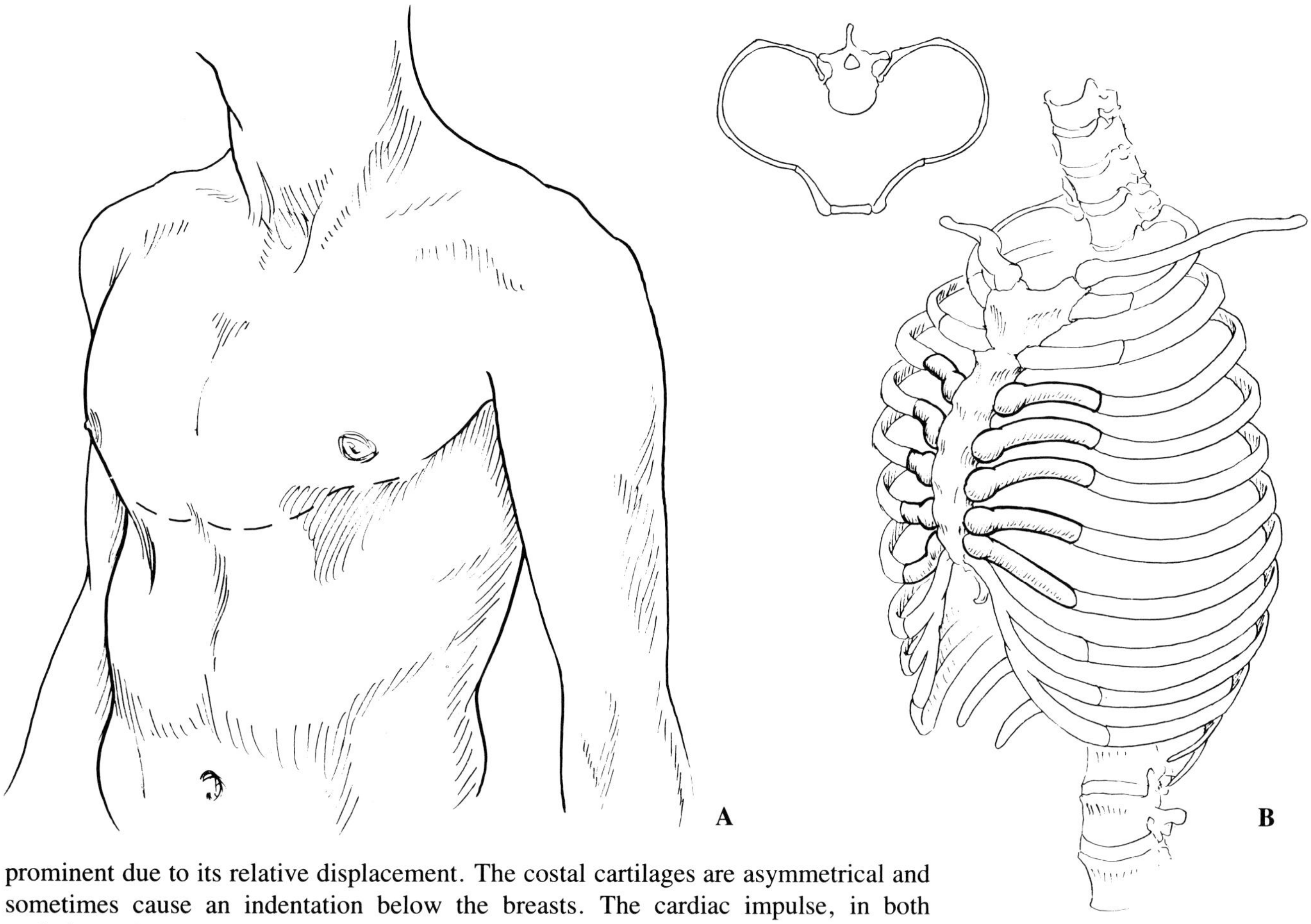

prominent due to its relative displacement. The costal cartilages are asymmetrical and sometimes cause an indentation below the breasts. The cardiac impulse, in both variations of carinatum, is usually at the expected location.

FIGURE 15.9A In the keel type of pectus carinatum, the sternum appears arched forward. The incision is shown.

FIGURE 15.9B The defect is caused by the costal cartilages being pinched in on either side of the sternum.

Laboratory Studies The chest x-rays show the characteristic sternal deformity associated with either one of these two conditions. This sternal prominence is more easily seen on lateral radiographs. Occasionally, the cardiac silhouette may seem large on the anteroposterior view due to the depressed sternum.

Computerized tomographic scanning usually shows the heart in its normal position and without evidence of compression. Although there may be some encroachment on the cardiac area in patients with the pouter pigeon type of deformity, this is the exception rather than the rule.

Other special studies have not been of great use in defining the abnormality. Standard preoperative tests are assessed as described in Chapter 4.

Surgical Correction A useful incision for the correction of either of the carinatum deformities follows a transverse course at the level of the lower sternal body, which is bowed slightly upward and which extends to both anterior axillary lines. As in the repair of pectus excavatum, the muscles are reflected off the costal cartilages, and the pectoralis major is dissected free superiorly. The rectus abdominis muscles are elevated and reflected inferiorly, and the xiphoid process is left in its normal position. The costal cartilages are excised as described for pectus excavatum. In the case of the pouter pigeon type, osteotomies are performed to straighten the Z (Figure 15.10). With the keel deformity, after the deformed cartilages have been excised, the deep (posterior) perichondrium, which has been left in place, is imbricated on itself so that the redundant tissue is shortened (Figure 15.11). This tailoring (or reefing) tightens the perichondrium to conform to a more natural chest wall contour. A soft, suction drain is inserted and the incision is closed in layers.

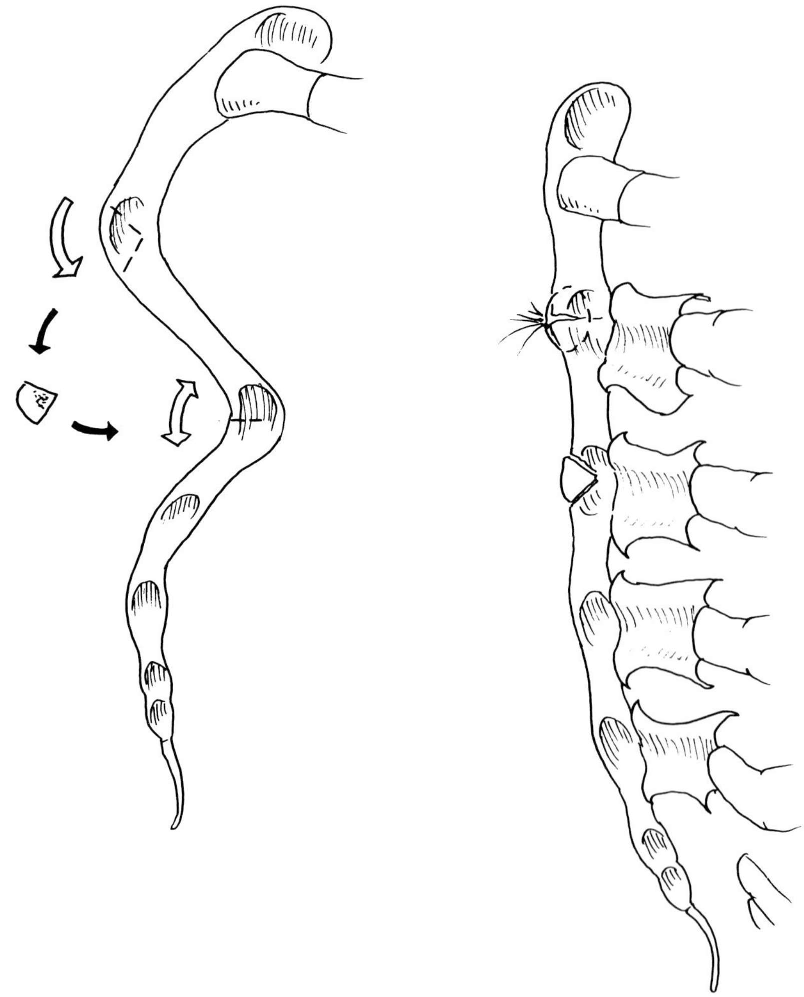

FIGURE 15.10 Osteotomies are performed to correct the Z deformities of the pouter pigeon type: a closing wedge osteotomy superiorly and an opening wedge osteotomy inferiorly.

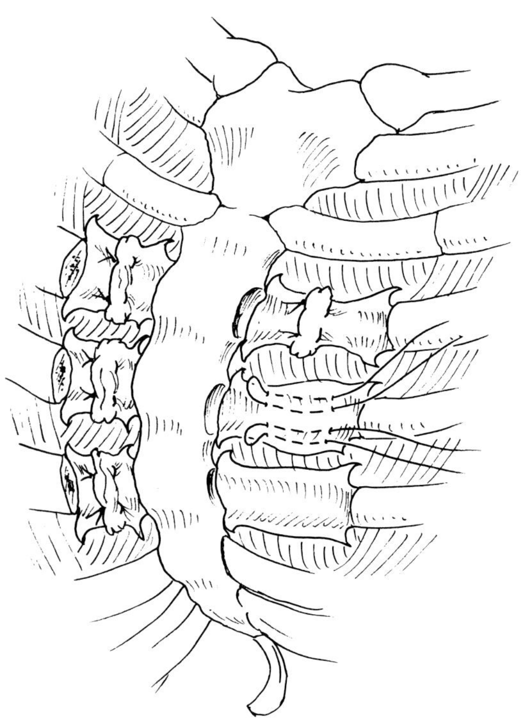

FIGURE 15.11 In correcting the keel deformity, the perichondrium is imbricated to tighten redundancy and create a natural chest wall contour.

Sternal Clefts

Sternal clefts generally fall into three categories: (1) superior, (2) distal, and (3) total (Figure 15.12). They are thought to form as a result of aberrant union of the primitive sternal bars. The mechanisms by which they are thought to occur have been discussed in Chapter 2. The true incidence is not well established since they are somewhat rare and most reported clefts are documented as individual cases. Collected series are few.

Before the repair of sternal clefts, a careful evaluation is performed to rule out the existence of other serious anomalies. This is particularly true in the distal (incomplete) clefts since they are often associated with cardiac defects. True ectopia cordis is an extremely rare condition, which can be associated with sternal clefts, but few successfully repaired cases have been documented.

Timing the Repair

The most opportune time for the repair of the complete cleft is in infancy, shortly after the cleft is recognized. Reconstruction is most successful at this time since the sternal elements are so pliable. When the child is older, the cartilaginous and ossified components of the ribs become somewhat fixed. When they are mobilized under such conditions, even with the use of chondrotomies and osteotomies, one-stage closure is not only difficult but can cause compression of the heart and decreased cardiac output due to the relatively fixed intrathoracic volume. In such older individuals, the repair may require insertion of a prosthetic mesh and muscle flaps for protection of the mediastinal structures, cosmetic improvement, and avoidance of uncompensated encroachment of the intrathoracic volume.

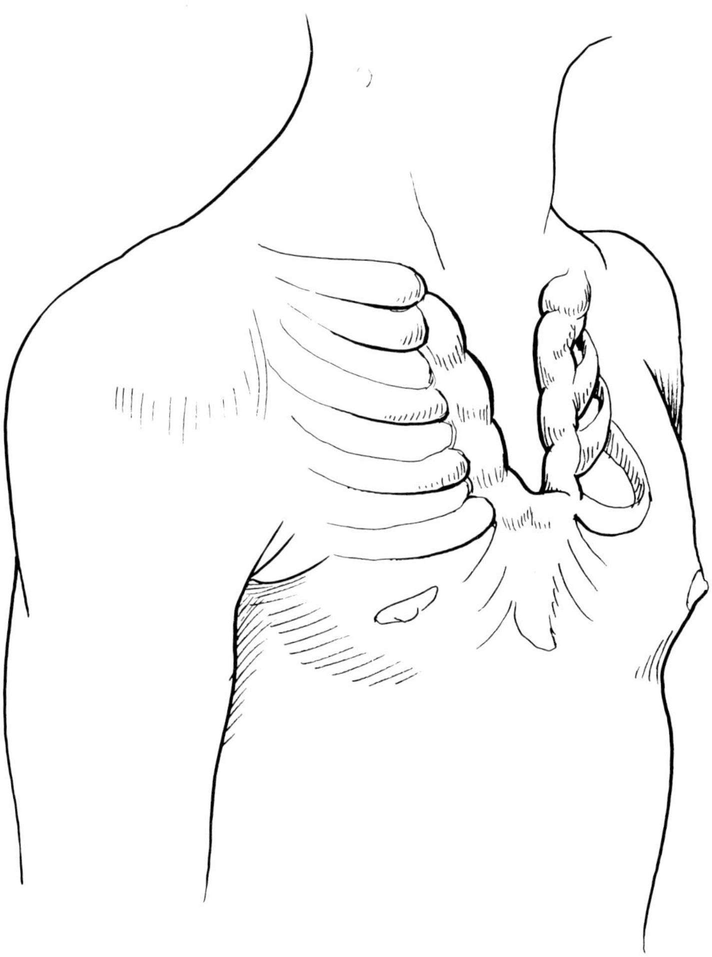

FIGURE 15.12 The superior type of sternal cleft is shown.

For the partial clefts, immediate repair is not mandatory. They, too, are usually reconstructed for cosmesis and for protection of the heart and great vessels. However, the urgency is not as great as with the complete clefts since the mediastinal structures are not as vulnerable to injury. Even though the heart may appear to be somewhat eccentrically situated with these defects, it is generally in its normal anatomic location.

Technique

Complete clefts usually can be safely repaired in the newborn period. With a midline exposure, the two lateral sternal bars are centrally approximated with permanent sutures. Blood pressure and cardiac output are closely monitored throughout the operative and perioperative period in order to detect evidence of compression of the heart or great vessels. Usually, the primary closure can be safely completed without such untoward events.

In the older child, lateral chondrotomies may be necessary to approximate the sternal bars effectively, and cardiac compression is more likely to supervene. There is still some controversy as to the repair of these defects if they are initially seen in early adolescence. Unfortunately, little experience is available concerning such late repair. One approach would be to allow the individual to attain full growth before repairing an asymptomatic cleft. Once the child has reached adult proportions, the repair is accomplished using whatever is necessary to stabilize the chest wall and restore a more natural-appearing sternum.

Prosthetic mesh and mobilization of the pectoralis muscles (both for protection and to provide bulk) may be required (Figure 15.13). Chondrotomies can be tailored to the individual deformity and used to attain optimum positioning of any portions of the sternal components that are present. This approach can also be done earlier, but subsequent growth usually necessitates revisions of the reconstruction especially when prosthetic materials are used. Occasionally, a combination of defects arises (Figure 15.14) in which multiple techniques are required to correct the deformity.

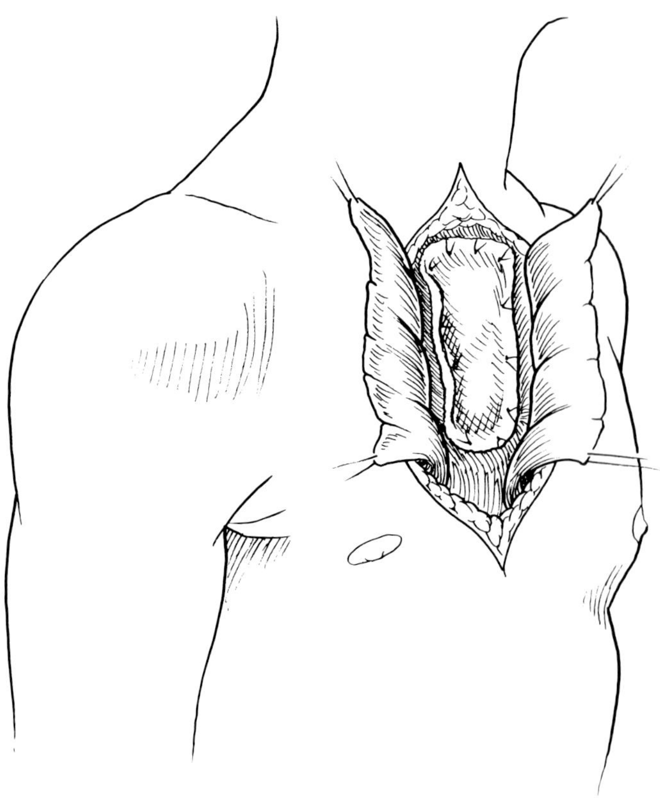

FIGURE 15.13 Prosthetic mesh and pectoralis muscle mobilization may be used to correct the defect in older patients.

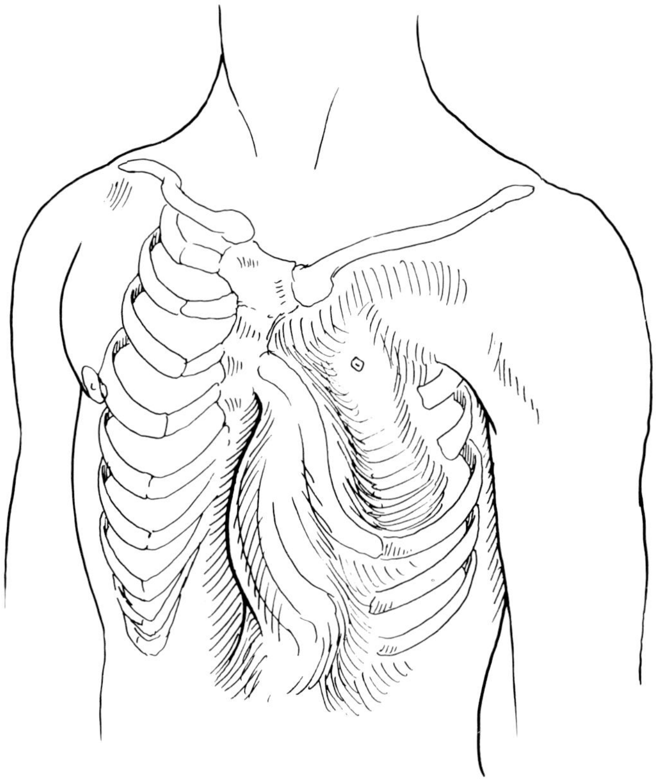

FIGURE 15.14 A combined defect including Poland's syndrome with components of pectus carinatum and an inferior cleft is shown. In this patient, the sternum is repaired in one stage, and the defects associated with Poland's syndrome are repaired later.

16

The Dehisced Median Sternotomy Incision

Median sternotomy is the incision of choice for most cardiac operations and for access to many mediastinal lesions. Although a dehiscence of this incision is infrequent, it can be a devastating complication, which carries with it the threat of mediastinitis and systemic sepsis. Initial management involves control of the infection through early and aggressive wound debridement. Later care centers on stabilization of the sternum, obliteration of any cavitary defect with healthy tissue, and the provision of serviceable skin coverage. In this chapter, the general management of sternal dehiscence is discussed along with several options for reconstruction.

Initial Evaluation and Preoperative Assessment

The patient usually presents with a history of early suture abscesses or granulomas and of the surgeon's efforts to remove these foreign materials from the wound. The infections are a source of pain and tenderness and are often manifested by intermittent fever, draining sinus tracts, sternal instability, and gradual protrusion of underlying foreign material (e.g., sternal sutures or pacer wires). The sternum may be grossly unstable with tenderness extending onto the adjacent rib cartilages.

Physical examination typically shows a poorly healed median sternotomy incision, with patchy erythema and one or more draining tracts. Palpation elicits an area of tenderness, which correlates well with the margins of infected bone and cartilage, and sinus tracts may be evident. These openings should not be aggressively probed since they may overly enlarge vessels or cardiac structures. The sternal halves may be mobile, and local pressure sometimes produces fresh drainage (or bubbling) of purulent material from the openings in the incision.

Laboratory studies are routinely obtained as needed. They may include a coagulation screen, complete blood count, and chemical profile that includes total protein and albumin determinations. Serum protein and albumin levels can be relatively low in patients who have lingering sternal infections and may reflect a caloric imbalance. This should be corrected by vigorous nutritional support as outlined in Chapter 4.

A computerized tomographic scan may offer useful information regarding the lateral extent and depth of the infected tissues. A gallium scan may also be helpful since positive areas correlate well with localized osteomyelitis and chondritis. After the necessary studies have been evaluated, the treatment plan is initiated with an early and wide debridement to eradicate the infection.

The Debridement

The first step in any successful reconstruction is a thorough debridement. This is a radical procedure designed to extirpate residual infection anywhere in the previous operative field.

The neck, anterior chest, and abdominal wall are prepared and draped as for a cardiac operation. Both femoral areas are included, in the eventuality that one of the cardiac chambers is entered and cardiopulmonary bypass becomes necessary to repair the opening. This is more of a possibility in extensive and chronic infections in which the substernal tissues are fused to the epicardium.

The incision is opened widely starting at the most prominent of the draining sinuses over the sternum. The old wire sutures are removed and a vigorous debridement is carried out. Sinus tracts are followed down to the heart if necessary and excised. Areas of loculated pus are sought out and opened, and any nonviable tissue is removed. No infected cartilage should be left since it behaves like an infected foreign body due to its poor vascularity. Such cartilage results in chronic drainage and failure of the reconstructive effort if allowed to remain in place.

The presence of foreign material such as pacemaker wires must also be dealt with. Most of these can be safely removed. Obviously, Dacron pledgets that are fixed to the apex of the heart or other such vital structures must be left undisturbed. After the debridement, granulation tissue usually grows over these pledgets so that their excision is unnecessary.

New drainage is established with large-bore mediastinal tubes, and provision is made for continuous irrigation of the resulting postdebridement cavity. If this is deemed necessary, it may be done with an antiseptic solution (such as half-strength povidone-iodine) through inflow and outflow catheters.

The sternum is then reapproximated over the irrigation catheters, and the subcutaneous tissue and skin are packed open for delayed closure. Since the remaining sternum may be friable, extra care is warranted if a closure of the intact portions is attempted. The usual sternal wires may cut through. Therefore, the wires may be more effective if placed in figure-of-eight fashion. Alternatively, the closure may be accomplished with Parham bands (such as are sometimes used in orthopedic surgery) or polyethylene strips.

However, if a large quantity of necrotic sternum or purulent material is encountered during the debridement, it is safest to pack the entire wound open, without reapproximation of the sternal halves. Closure of the sternum may, in fact, be impossible due to edema or to the large cavitary defect remaining after removal of infected bone and cartilage.

During the postoperative period, the packing is changed once every 8-hour shift and replaced. Each day, the surgeon inspects the wound, which is debrided as the cotton-gauze dressing is carefully removed. Small, shallow defects, with large portions of viable sternum still intact, may close by secondary intention. If the defect is relatively large (as is often the case), and if healthy granulation tissue is not forthcoming by the fifth postoperative day, the patient is returned to the operating room for further debridement. This sequence is repeated until the wound is thoroughly cleansed. When the bed of the cavity is filling with healthy granulations, it is ready for permanent coverage with skin grafts or soft-tissue flaps.

Although skin grafts may be effectively used to provide early healing, the first choice is reconstruction with well-vascularized flaps. Such flaps provide better protection to underlying structures and, due to their excellent blood supply, are more resistant to infection. They also allow secure, primary healing to take place, even under adverse local conditions. In addition, they provide increased durability and better cosmesis than skin grafts alone are able to provide.

Reconstruction

The goals are to fill the defect with healthy tissue so that the wound will heal securely; to provide thick, stable, and durable coverage that protects the underlying structures; and to provide a natural contour to the defect so that the appearance is acceptable. Ideally, they should be accomplished in one operative procedure. These criteria are best met through the transposition of well-vascularized flaps from adjacent areas of the body. The first choice is muscle tissue due to its excellent blood supply and thickness. The second choice is omentum.

If the defect is limited to a central, longitudinal trough, and if the internal thoracic artery (and its terminal vessel, the superior epigastric artery) on one side is still intact after the debridement (arteriography may be necessary to assess the patency of the vessel), the flap of choice is the unilateral rectus abdominis muscle. This strip of tissue can be easily and rapidly mobilized (as described in Chapter 11) and rotated on its

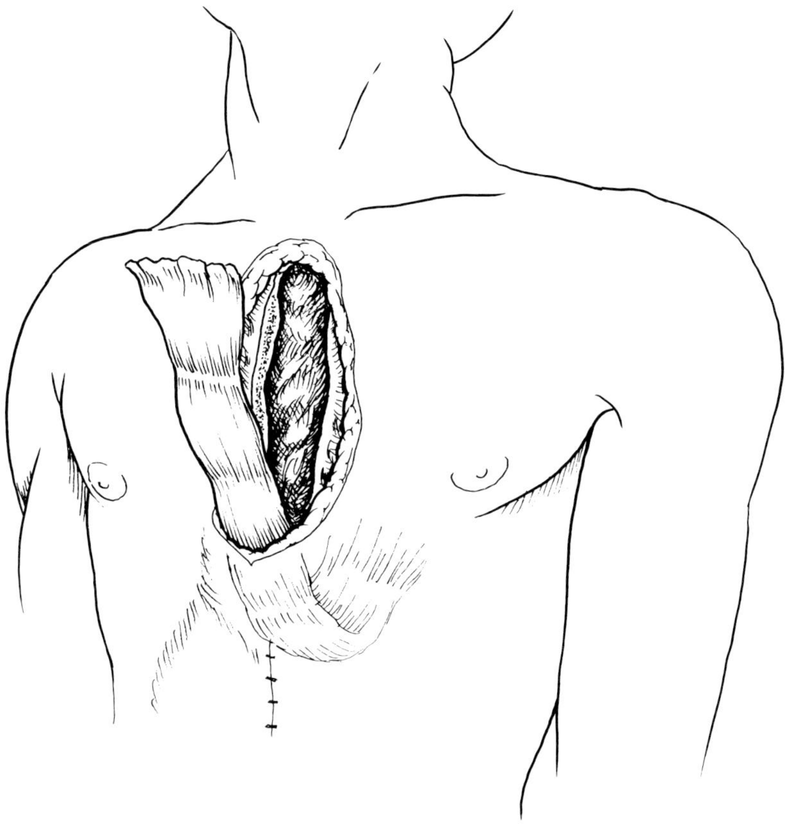

FIGURE 16.1 The unilateral rectus abdominis muscle flap is the tissue of choice for a central sternal trough defect when the internal thoracic artery remains intact after debridement.

superior pedicle to fill the defect (Figure 16.1). Both muscles can be used, but this is usually not necessary (see Chapter 11 for precautions). The muscle can be positioned to fit the cavity, and the skin at the margins of the defect mobilized to complete the closure. If additional skin is needed, a meshed skin graft can be applied to the surface of the muscle. Since the graft is applied to a thick pad of muscle, it can be expected to provide excellent serviceability. The rectus muscle is the flap of choice for longitudinal and lower sternal defects.

If the defect is limited to the upper two-thirds of the sternum, the pectoralis major muscle may be used (Figure 16.2). This defect is not as common as the longitudinal cavity.

The pectoralis major muscle is mobilized (as described in Chapter 9), based on its primary blood supply, the thoracoacromial artery, and moved medially to fill the defect (Figure 16.3). Its humeral insertion is divided if additional mobility is necessary, and both muscles can be effectively used to provide more bulk (Chapter 9, Figure 9.22). The adjacent skin can usually be mobilized for closure over the muscle. An alternative method, which uses the pectoralis muscle based on its medial (internal thoracic artery) blood supply has been described (Chapter 9, Figure 9.5). This is less satisfactory since the internal thoracic artery may be ablated by the debridement or compromised by sternal sutures. This option also requires folding of the muscle on itself, which may place excessive tension both on the closure and on the pedicle. Perhaps the biggest disadvantage to this technique is that it requires division of the primary blood supply to the muscle, the thoracoacromial artery.

The latissimus dorsi muscle flap may also be considered for upper sternal defects, but this is usually not necessary due to the closer availability of the other options discussed in this chapter. If selected, it is mobilized and transposed as described in Chapter 8.

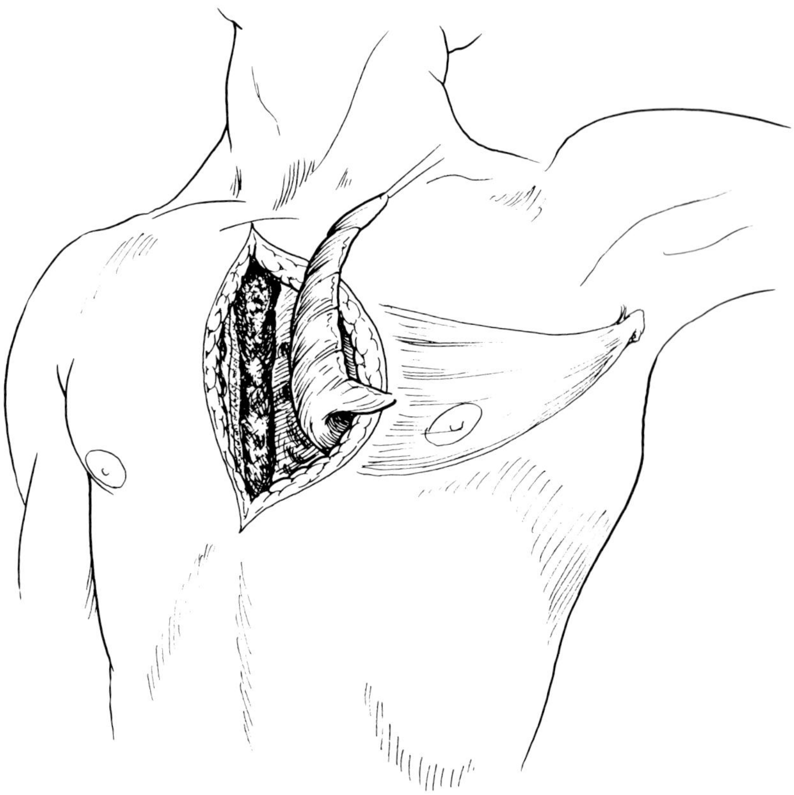

FIGURE 16.2 An upper sternal defect may be filled with a unilateral pectoralis major muscle flap. Usually, however, both muscles are required to adequately fill the defect with healthy tissue.

FIGURE 16.3 The humeral insertion of the pectoralis muscle may be divided for mobility, and both pectoralis major muscles may be used for added bulk.

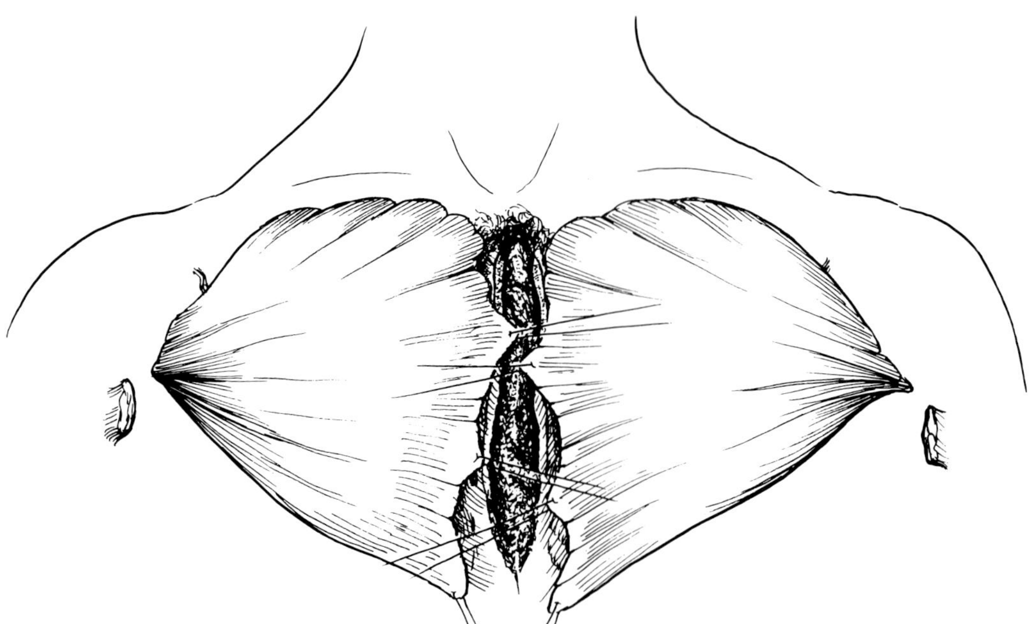

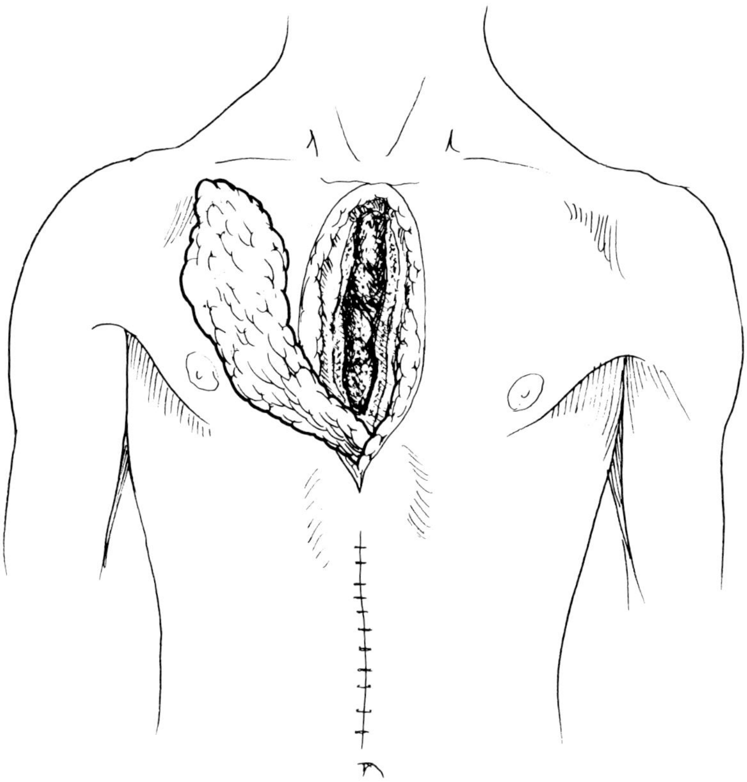

FIGURE 16.4 The omentum provides healthy tissue to fill a large sternal defect when compromise of the internal thoracic arteries makes the rectus muscles unusable.

When confronted with a large, cavitary defect, it may be impossible to use the rectus abdominis muscle because of interruption of the internal thoracic artery. The next choice is the omentum. As noted in Chapter 10, it provides well-vascularized tissue and has an excellent range of coverage (Figure 16.4). It readily accepts skin grafts and can be folded to fill irregular contours at the base of the sternal cavity. Since it requires a laparotomy, however, it should be considered as a second alternative.

The stability of the sternum is usually well restored by the fibrosis that accompanies the widespread inflammation in the area. When the shell-like cavity has been cleansed and filled with healthy flap tissue, there is no need for additional support such as bone grafts or prosthetic material. In fact, such material may be contraindicated due to the contaminated nature of the previous infection and open wound.

Index

Note: Italicized page numbers indicate illustrations or tabular material.

C

D

R